LIVING WITH EPILEPTIC SEIZURES

LIVING WITH
EPILEPTIC SEIZURES

By

SAMUEL LIVINGSTON, M.D.

Assistant Professor of Pediatrics
The Johns Hopkins University School of Medicine
Physician-in-Charge
The Johns Hopkins Hospital Epilepsy Clinic
Associate Attending Physician in Pediatrics
Assistant Physician in Internal Medicine
Physician-in-Charge of The Epilepsy Clinic
Sinai Hospital
Baltimore, Maryland

Assisted by

Irving M. Pruce, B.S.

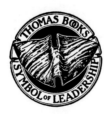

CHARLES C THOMAS • PUBLISHER
Springfield • Illinois • U.S.A.

Published and Distributed Throughout the World by

CHARLES C THOMAS • PUBLISHER

BANNERSTONE HOUSE

301-327 East Lawrence Avenue, Springfield, Illinois, U.S.A.

© *1963, by* CHARLES C THOMAS • PUBLISHER

Library of Congress Catalog Card Number: 63-9639

With THOMAS BOOKS careful attention is given to all details of manufacturing and design. It is the Publisher's desire to present books that are satisfactory as to their physical qualities and artistic possibilities and appropriate for their particular use. THOMAS BOOKS will be true to those laws of quality that assure a good name and good will.

Printed in the United States of America

Dedicated to

THE LATE FRANCIS F. SCHWENTKER

whose sincere interest and constant encouragement were responsible for my endeavors in the field of epilepsy

and

THE FIFTEEN THOUSAND EPILEPTIC PATIENTS

who supplied me with most of the information contained in this book

and

ROBERT E. COOKE

Professor of Pediatrics, the Johns Hopkins University School of Medicine, Director of the Department of Pediatrics and Pediatrician-in-Chief, The Johns Hopkins Hospital, whose sincere interest in my work in the field of convulsive disorders has been manifested by the complete free hand which he has allowed me in the medical and administrative management of The Johns Hopkins Hospital Epilepsy Clinic.

PREFACE

THE primary purpose of this book is to present pertinent information relative to epilepsy to non-medical persons such as patients and/or their parents, educators and counselors, as well as to the medical profession.

My knowledge and learning of epilepsy was acquired mostly from intimate follow-up studies of approximately 15,000 epileptic patients over the course of the past twenty-six years.

I have the impression that many physicians believe that my experience with epilepsy has been limited entirely to children. This definitely is not true. Many of these 15,000 patients are adults. Some of them have been under my care since early childhood; others were referred to me when they were adults. Epilepsy made its initial appearance in some of these latter patients during adulthood.

These 15,000 patients were obtained from the following sources: The Epilepsy Clinic of The Johns Hopkins Hospital, The Epilepsy Clinic of Sinai Hospital, Baltimore, Maryland and referrals from practically every area in the United States and also the South American countries. An additional source consisted of patients who attended Epilepsy Clinics conducted under my supervision in various counties in the State of Maryland. Patients residing in these counties are sent initially to the Epilepsy Clinic of The Johns Hopkins Hospital for diagnostic investigations and are subsequently followed in their respective county clinics by one of my associates. I believe that these 15,000 patients represent an excellent cross-section of the over-all epileptic population.

When I first started to write this book, it was my primary intention to discuss only the socio-economic aspects of epilepsy at the level of the non-medical reader. Subsequently, however, I thought it best to include all aspects of the disorder of epilepsy in this book. It has been my experience that a complete understanding of epilepsy by the patient and/or his family is one of the most important factors in the management of this disorder and that, by and large, the best results are obtained in those individuals whose parents and families have an understanding of all aspects of epilepsy, including diagnostic, therapeutic and prognostic. I believe that this is true of epilepsy more than most illnesses and its importance is amplified by the fact that epilepsy is one of the most common, if not the most common, of all the medical disorders which tend to be chronic. I believe that a book written in this fashion would relate the complete message concerning the disorder of epilepsy to all persons who are confronted with this problem.

My experiences have taught me that many competent physicians are not aware of the many obstacles with which the epileptic is confronted and also of the many services which are available to the epileptic. Although some sections of this book are written in an essentially non-technical form, I do believe that the information contained therein will be of significant value to many practicing physicians.

Perhaps it may be said that certain sections of this book, particularly the one dealing with antiepileptic drugs, are too scientific and contain information which should not be included in a book recommended for patients. However, I believe it is exceedingly important and helpful for the epileptic patient, his parents and family to know as much as possible about the various therapeutic agents and of the recent advances made in the treatment of epilepsy. The practice of hiding or concealing therapeutic measures from non-medical persons is gradually disappearing with the passage of time. Certainly, these aspects of other disorders such as cancer, diabetes, heart disease, mental retardation, and cerebral palsy are presented to the general public through media such as radio, newspapers, magazines and television. However, very rarely have I seen or heard significant information relative to epilepsy publicized in these manners. This may be due to many reasons such as lack of knowledge of epilepsy, both by non-medical persons and the medical profession and probably, and most significantly, due to the fact that epilepsy is still a stepchild of medicine and is still considered by many to be a hopelessly incurable and shameful disorder. It is well known that for many years, mental retardation was "hidden in the closet." It is of interest to note, however, that within recent years mental retardation has come partially out of the "closet." However, by and large, epilepsy is still hidden deep in this same closet. Today many parents and families are not too reluctant to disclose the fact that a member of the family is mentally retarded, but this definitely is not true with respect to epilepsy.

Therefore, in order to "win the battle for epilepsy," I believe that patients, their parents and families and physicians must know more about epilepsy and I do hope that the information contained in this book will assist in the endeavor to eliminate the many unwarranted stigmas associated with epilepsy and also the attitude that epilepsy is a shameful, hopeless and incurable disease. I believe that it will not be too long before the epileptic is removed from the class of a second rate citizen.

SAMUEL LIVINGSTON

ACKNOWLEDGMENTS

I WISH to express my sincere gratitude to Dr. Edwards A. Park, Professor Emeritus of Pediatrics of The Johns Hopkins University School of Medicine, who, in 1936, suggested that I work in the Epilepsy Clinic of The Johns Hopkins Hospital with Dr. Edward M. Bridge. Dr. Bridge, who was Director of the Epilepsy Clinic at that time, together with Dr. Laslo Kajdi, directed my initial endeavors in the field of epilepsy.

The late Dr. Francis F. Schwentker, former Professor of Pediatrics of The Johns Hopkins University School of Medicine, was instrumental in obtaining additional financial assistance which enabled me to enlarge the facilities and personnel of the Epilepsy Clinic. He also encouraged me to write my first book on convulsive disorders entitled *The Diagnosis and Treatment of Convulsive Disorders in Children*, (Charles C Thomas, Publisher, Springfield, Illinois, 1954).

I am especially indebted to Dr. Lydia L. Pauli and Dr. Dennis Whitehouse for reading this entire manuscript and making many excellent suggestions. Dr. Pauli has been associated with me in the Epilepsy Clinic for approximately ten years and Dr. Whitehouse has just recently become a member of this Clinic.

I wish to offer thanks to Dr. A. Earl Walker, Professor of Neurological Surgery of The Johns Hopkins University School of Medicine for reviewing the section of this book entitled Surgical Treatment of Convulsive Disorders.

To my wife I am indebted for secretarial and editorial assistance and especially for her tolerance during my writing of this book.

I am also grateful to my secretaries, Mrs. Mollye Livingston and Mrs. Mary Kavanagh for performing the arduous task of typing the initial drafts of the contents of this book.

It is impossible to make appropriate acknowledgment to the following individuals who, directly or indirectly, have helped to provide the knowledge which is the basis of this book.

Edward L. Binder, Chief, Evaluation Policy Section, Division of Disability Operations, Bureau of Old-Age and Survivors Insurance, Social Security Administration

Alice D. Chenoweth, M.D., Chief, Program Services Branch, Division of Health Services, Children's Bureau, Department of Health, Education, and Welfare.

Mrs. Virginia Cosden, Dietitian, the Nutrition Clinic of The Johns Hopkins Hospital.

Robert D. Garrett, Secretary, Medical Advisory Board of the Department of Motor Vehicles, State of Maryland (retired 1961).

Miss Mary Lou Gedel, Dietitian, the Nutrition Clinic of The Johns Hopkins Hospital.

Mrs. Ellen R. Grass, President, The American Epilepsy Federation.

Dr. Charles Kram, Executive Director, The Federal Association for Epilepsy.

L. Gordon LaPointe, M.D., Vice-President and Medical Director, The Manhattan Life Insurance Company, New York, New York.

Joseph Lerner, M.D., Chief Consultant in Psychiatry and Neurology, Division of Disability Operations, Bureau of Old-Age and Survivors Insurance, Social Security Administration.

Arthur J. Lesser, M.D., Medical Director, Division of Health Services, Children's Bureau, Department of Health, Education, and Welfare.

Clement Martin, M.D., Medical Director, Continental Casualty Company, Chicago, Illinois.

Nathan E. Needle, M.D., Medical Director, Department of Personnel, State of Maryland.

Lt. Colonel Matthew D. Parrish, Assistant Chief Consultant of Psychiatry and Neurology, United States Army.

Mrs. Margaret Rider, Dietitian, the Nutrition Clinic of The Johns Hopkins Hospital.

Dr. Frank Risch, Director, Epi-Hab U.S.A., Inc., and Epileptic Rehabilitation Service, V. A. Center, W. Los Angeles, California.

Dr. Harry Sands, Director of Program, United Epilepsy Association.

W. H. Scoins, M.D., Chief Medical Director, The Lincoln National Life Insurance Company, Fort Wayne, Indiana.

F. R. Stearns, M.D., Vice-President and Medical Director, Security Benefit Life Insurance Company, Topeka, Kansas.

Jean Rose Stifler, M.D., Chief, Division for Crippled Children and Heart Disease Control, Maryland State Department of Health.

W. Bird Terwilliger, Assistant Director, Division of Vocational Rehabilitation, State of Maryland.

Mrs. Eileen Trawinski, Dietitian, the Nutrition Clinic of The Johns Hopkins Hospital.

Dr. George N. Wright, Program Director, The National Epilepsy League (resigned 1962).

The editorial and administrative staffs of Charles C Thomas, Publisher have also been helpful and cooperative.

SAMUEL LIVINGSTON

CONTENTS

LIVING WITH EPILEPTIC SEIZURES

Chapter 1

GENERAL CONSIDERATIONS OF SEIZURE DISORDERS

WHAT IS A SEIZURE?

A SEIZURE is not a disease; it is merely a symptom of a disease. The general public almost always associates a seizure with the specific disorder of epilepsy, but this assumption definitely is not true. There are many diseases in which seizures may be one of the symptoms such as brain tumors, infections of the brain and biochemical disorders.

Many words such as convulsion, spell, fit and attack are used synonymously with the term seizure by both the laiety and the medical profession.

A seizure may be briefly described as an episode of impairment of consciousness, which may or may not be associated with convulsive movements. Some degree of impairment of consciousness almost always occurs in association with all types of seizures except focal seizures. In most instances patients with focal seizures do not manifest evidence of disturbances of consciousness.

It is important to understand what is meant by "impairment of consciousness." With a seizure, an individual may go into a state of complete unconsciousness, that is, he may appear almost lifeless except for breathing movements. On the other hand, consciousness may be only slightly impaired, so that he may appear merely to be staring vacantly into space for a few seconds. Then again, he may be able to walk about or even talk, but usually in a disoriented fashion. However, during these episodes he is generally not completely aware of his surroundings.

The general public thinks of a seizure almost exclusively as manifesting itself by such disturbances as violent shaking movements, foaming at the mouth, biting of the tongue, thrashing of the

3

arms and legs or unconsciousness. The convulsive form is unquestionably the most common type of seizure. However, a seizure may present itself in many forms and these are described in detail in the section of this book entitled Classification of Epileptic Seizures (Chapter 4).

The duration of a seizure varies considerably, lasting from a few seconds to hours or even days.

WHAT CAUSES SEIZURES?

A seizure is a manifestation of disturbed brain function and can be produced in any individual upon exposure to stimuli which exceed his convulsive threshold.

For example, convulsions can be produced when electrical currents are applied to the head of an individual receiving electroshock therapy for certain psychiatric disorders, and also when excessive amounts of certain drugs are ingested or injected into the blood circulation. In other words, one could say that every person is prone to have a seizure or convulsion under certain circumstances.

It is also known that seizures occur in some individuals who suffer with certain medical disorders. For example, some people will experience convulsions when the blood sugar content falls below a certain level; these are known as hypoglycemic convulsions. Convulsions also occur in some individuals when the blood calcium content falls below a certain level; these are known as hypocalcemic convulsions.

Convulsions also occur in some persons with conditions such as brain tumors, infections of the brain, and after brain damage, sustained either at birth or from a direct blow to the head.

Convulsions are also encountered in association with fever and in association with severe breath-holding spells in some children.

The fact, however, that all individuals who suffer with the conditions heretofore mentioned do not have convulsions suggests very strongly that there are other factors involved in the causation of seizures which, at the present time, are not known. One explanation is that certain people have an inherent abnormally low convulsive threshold or a so-called predisposition to seizures.

WHAT IS EPILEPSY?

The derivation of the term "epilepsy" according to Webster's New International Dictionary (unabridged) is as follows: French—épilepsie, from Late Latin—epilepsia, from Greek—epilepsia a seizure, the "falling sickness," from epi—lambanein to take besides, seize, attack, from epi upon, besides plus lambanein, to take. Thus, a person was supposedly "seized" by the capricious gods and this led the Romans and others to label epilepsy "the sacred disease."

Hippocrates, the great Greek physician, is credited with the first study of epilepsy, about 400 B.C. He reported: "It is thus with the disease called 'sacred.' It appears to me to be in no way more divine nor more accursed than other diseases, but like them, has a natural cause from which it originates. The brain is the seat of this affection. . . . ." In his treatise on epilepsy, Hippocrates stated that "its origin, like that of other diseases, lies in heredity."

According to the New Testament (St. Luke 9:39) epilepsy was regarded as a form of demonic possession, as evidenced by the well known passage: "And, lo, a spirit taketh him, and he suddenly crieth out; and it teareth him that he foameth again, and bruising him hardly departeth from him."

Fallacious concepts of epilepsy persisted down through the ages until Dr. John Hughlings Jackson, the English neurologist of the late nineteenth century, scientifically defined the epileptic seizure as being a state produced by a "sudden, violent, disorderly discharge of the brain cells."

Today most physicians use the term epilepsy as a diagnosis in cases where patients suffer with seizures and where no definite disease can be demonstrated with the available diagnostic techniques.

When, however, the physician is able to discover a specific condition such as a brain tumor, hypoglycemia or infection of the brain, the patient is then classified as having a seizure related to the respective medical disorder. On the other hand, when the physician is unable to determine a specific medical disorder, the patient is then classified as having a seizure disorder of undetermined cause or epilepsy.

Some physicians define epilepsy as a recurrent illness and therefore do not assign the diagnosis of epilepsy until the patient has had "many" seizures. It is true that epileptic seizures have a tendency to recur in many patients. However, I believe that a tentative diagnosis of epilepsy should be entertained in all patients who suffer with a seizure of undetermined etiology. This is the best attitude to assume from the standpoint of treatment, since my experience has taught me that the best results are obtained in those patients in whom treatment is started early. My method of management of a patient after his first epileptic seizure is described in the section of this book entitled Medical Treatment of Epilepsy (Chapter 8).

The epilepsies are classified by many physicians into two groups. When the seizures occur following permanent brain changes or damage, it is called secondary, organic or symptomatic epilepsy. The recurrent seizures which may follow brain injuries or infections of the brain such as meningitis and encephalitis, or disturbances of the brain which occur with lead intoxication (lead encephalitis) are examples of so-called secondary epilepsy. Recurrent seizures which follow injuries to the brain are also sometimes called post-traumatic epilepsy.

When seizures occur in patients in whom the physician is unable to demonstrate specific evidence of a cerebral disturbance, the disorder is frequently labeled as idiopathic epilepsy. This condition is also known as cryptogenic, essential, pure, primary, true or genetic epilepsy.

FACTORS WHICH PREDISPOSE SOME INDIVIDUALS TO EPILEPSY

In some writings on epilepsy it is stated that the cause of epilepsy in some cases is known, while in others it is not known. Some physicians consider head injuries sustained either at birth or subsequently and infections of the brain, such as meningitis and encephalitis, as conditions which cause epilepsy. In these cases, they classify the seizure disorder as secondary or organic epilepsy, with the recurrent seizures being caused by the brain damage produced by the injury or infection.

Certainly it is quite likely that the brain damage sustained by these patients played some part in the development of their epileptic disorders. Nevertheless, I do not believe that it is the sole or only cause of their recurrent epileptic seizures.

It is generally recognized that acute brain damage, either from trauma or infection, is frequently accompanied by a seizure. Residual brain damage, on the other hand, cannot be the sole cause of subsequent recurrent epileptic seizures since the residual brain damage is always present, but the seizures occur only periodically. If the residual brain damage were the only cause of recurring epileptic seizures, the afflicted individual would be in a constant state of seizures since the brain damage is present at all times. I have seen many patients whose clinical histories were almost identical with Case History Number One. Certainly the sequence of events which occurred in this patient strongly indicates that brain damage, per se, was not the sole cause of his recurrent epileptic seizures.

Case History Number 1

J. H. is a seven year old white boy who was in perfect health and had no illnesses or sustained no injuries in the past which indicated that his brain was affected in any significant manner. When he was four years old he was struck by an automobile while playing outside and received serious injuries to his head. He sustained a fractured skull and remained in an unconscious state for several weeks thereafter. He recovered from his injuries and was in excellent health, except that he was left with a partial paralysis of the right side of his body. He had experienced no seizures or convulsions at the time of his head injury. However, about one year later he had a generalized convulsion lasting approximately ten minutes and subsequently he continued to have similar seizures about once or twice a month.

In view of the fact that this child was left with a right-sided paralysis, there is no doubt that he suffered irreversible brain damage at the time of his accident. It is reasonable to assume that the convulsions which first appeared about one year after the accident, and which have been recurring periodically, were not due solely to the brain damage which he sustained in association with his accident at four years of age. Obviously, other factors which were at least partially responsible for this patient's recurring seizures must have been involved. It is reasonable to assume that in all probability this child would not have developed recurrent epileptic seizures if he had not been struck by the automobile. One can theorize that the automobile accident rendered this patient prone to recurring seizures by lowering his convulsive threshold.

The fact that recurring epileptic seizures do not develop in all patients who sustain similar brain damage, for example, in babies who sustain injury to the brain at birth, also suggests that brain damage is not the sole cause of recurrent epileptic seizures.

However, since recurrent seizures do occur very frequently in individuals subsequent to sustaining brain damage, I prefer to classify brain damage not as a complete cause, but rather as a pre-disposing factor to epilepsy. I think that it is reasonable to assume that a given individual may never have developed epilepsy had he not sustained brain damage. However, one can never be completely certain of this. An appropriate explanation for the part which brain damage plays in the causation of epileptic seizures is that in some manner it lowers the individual's convulsive threshold.

It is my belief that the specific factor or factors which are com-pletely responsible for the development of recurrent epileptic seizures are not known at this time. It is also quite likely that the specific cause or causes of the recurrent seizures of so-called secondary or organic epilepsy are essentially the same as those in patients with so-called idiopathic epilepsy.

On the other hand it is usually stated that there is no associated brain lesion in patients with idiopathic or cryptogenic epilepsy. This assumption also is not completely justified.

It seems quite obvious that there must be some type of cerebral disturbance present in all patients who suffer with recurrent epileptic seizures. Actually all the physician can justly state when he classifies a patient as having idiopathic epilepsy is that he was unable to demonstrate the presence of abnormalities of the brain. The brain abnormalities may be so minor as to be undetectable with the techniques currently available.

Many hypotheses have been advanced in regard to the cause of epileptic seizures. Among these causes are disturbances which produce defects in the physiological, metabolic, enzymatic or chemical systems of the brain. No significant evidence has been presented to my knowledge which definitely proves that any one or a combination of such cerebral abnormalities is unquestionably the cause of epileptic seizures. The part that hereditary factors play in the development of epilepsy is discussed in another section of this book entitled Heredity and Epilepsy (Chapter 16).

AGE OF ONSET OF SEIZURE DISORDERS

Every individual is subject to a seizure or convulsion at any age from birth to death. All races are equally subject to this disturbance and there is no true sex incidence.

With certain illnesses or disorders, such as infections of the brain (meningitis or encephalitis) or the ingestion of poisons, convulsions may occur at any age.

However, with certain other disorders convulsions occur with greater frequency in certain age groups. For example, a brain tumor is more likely to be associated with a seizure in an adult than in a young child.

On the other hand, fever convulsions and breath-holding convulsions occur almost entirely in young children and are rarely observed in the older individual. A convulsion appearing as a result of lead intoxication is also more likely to be observed in the young child than in the older person.

It is important that every individual who suffers with a seizure be investigated completely for all of the known causes of convulsions. The age of onset of the first seizure often leads the physician to a presumptive diagnosis of the cause, since certain convulsion-provoking conditions occur more frequently at one age than at another. However, this factor must be used as supportive and not definite evidence of the cause.

The greatest number of patients are afflicted with epilepsy during early childhood and approximately 90% of all patients develop their initial symptoms before the age of 20. Therefore, convulsions of undetermined etiology appearing during early childhood definitely should direct the physician's attention to a diagnosis of an epileptic disorder.

I have been impressed with the fact that some physicians are exceedingly reluctant to consider a diagnosis of an epileptic disorder when convulsions appear for the first time during adult life. This is unquestionably the soundest medical approach for the physician to assume, since convulsions appearing during adulthood are more likely to be manifestations of an intracranial neoplasm than those appearing initially during childhood. However, an analysis made in our clinic of a large group of patients whose attacks began after 20 years of age, indicates that the initial onset of epilepsy during adult life is not uncommon.

I would like to call attention to a news column (*The Baltimore Sun*, September 11, 1962) in which Helen Erskine quoted the United Epilepsy Association as stating that it is practically impossible to develop epilepsy at 32 years of age. This was in answer to a question referred to her by a 32 year old individual who suffered with seizures. I believe that Helen Erskine desired to relate to this individual that it is practically impossible to develop epilepsy during adulthood. This definitely is not true. This statement certainly could give a patient who became afflicted with a convulsive disorder during adult life some reason to question a physician's diagnosis of epilepsy. Such a patient may be inclined to suspect that his convulsion was due to a disorder more serious than epilepsy, such as a brain tumor

Although epilepsy may make its initial appearance at any time during childhood, there are two specific times at which it is more likely to occur: during the first few years of life and at the onset of puberty. The initial appearance of epilepsy during the latter period is observed much more frequently in females than in males.

The high incidence of epilepsy during the first few years of life is thought to be related to cerebral damage occurring either prenatally or at birth. The factors which predispose to the relatively high incidence of epilepsy during adolescence are not known. However some physicians have postulated that the many complex chemical and physiological changes which take place in the body at this time may predispose an individual to epilepsy. The chances of developing epilepsy after passing through adolescence are relatively small, unless the individual subsequently sustains brain damage either from trauma or infection. This brain damage may predispose the individual to epilepsy.

FREQUENCY OF EPILEPSY

There is no doubt that epilepsy is an exceedingly common disease. There are no accurate figures available on the actual number of epileptics in the general population. This is due to a number of factors. Firstly, epilepsy is not a condition which must be reported by the physician to the health department, as must be done with many other disorders; secondly, since it is now known that epilepsy may take a variety of forms other than the true convulsive type, many individuals suffer with epilepsy unknown to both themselves and their physicians; and finally it is well known that many individuals conceal the fact that they have epilepsy.

Case Histories Numbers 2 and 3 are examples of the lengths to which some individuals will go in order to conceal their epileptic disorder.

Case History Number 2

A wealthy and socially prominent, middle-aged woman, who suffered with epileptic seizures, received treatment and medication from a hospital dispensary rather than from her family physician and neighborhood pharmacy. In order to conceal her identity, she gave a fictitious name and address and wore very shabby clothing to the dispensary. Eventually, her real identity was discovered and when asked why she resorted to such extreme measures to conceal the nature of her illness, she offered the following reasons: she feared that she may be seen in her physician's office by some of her friends and questioned as to why she was consulting the physician; she did not want her physician to know that she had epilepsy; by the nature of the medication which she was taking, she felt that her neighborhood pharmacist would in all probability be cognizant of her disorder; she felt that any one or a combination of these factors might endanger her social position in the community.

Case History Number 3

A fifty year old man suffered with cataracts and was being treated for this condition by an ophthalmologist. The patient was so intent upon keeping his epileptic disorder unknown that he resorted to a mail order house for treatment. He visited the eye doctor quite frequently, but did not disclose the fact that he had epilepsy until the day that the ophthalmologist scheduled him for surgical removal of the cataracts. Realizing that he might have a convulsion while on the operating table, the patient became very frightened and informed the doctor of his epileptic seizures.

Nevertheless, despite these barriers to the obtention of correct figures on the incidence of epilepsy, the number of known epileptics is increasing with the passage of time. This is due in great measure to the introduction of electroencephalography as an adjunctive diagnostic tool with the result that the physician has become more aware that epilepsy can manifest itself clinically in many forms other than the classical convulsive seizure.

In addition, a better public understanding of the nature of the disorder has led to a decrease in the stigmas associated with epilepsy, although this, of course, is still woefully short of the mark. This has resulted in a greater willingness among epileptics to reveal their condition.

The repeal, in some communities, of laws prohibiting epileptics from marrying, driving automobiles and other activities, has also eliminated some of the barriers which have caused individuals to conceal their condition from public authorities.

The incidence of epilepsy is such that I believe it rates second among all medical disorders which have a tendency to chronicity, being surpassed only by mental retardation. Many general figures on the incidence of epilepsy have been quoted. The most common figure is that one in 100 individuals in the United States suffer with epileptic seizures. A recent survey conducted by Eisner and coworkers in our clinic indicated that one out of every fifty persons will develop some form of epilepsy during his lifetime. In a publication covering a five year study of 845 children, Miller and coworkers reported the incidence of recurrent convulsions to be one in fifty-three.

It has been further estimated that one out of ten persons in the population at large has a dysrhythmic electroencephalogram; some of these persons apparently have unrecognized seizures.

According to a recent brochure published by the American Epilepsy Federation the incidence of epilepsy in the United States as compared to that of some other conditions is as follows:

Epilepsy	1,700,000
Cancer	1,100,000
Cerebral Palsy	550,000
Tuberculosis (active)	400,000
Infantile Paralysis (1953, pre-Salk)	35,968

Epilepsy also affects many more people than some of the more publicized disorders which have a tendency to be chronic, such as diabetes, muscular dystrophy, multiple sclerosis and blindness.

BIBLIOGRAPHY

Eisner, V., Pauli, L. L., and Livingston, S.: Hereditary Aspects of Epilepsy. *Bull. Johns Hopkins Hosp.*, *105:*245, 1959.

Eisner, V., Pauli, L. L., and Livingston, S.: Epilepsy in the Families of Epileptics. *J. Pediat.*, *56:*347, 1960.

Miller, F. J. W., Court, S. D. M., Walton, W. S., and Knox, E. G.: *Growing Up in Newcastle Upon Tyne.* London, Oxford University Press, 1960, pp. 164-165.

Livingston, S.: Etiologic Factors in Adult Convulsions. An Analysis of 689 Patients Whose Attacks Began After Twenty Years of Age. *New England J. Med.*, *254:*1211 1956.

Chapter 2

DIAGNOSIS OF SEIZURE DISORDERS

A SEIZURE, particularly the first one, should be regarded as a serious sign, since it might be one of the manifestations of disorders requiring immediate definitive treatment, such as meningitis, encephalitis or drug intoxication. *A diagnosis of epilepsy should, therefore, not be made until the patient has been thoroughly investigated for such disorders and no specific cause for the seizures can be discovered with the diagnostic techniques currently available.* Table 1 lists some of the disorders which are associated with seizures or spells of various types.

Many physicians do not diagnose a disorder as epilepsy until a patient has had "many" seizures of undetermined cause. I assign a diagnosis of epilepsy to all patients who have seizures of undetermined etiology, regardless of whether they have had only one seizure or many. In the case of a patient who has had one seizure of undetermined etiology, I make a tentative diagnosis of epilepsy and continue with this diagnosis unless the passage of time proves that the seizure was a manifestation of some other disorder. My opinions on the management of a patient with one seizure are discussed in detail in another section of this book entitled Medical Treatment of Epilepsy (Chapter 8).

Arriving at the proper diagnosis depends upon correct interpretation of many factors gathered from the patient's history, his examination and various laboratory procedures.

1. CASE HISTORY

The case history frequently provides important diagnostic information. In fact, it has been my experience that a diagnosis can be made in the vast majority of individuals on the basis of the case history alone.

TABLE 1

DISORDERS WHICH ARE ASSOCIATED WITH CONVULSIONS OR SPELLS OF VARIOUS TYPES

1. Intracranial infections, e.g., meningitis, encephalitis, cerebral abscess.
2. Intracranial hemorrhage, such as caused by direct injury to the brain substance (at birth or other trauma), rupture of cerebral blood vessel (from disease such as arteriosclerosis or defect such as aneurysm).
3. Subdural hematoma.
4. Concussion of the brain, e.g., acute trauma to the head.
5. Metabolic disorders, e.g., tetany (hypocalcemia, alkalosis), hypoglycemic states, phenylpyruvic oligophrenia, hypernatremia.
6. Renal disorders, e.g., uremia.
7. Breath-holding spells (in children).
8. Emotional (functional) disorders, e.g., simple fainting spells, hysterical convulsions.
9. Parasitic brain diseases, e.g., toxoplasmosis, malaria, hydatid cyst, cysticercosis.
10. Narcolepsy and Cataplexy.
11. Allergy (?).
12. Intracranial neoplastic diseases, e.g., brain tumors.
13. Hypertension and cerebral arteriosclerosis.
14. Syncopal attacks, e.g., carotid sinus syndrome, Stokes-Adams disease, Menière's syndrome.
15. Toxic
    a. Drugs, e.g., when taken in excess or if sensitivity is present, many of the commonly used drugs such as ACTH, atropine, Benadryl, boric acid, caffeine, cortisone, epinephrine, penicillin, Thorazine and Compazine will cause convulsions.
    b. Acute lead encephalopathy.
    c. Kernicterus.
    d. Immunizations, particularly pertussis (may also be due to fever).
    e. Roseola infantum (may also be due to fever).
    f. Shigella gastroenteritis (may also be due to fever).
16. Cerebral degenerative diseases, e.g., Schilder's disease.
17. Congenital cerebral defects, e.g., tuberous sclerosis, Sturge-Weber syndrome, hydrocephalus, cerebral aplasia.
18. Fever in young children (usually associated with infections such as tonsillitis or otitis media), e.g., simple febrile convulsions.
19. Alcoholism.
20. Neurosyphilis.
21. Anoxia, e.g., anesthetics.
22. Eclampsia.
23. Tetanus.
24. Epilepsy.

The physician should inquire if the seizure was the patient's first. The age of onset of the first seizure may give the physician a clue as to the proper diagnosis, since it is known that certain disorders associated with convulsions are more prone to occur in different age groups. For example, a convulsion is more likely to be a manifestation of a brain tumor in an adult than in a child.

It is important for the physician to know if there was an associated elevation of temperature. Convulsions occurring in association with fever should direct the physician's attention to the three most likely disorders: (a) an intracranial infection such as meningitis or encephalitis; (b) epilepsy triggered off by fever; (c) simple febrile convulsions. This latter disorder occurs almost entirely in young children and is discussed in detail in another section of this book entitled Disorders Stimulating Epilepsy (Chapter 6).

The possibility of drug intoxication or the ingestion of toxic substances such as lead should be investigated.

The physician should also endeavor to ascertain if the patient recently sustained any injury to the head.

A history of similar convulsions in the past should always suggest the possibility of disturbances which are associated with recurrent seizures, such as brain tumors, hypoglycemia and epilepsy.

Sometimes the character of the seizure itself provides a clue to the underlying disturbance. A focal seizure, for example, should always suggest the possibility of a local lesion in the brain such as a brain tumor.

A history of seizures occurring only in association with sleep or only in association with the menstrual period is suggestive evidence in favor of epilepsy.

It is important that the physician ask the patient if he is aware of any circumstances which may be related to the occurrence of his seizures, regardless of how trivial they may appear. The observations of the patient may supply the physician with valuable information which can be utilized in the diagnosis and treatment of the case.

2. PHYSICAL AND NEUROLOGICAL EXAMINATION

A complete physical and neurological examination is imperative. This is obvious to all physicians and the details of these examinations need not be presented in this book.

3. LABORATORY PROCEDURES

When the history or physical examination does not produce conclusive evidence of a specific diagnosis, laboratory procedures should be performed including the following.

Blood Examinations

Blood calcium and phosphorus determinations;

Studies of carbohydrate metabolism, such as fasting blood sugar determinations and glucose tolerance test;

Blood lead level determinations, when indicated as, for instance, when there is a history or suspicion of pica, involving the eating of substances such as paint, plaster or wall paper.

Urine Examinations

Urine examination for protein and cellular elements;

Urine test for phenylketonuria;

Urine examination for evidence of lead intoxication, when indicated.

Cerebrospinal Fluid Examinations

The cerebrospinal fluid should be examined in all patients who present the following findings: (a) those in whom the convulsive seizure is associated with clinical evidence of an intracranial infection such as meningitis or encephalitis; (b) those in whom the convulsive seizure is associated with an elevation of temperature and in whom the physical examination fails to reveal evidence of an extracranial infection such as otitis media or tonsillitis. This applies even when there is no clinical evidence of meningeal or cortical irritation; (c) those who present definite signs or symptoms suggestive of central nervous system diseases, with necessary caution in the presence of increased intracranial pressure.

Subdural Puncture

A subdural puncture should be performed when a diagnosis of subdural hematoma is considered. The signs and symptoms of a subdural hematoma are variable. It should always be suspected in an individual who, subsequent to a cranial injury complains of vomiting, headache of increasing severity, lethargy or symptoms suggestive of compression of the brain.

Electroencephalographic Examination

This subject is discussed in detail in another section of this book entitled Electroencephalography (Chapter 3).

Cranial Roentgenography

In the majority of instances routine x-rays of the skull do not reveal any abnormality of the brain. However, as it is impossible to predict when such examinations might be of value and since it is a completely innocuous procedure, it is my policy to perform this examination routinely. I recently saw two patients who were being treated elsewhere for epilepsy without having had a roentgenographic examination of the skull. A routine x-ray of the skull provided the initial clue as to the proper diagnosis in each of these patients: one patient had an operable brain tumor and the other had tuberous sclerosis.

Pneumoencephalography or cerebral arteriography or both should be performed on those patients in whom an intracranial neoplasm or cerebral vasular anomaly is suspected.

Pneumoencephalography consists of replacing the spinal fluid with air or oxygen and taking x-rays of the head to outline the size, shape and position of the various cavities in and above the brain substance. This procedure is most frequently carried out by injecting the air or oxygen into the spinal canal, but in certain specific instances the air is injected directly into the brain cavities. It has been my experience that pneumoencephalography is an essentially innocuous procedure when performed by competent physicians. It is important for the patient to be told that following a pneumoencephalographic examination he may experience a severe headache which may persist for three or four days or so. I generally explain to my patients that the headache is caused by the air which was introduced into the brain cavities and that it usually takes about three or four days for the air to disappear. The headache is usually less severe when the patient is in a recumbent position and becomes more pronounced when he sits up.

Cerebral arteriography consists of taking x-rays of the skull after some opaque substance such as Diodrast has been introduced into one of the carotid or vertebral arteries. When the procedure is properly performed the shape and location of the arterial and venous systems of the brain are visualized. Thus, deformities of the cerebral vascular system, produced by vascular anomalies and tumors, can be detected.

Chapter 3

ELECTROENCEPHALOGRAPHY

THIS chapter consists essentially of a discussion of some of the many questions which I have been asked by patients and their parents or guardians, educators, counselors, nurses and also many physicians in regard to electroencephalography. Those individuals interested in a more scientific discussion of electroencephalography may refer to some of the standard text books on this subject which which are listed in the bibliography at the end of this chapter.

WHAT IS ELECTROENCEPHALOGRAPHY?

Electroencephalography is a laboratory examination which is employed primarily to study the electrical activity of the brain. This examination is commonly called the "brain wave test."

Electroencephalography dates back to 1875, when Dr. Caton discovered evidence of electrical activity in the brains of living animals. However, it was not until 1929 that the first recordings of electrical activity of the human brain were published by Dr. Hans Berger. Since Dr. Berger reported his original observations, considerable work has been done in the development and exploitation of the technique of electroencephalography by such investigators as the Gibbses, Jasper, Lennox and Walter. Today, electroencephalography is one of the most important tests available for the diagnosis of seizure disorders. Its most significant value, however, is in the study of the disorder of epilepsy.

The electroencephalogram or "brain wave" is a written record of the electrical currents which are constantly being generated in tiny amounts in the brains of all individuals. An instrument called an electroencephalograph registers this activity in the form of a wavy line traced on a moving strip of paper. The electroencephalograph determines the electrical activity of the brain in essentially

19

the same manner as the electrocardiograph determines the electrical activity of the heart. The former test is frequently referred to as an EEG and the latter as an EKG or ECG.

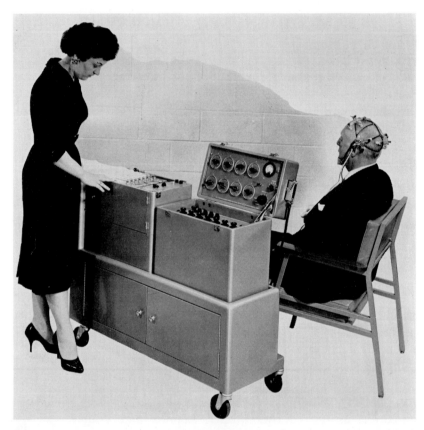

Figure 1. Photograph of technician performing a brain wave test on patient using the Offner Type T Electroencephalograph. The electroencephalograph shown in this photograph was selected for two reasons: (1) it is one of the newest types available, and (2) and more important for the purpose of this book, it illustrates to the patient that an electroencephalographic examination is a completely innocuous procedure. This latter point is emphasized, since many patients, including adults, have stated that they "suffered many anxious moments" prior to the performance of their electroencephalographic examination. (Manufactured by Offner Division of Beckman Instruments, Inc., 3900 River Road, Schiller Park, Illinois.)

HOW IS A BRAIN WAVE TEST CARRIED OUT?

The EEG machine is so sensitive that it is capable of picking up outside electrical signals which may interfere with the obtention of an accurate brain wave recording. In many instances, therefore, the EEG laboratory is constructed so as to exclude all external electrical interference. For example, the EEG machine itself may be located in one room while the patient will be "connected" to its leads in another room which is completely insulated by a "cage" of copper screening.

Newer equipment, however, such as the Offner Type T Electro-encephalograph (Figure 1) has largely eliminated the need for such extreme measures. Today, only relatively simple precautions are required to obtain clean, interference-free tracings under most conditions. Not only does this new equipment eliminate the need for special rooms in the hospital, but, being portable, it makes possible the taking of recordings on the wards or in remote locations when necessary.

In a brain wave test, small metal discs called electrodes are attached to various places on the patient's scalp. These discs may be secured to the scalp either with a sticky substance known as collodion, or a paste containing bentonite; or they may be held in place by a cap or a headband. Before putting the discs on the patient's scalp, the technician may apply a little fluid—usually acetone—to the appropriate areas of the head in order to remove substances, such as the natural oil of the hair, which may interfere with obtaining a satisfactory examination.

The technician will frequently ask the patient for information concerning his medical history and for information about medication which he has been taking.

The test is most frequently carried out with the patient in a reclining position on a bed or a couch. However, it may be performed with the patient in a seated position in an easy chair. When the test begins, the technician instructs the patient to keep his eyes closed and to relax as much as possible.

The lights in the laboratory probably are dimmed when the examination begins. During the course of the examination, the technician may enter the room and put additional discs on other parts of the scalp or reapply some of the discs which might have become loose.

A routine recording usually takes about twenty minutes, during which time the patient lies or sits in a relaxed state with his eyes closed. However, the test may take longer if the patient requires additional time to relax properly or if the technician or the physician uses additional techniques.

Another part of the examination which is considered routine is the so-called hyperventilation phase of the test. For this portion of the examination, the patient is instructed to breathe deeply for approximately four minutes. During this period of time, the EEG machine is allowed to operate and to produce a brain wave recording. The patient may experience a sensation of dizziness, numbness or tingling in the extremities during this period of deep breathing. This is no cause for alarm, as it is a perfectly normal reaction. The hyperventilation phase of the test is particularly important, since, at this time some patients will have a seizure which will be recorded on the EEG machine. This tracing will supply the physician with some very valuable information with regard to diagnosis and treatment of the case.

During the course of the test, the patient may also be asked to open and close his eyes several times. The character of the waves which are recorded on the tracing change with the opening and closing of the eyes and this may also give the physician some valuable information.

Sometimes the patient may be given a small quantity of sedative to help him relax while the examination is taking place, and, on occasion, larger doses may be given in order to induce sleep.

Sleep produces changes in the EEG recordings of every individual, whether he be a person with a seizure disorder or not. Often, a patient will have a normal electroencephalogram during the waking state and show abnormalities either during a drowsy state or during the sleep period. This is frequently a meaningful factor in the electroencephalographic examination, because it assists the physician in determining the type of seizure disorder with which an individual patient suffers.

There are other procedures which the physician employs in an attempt to elicit abnormalitles in the electroencephalogram. One of the commonly used methods is the so-called photic stimulation test. This consists of having the patient focus his eyes at a special light which flickers very frequently. In some patients this will produce certain changes in the brain wave pattern which are of diagnostic value to the physician. Sometimes other procedures, such as injection of medication into the veins, are employed to bring about changes in the brain wave pattern.

With older children and adults, the electroencephalographic examination is most frequently carried out without too much trouble. However, with many children and particularly with the younger child, it may be a more difficult problem. In order to conduct the test properly, it is necessary that a patient remain perfectly still for about twenty minutes, since movements will sometimes be reflected in the EEG tracing and will interfere with a proper reading.

With children of under two or three years of age, it is almost always necessary to administer sedative medication in order to obtain a satisfactory record. Most children of this age group will not lie still for the required time. Also, some of the younger children are so fearful that they cannot be calmed by verbal persuasion. The hyperventilation phase of the test frequently cannot be carried out in the younger child, since he will not cooperate satisfactorily for this procedure.

It is almost always necessary with very young children to administer sedative medication rectally or by hypodermic injection since most of them are unable to swallow tablets or capsules or even liquids. With older children, medication is given by mouth, or rectally or by hypodermic injection, depending upon the child's reaction.

HOW SHOULD A PATIENT PREPARE FOR A BRAIN WAVE TEST?

There are certain preparatory steps which a patient should perform preliminary to taking an electroencephalographic examination. If the test is to take place in the morning, for example, the head should be washed thoroughly with soap and water the preceding night. No oily substances, such as tonics or creams, should be put on the head before the test is performed. No medication except the patient's regular antiepileptic drugs should be taken unless specific instructions are given by the physician. And, unless he has been told by the physician to do otherwise, the patient should conduct himself in his regular fashion on the morning of the test.

Where a child will require rectal administration of sedative medication in order to perform the brain wave test, it is usually advisable that the parents give him an enema, either the night or the early morning before the test is performed in order to cleanse the lower bowel of all fecal matter. This will permit the sedative medication to be more quickly absorbed and to act more quickly.

The electroencephalographic examination is both simple and painless. All the patient must do is sit in an easy chair or recline on a bed or couch while small, flat discs (electrodes) are attached to various parts of his head. In some instances, electrodes are also placed on the lobe of each ear. The electrodes are held in contact with the skin of the scalp with the use of the sticky or pasty materials described previously; when they are applied to the lobes of the ears, the electrodes are frequently secured with a small clamp. Fine wires extend from these discs to a radio-like box which amplifies the currents received from the brain. These amplified currents move a series of pens on a moving roll or pad of paper and record the currents as a series of wavy lines (brain waves).

WHAT CAN A BRAIN WAVE TEST DO? HOW CAN IT HELP THE PHYSICIAN?

It is important that the patient understand what an EEG can do and what it cannot do. The EEG machine cannot hurt or influence a person's brain in any way. It cannot read the mind; it cannot determine whether a person is emotionally or mentally ill; it cannot give electric shocks; it is not a form of treatment; it does not cure and it does not hurt. Brain waves do not reflect thoughts, intelligence or disposition.

Many individuals have the impression that the electroencephalograph is capable of measuring the intelligence of a patient. This definitely is not true. I have also had many patients who stated that they did not experience a recurrence of seizures after having a "treatment" with the electroencephalograph and, therefore, assumed that the EEG "cured" them. The patient should definitely understand that the EEG machine is a diagnostic and not a therapeutic medium.

The information which a physician receives from a brain wave examination can frequently help him in making the correct diagnosis. This information may also be of value in determining the type of treatment which should be employed. In some instances, it may supply the physician with information as to the prognosis of the individual case.

Every person has his own individual brain wave pattern and this pattern, as stated previously, may vary with the patient's state at the time it is taken. That is, the brain wave pattern is different if taken while the patient is awake; it is different if taken while the patient is restless and apprehensive; it is different if taken while the patient is drowsy; and then again, it is completely different if taken while the patient is deeply asleep.

Generally, most patients with seizure disorders will show brain waves which are different from those of so-called normal people. Figure 2 shows a section of an EEG tracing obtained from a normal eight year old child, and Figure 3 shows a section of an EEG tracing obtained from a seven year old child with petit mal epilepsy. (See pages 26 and 27).

In addition, the type of abnormal waves which an epileptic will record depends upon the type of epilepsy with which he suffers. In other words, those patients with petit mal epilepsy, for example, will show a different abnormal pattern from that of patients with grand mal or psychomotor types of epilepsy.

The physician makes the correct diagnosis by considering the type of brain wave pattern together with the patient's clinical symptoms and the results of other laboratory procedures. I would like to emphasize this fact and I make the following statements primarily because of my experiences with many attorneys who requested that I perform an electroencephalographic examination on one of their clients. Invariably, their attitude was that the performance of this examination was all that was necessary in order to arrive at the proper diagnosis and prognosis of their client. I

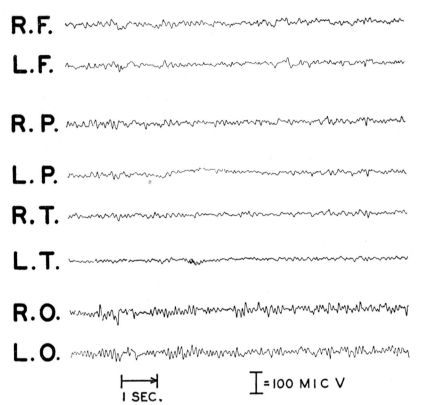

R.F.

L.F.

R. P.

L. P.

R. T.

L. T.

R. O.

L. O.

├──→┤   1 SEC.   𝕀 = 100 MI C V

Figure 2. Shows sample of EEG tracing of normal female, age eight years.

would like to repeat that electroencephalography is a valuable tool, but a diagnosis should never be made until after the information provided by the electroencephalographic examination is properly evaluated and considered together with the clinical history, the results of the physical and neurological examinations, appropriate roentgenograms, blood examinations and other special tests. I am in complete agreement with Dr. P. C. Bucy who stated in an editorial published in the *Journal of the American Medical Association* in 1956, "We have not yet achieved 'push button' medicine, and the electroencephalograph is not neurology's 'diagnostic machine.'"

In some seizure disorders, for example, in petit mal epilepsy, the brain wave pattern is almost always abnormal. The electro-

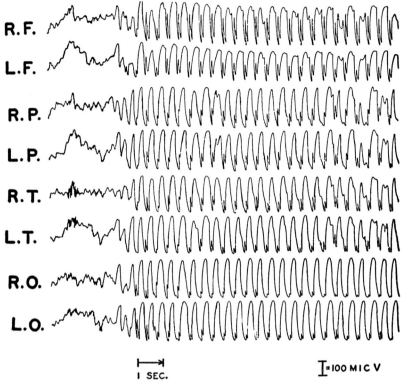

R. F.

L. F.

R. P.

L. P.

R. T.

L. T.

R. O.

L. O.

I SEC.   I = 100 MIC V

Figure 3. Shows sample of EEG tracing of female, age seven years, with petit mal epilepsy. Note the characteristic abnormalities (3 per second spike and wave forms).

encephalogram of patients with petit mal epilepsy presents the most characteristic abnormalities of all the epilepsies. Figure 3 shows a sample of EEG abnormality found in petit mal epilepsy, and Figure 2, for comparison, shows a sample of tracing of a normal child of similar age.

In certain other forms of seizure disorders, such as in grand mal convulsions, the brain waves may be normal. This is particularly true in the case of children and especially so in the case of very young children. Therefore it is important that the patient realize that the electroencephalogram may reveal normal findings in spite of the fact that he suffers with convulsions. Because of this, in some instances, the physician may want to perform another electroencephalogram to see whether he can elicit abnormalities in the repeat test.

It is of interest to note also, that several investigators have reported the occurrence of abnormal tracings in five to ten per cent of a group of people none of whom exhibited signs or symptoms of a seizure disorder. It may be that these individuals will subsequently develop seizures.

The electroencephalogram is of particular importance to the neurosurgeon. It frequently supplies valuable information which may assist him in locating brain tumors and other disturbances of the brain which, in some instances, can be corrected by surgical removal.

Within recent years considerable advances have been made in the surgical treatment of epilepsy by such noted physicians as Dr. Wilder Penfield and Dr. A. Earl Walker. The electroencephalogram has been largely responsible for the advancements made in this field. Since the introduction of the electroencephalogram, the neurosurgeon is sometimes able to localize certain areas of the brain which contain the so-called epileptic "foci," something which previously was most difficult to achieve. If the "disturbed" portion of the brain is in an area which can be removed, that is, if it is not in a so-called vital area, the patient can sometimes be relieved of his seizures.

The neurosurgeon utilizes the electroencephalograph right in the operating room and places the electrodes directly on the cortex of the brain. They are held in place by various types of so-called cortical electrode holders.

Since the brain wave examination sometimes supplies information as to the prognosis of the patient's disorder, the physician may request that brain wave tests be repeated periodically during the course of treatment so that he can compare the results of the various examinations.

It must be stressed that the electroencephalographic examination is not always a complete indicator of a patient's progress. He should also understand that the EEG has many limitations and that it does not always provide a positive answer. In some of my patients, for instance, the EEG became more normal concurrent with improvement in seizures; whereas, in others, the EEG became more abnormal even though the patient had fewer or no seizures. Also, many of my patients continue to have EEG abnormalities in spite of the fact that they have been free of seizures for periods of from fifteen to twenty or twenty-five years. It is generally known that in some children the EEG tends to revert to normal as they approach adolescence regardless of their clinical progress.

Nevertheless, the electroencephalogram is an exceedingly valuable instrument for the research laboratory and probably has done more to clarify some of the problems of seizure disorders, particularly epilepsy, than any other discovery of the past twenty-five years.

BIBLIOGRAPHY

Bernstine, A. L.: *Fetal Electrocardiography and Electroencephalography.* Springfield, Ill., Thomas, 1961.

Brechner, V. L., Walter, R. D., and Dillon, J. B.: *Practical Electroencephalography for the Anesthesiologist.* Springfield, Ill., Thomas, 1961.

Davidoff, L. M., and Dyke, C. G.: *The Normal Encephalogram.* 3rd edition. Philadelphia, Lea & Febiger, 1951.

Faulconer, A., and Bickford, R. G.: *Electroencephalography in Anesthesiology.* Springfield, Ill., Thomas, 1960.

Fois, A.: *The Electroencephalogram of the Normal Child.* Springfield, Ill , Thomas, 1961.

Gibbs, F. A., and Gibbs, E. L.: *Atlas of Electroencephalography.* Cambridge, Mass., Addison-Wesley Press, 1952.

Hill, D., and Parr, G.: *Electroencephalography.* London, MacDonald, 1950.

Hill, D., and Parr, G. (Editors): *Electroencephalography: A Symposium on its Various Aspects.* London, MacDonald, 1952.

Lennox, W. G.: *Epilepsy and Related Disorders.* Vol. 2. Little, Brown & Co., Boston, 1960, pp. 772-784.

Livingston, S.: *The Diagnosis and Treatment of Convulsive Disorders in Children.* Springfield, Ill., Thomas, 1954, pp. 144-172.

Livingston, S.: Convulsive Disorders in Infants and Children, in *Advances in Pediatrics.* The Year Book Publishers, Chicago, 1958, pp. 145-151.

Livingston, S.: Valor y Limitaciones de la Electroencefalografia en el Diagnostico, Tratamiento y Pronostico de la Epilepsia en los Ninos, El Dia Medico, Edicion Especial, Mayo 1962, pp. 907-913.

Meyer, J. S., and Gastaut, H.: *Cerebral Anoxia and the Electroencephalogram.* Springfield, Ill., Thomas, 1961.

Schwab, R. S.: *Electroencephalography in Clinical Practice.* Philadelphia, Saunders, 1951.

Stewart, L. F.: *Introduction to the Principles of Electroencephalography.* Springfield, Ill., Thomas, 1961.

Strauss, H., Ostow, M., and Greenstein, L.: *Diagnostic Electroencephalography.* New York, Grune & Stratton, 1952.

Chapter 4

CLASSIFICATION OF EPILEPTIC SEIZURES

AN EPILEPTIC seizure may vary considerably in its clinical manifestations. However, one feature common to most seizures is a sudden loss or impairment of consciousness. This may or may not be associated with frank convulsive movements and other abnormal motor or psychic performances. Tongue biting, urinary and/or fecal incontinence occur in some patients, especially those with grand mal seizures. When urinary incontinence occurs in association with major spells, it generally does not present too great a problem because the violent nature of the attack itself attracts most attention. On the other hand, when urinary incontinence occurs with the less violent seizures, such as petit mal spells or short psychomotor seizures, it may cause the patient considerable embarrassment.

Most patients usually have only one type of epileptic seizure. When a patient has more than one type, it is sometimes called mixed epilepsy.

The following classification of epileptic seizures is the one currently employed at the Epilepsy Clinic of The Johns Hopkins Hospital.

GRAND MAL SEIZURES

A grand mal seizure is also sometimes called a major motor seizure, a major seizure or a "big" seizure. Grand mal seizures are the most frequent of the epileptic attacks.

A typical attack consists of a sudden loss of consciousness and generalized tonic and clonic movements. If the patient is standing when he loses consciousness, he falls with boardlike rigidity (tonic phase) in whatever direction he happens to be leaning. The tonic rigidity soon changes to very rapid generalized jerking movements of the muscles (clonic phase). During the convulsive phase, the patient may bite his tongue or may lose control of his urine or bowels. Some patients may issue a loud cry or shriek before the onset of a seizure. The patient's breathing is frequently labored and jerky and at times it may appear as if the patient has stopped breathing completely. The patient's face may present a somewhat bluish color, particularly at those times when the breathing is very shallow or momentarily suspended. These jerking movements of the body gradually diminish and finally disappear, and the patient then relaxes.

When the seizure is brief, the patient is usually able to resume normal activity within several minutes after the seizure has subsided. However, at the end of a protracted seizure, the patient usually passes into a deep sleep or coma. Upon recovery from this so-called post-convulsive sleep or coma, the patient may present a variety of irregular and inconsistent signs or symptoms which are designated as post-convulsive phenomena. Generalized weakness, nausea, vomiting, severe headaches, soreness of muscles, generalized fatigue, restlessness, increased irritability and various types of abnormal behavior are common post-convulsive phenomena. Impaired speech, mental confusion and transient paralysis of the muscles also occasionally occur. These so-called post-convulsive disturbances may last for a moment or so, or they may persist for as long as a week.

The duration of a grand mal attack varies from less than one minute to as long as thirty minutes or even longer. They may recur many times a day, or occur only once in several years.

Sometimes a patient may go into a state of constant convulsions, that is, the patient may have a series of recurrent grand mal convulsions between which he does not completely gain consciousness. The individual convulsions themselves may only last for two or three minutes, but they may recur continuously and the patient does not regain consciousness between each individual convulsion. This condition is known as status epilepticus. The patient may remain in this state for several hours or so and even for days in some instances. This form of epilepsy is a definite medical emergency and patients with such a condition should receive immediate medical treatment.

PETIT MAL SEIZURES

Petit mal spells are always of very short duration, usually lasting five to ten seconds and rarely for much longer than 20 seconds. During these spells the patient generally becomes pale and his eyes appear as though they are staring vacantly into space. He is in a state of loss of consciousness for a brief period of time. In some instances, the spell involves only a blank staring into space for several moments. In other instances, the eyes may roll back into the head and there may be slight jerking movements of the head, eyes or the upper extremities. With these spells, the patient may stagger or sway a little but rarely falls. Occasionally, there may be smacking movements of the lips or urinary incontinence. After the attack is over, the patient is usually alert and able to continue what he had been doing before the spell occurred.

As a rule, petit mal spells occur most frequently in the first few hours after arising, and usually are relatively infrequent during active exercise. Petit mal spells frequently have a high degree of recurrence, some patients experiencing as high as 50 to 100 such spells daily. They occur almost entirely in children, particularly girls, between the ages of four and eight years. Petit mal spells have a tendency to disappear in many patients as they grow older, even without treatment, and in some instances they disappear completely when the patient goes through puberty.

Some patients subsequently develop other types of epileptic seizures, especially grand mal attacks. These other attacks may appear during early childhood but most frequently appear at puberty or later in life.

Some patients with petit mal epilepsy have attacks so frequently that they are unable to regain consciousness between individual attacks. This condition is known as petit mal status.

I know of many instances where school teachers and also parents reprimanded and punished children for sleeping in class and also for being inattentive at times. Actually, these children were having petit mal attacks at these times and were not responsible for their actions.

Because of the innocuous appearance of most spells of petit mal epilepsy, which consist essentially of just staring momentarily into space, this condition is frequently overlooked or neglected by the parents. I can mention several instances where a mother took her child to the pediatrician for a general checkup and, during the course of the routine examination of the lungs, in which the patient is asked to breathe in and out, the patient simply stopped and stared vacantly into space for several seconds or so. The pediatrician asked the mother, "How long has your child been staring like that?" The mother answered, "Oh, she's been doing that for the past two or three years. She frequently stares into space like that." The mother had no idea whatsoever that her child was suffering with petit mal epilepsy. The parents should consult a physician at the slightest suggestion of any petit mal spell because with this type of epilepsy, as with all other types, the sooner it is treated the better is the chance that a control of spells will be obtained.

I have had several patients whose petit mal spells were not particularly distressing. They just consisted of staring vacantly into space for four or five seconds. However, during this period of unconsciousness, these patients lost control of their bladders and wet their pants. These episodes occurred in school and although the patient's schoolmates actually were not cognizant of the fact that he had suffered a petit mal spell, the patient was caused considerable embarrassment when his schoolmates observed that he wet his pants frequently during the course of the day.

In most instances older male patients can avoid the emotional disturbance caused by urinary incontinence by wearing a urinary bag. Urinary bags are available in a variety of styles and sizes and may be readily obtained at surgical supply stores. In the case of older boys, the use of an athletic supporter containing absorbent disposable padding may prove helpful. In the case of females and very young males who experience loss of bladder control in association with their spells, the situation may be helped by having them wear rubber or plastic underpants containing disposable absorbent padding. One such garment is Staydry Panties, available to patients of all ages. Figure 4 is a photograph of a boy wearing Staydry Panties.

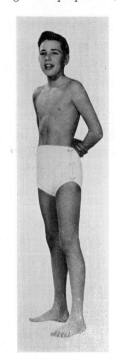

Figure 4. Photograph of boy wearing Staydry Panties. These panties contain thick, highly absorbent material with waterproof outer soft plastic covering. They are completely washable and may even be boiled and bleached. (Manufactured by Amira Products, Inc., Newburgh, N. Y.; Jolan Sales Co., 811 Fostertown Rd., Newburgh, N. Y. is the retail mail order outlet.)

PSYCHOMOTOR SEIZURES

A psychomotor seizure is a bizarre and variable type of epileptic attack. The term "psychomotor" as used at the present time refers to a seizure characterized by automatic, stereotyped movements, or a variety of abnormal behavior manifestations, associated with some clouding of consciousness and at least partial amnesia for the event. Psychomotor seizures are also referred to by some physicians as epileptic fugues, epileptic automatisms and temporal lobe epilepsy. This latter term, temporal lobe epilepsy, has been used because many patients with psychomotor epilepsy show abnormalities in their electroencephalograms which come almost entirely from the temporal lobe area of the brain.

Psychomotor epileptic seizures are observed most frequently in adults, but they do occur also in children. In some children, particularly the very young child, a psychomotor seizure consists only of a simple, isolated automatism such as smacking or chewing movements. In the older child and in the adult, the seizure often consists of a chronologic sequence of events involving brief phases. First, there may be an arrest or suspension of activity, such as staring or dazed expression; this is followed by repetitious, automatic, stereotyped, apparently purposeless, coarse and poorly coordinated movements; and finally, by repetitious, automatic reflections of disordered and confused psychic functioning, such as incoherent or irrelevant speech, rages and tantrums.

Numerous disturbances of varying complexity have been classified as manifestations of psychomotor epilepsy, e.g., fears, anxieties, sleepwalking, dreaming states, chewing and smacking movements of the mouth, wandering, belligerence, temper outbursts, staring expression, mental confusion, incoherent and irrelevant speech, rubbing or fumbling of the hands, mumbling or running wildly.

Some patients become exceedingly violent with a psychomotor attack and it is stated that serious crimes and even murder have been committed during a psychomotor attack. It has been suggested that it was during a psychomotor attack that Vincent Van Gogh cut off one of his ears.

Psychomotor attacks may be the only manifestation of epilepsy in an individual patient, but on the other hand, many patients will have psychomotor attacks in addition to other forms of epilepsy such as petit mal or grand mal. Although the manifestations of a psychomotor attack vary considerably from patient to patient, any individual patient will usually have the same form of attack.

Psychomotor seizures vary considerably in length. In some patients they persist only for a moment or so, while in others they may continue for hours or even days.

Since a wide variety of apparent behavior disturbances may be a manifestation of psychomotor epilepsy, the physician is often faced with the difficult problem of differentiating psychomotor epileptic seizures from some of the non-epileptic functional disturbances. For example, it may be difficult for the physician to determine whether the frequent temper tantrums, rages or sleepwalking of a child are really epileptic in origin or are a manifestation of a behavioral disorder. It is important that the patient be cognizant of this fact, since in many instances the physician may not be able to give him a specific diagnosis at the times of the first few visits. It may also be necessary that the physician have many electro-encephalograms performed before he arrives at the correct diagnosis.

In many cases, particularly those in which the findings of the electroencephalogram are not revealing, the physician may only be able to make a diagnosis of epilepsy in retrospect. It may be necessary for him to prescribe various drugs which are used for the treatment of epilepsy and to determine how the patient responds to these drugs before he is able to differentiate between a real epileptic disorder and a behavioral disorder.

Since psychomotor epilepsy is much less well-known and also less well-defined than the more easily recognized spells of grand mal or petit mal epilepsy, a brief resume of Case Histories Numbers 4 and 5 may be informative.

Case History Number 4

R. H. is a sixteen year old white female. Her father gave the following description of her spells.

"My daughter and I were sitting in the restaurant eating lunch and discussing our trip to Baltimore. Suddenly she stopped talking and complained of feeling funny in the stomach. Then she had a blank and dazed expression in her eyes which lasted for a moment or so. Then she began repeating the questions: 'Where am I'? 'What day is this?' 'What time is it?' She continued to repeat these questions in the same order for about fifteen minutes. Then she got up from the table and took a fork and began hitting it against the table and she continued to do this for about ten minutes. Following this she sat down again and then she seemed to relax and after this she came to herself. For a moment she appeared somewhat confused, but then recovered completely. I spoke to her frequently during the course of the spell, but she did not seem to hear me and she did not answer the questions. When she recovered completely, I asked her what happened and she had no recollection of the disturbance."

This patient's EEG revealed abnormalities consistent with an epileptic disorder. Her seizures responded to antiepileptic therapy.

Case History Number 5

A ten year old white girl, who gave a history of having had frequent major motor seizures from two to six years of age, had bi-monthly attacks occurring at night, during which she would first call out for her mother and then would begin to talk incoherently, continuously repeating meaningless expressions. She would also repetitiously pick at the bedclothing. During these episodes she would not answer questions directed to her by her parents. The attacks lasted fifteen to thirty minutes. After the spell she would go back to sleep and the following day have no recollection of the event. Two electroencephalographic examinations revealed normal brain wave patterns. Her seizures responded to antiepileptic medication.

MINOR MOTOR SEIZURES

The term "minor motor" may be somewhat misleading insofar as one may get the impression that because of the word "minor" the spell is of little significance. The words "minor motor" are attached to this spell because during the spell the patient makes motor movements of the body which are of very short duration in contrast to grand mal attacks, where the motor movements are usually of great magnitude. In fact, of all of the various types of epileptic seizures, minor motor seizures have the worst outlook and one can say that they represent the most serious form of epilepsy.

Minor motor seizures are designated by other terms such as infantile spasms, salaam attacks or lightning majors and they are also sometimes classified by some physicians as hypsarrhythmia (meaning "mountainous arrhythmia") because a specific EEG abnormality is found in most patients with this type of spell.

In contrast to petit mal spells which occur most frequently in children between four and eight years of age, minor motor seizures most often make their initial appearance early in life, usually in infants between ages of three and twelve months. In fact, minor motor epilepsy is observed almost entirely in the very young child.

The external manifestations of minor motor epilepsy vary somewhat, but the most typical and also the most frequent type consists of a sudden flexion of the head with simultaneous extension of the upper extremities and flexion of the thighs on the abdomen. This type of spell is frequently preceded by a short cry, laugh or giggle. I classify this type of spell as a massive myoclonic minor motor seizure.

I have seen many patients who were considered by their parents as having ordinary abdominal pain and also some patients who were diagnosed by physicians as having colic, when they actually suffered with minor motor epilepsy. This mistaken impression or diagnosis was entertained because the child would first give out a cry and then suddenly draw his thighs up on his abdomen as if he were in pain.

Another manifestation of a minor motor spell consists of a sudden nod of the head, usually forward, and another manifestation consists of an abrupt loss of all muscle control with consequent falls, usually forward. The patient is usually able to get up almost immediately and generally the return to consciousness is immediate. In some instances, however, he may appear somewhat disoriented for several seconds or so. The former type of spell is sometimes designated as the head-nodding spell and the latter type is sometimes designated as the akinetic or dropping spell.

As with the petit mal spell, minor motor seizures also recur very frequently during the course of the day. Some patients may have as many as 50 to 100 attacks daily and in many instances these attacks which, in themselves, only last for a few seconds or so, recur in rapid succession (series) lasting for five to ten minutes.

The akinetic or dropping form of minor motor epilepsy is associated with frequent personal injuries to the patient. The patient generally falls forward and the injury is usually to the forehead or to the chin. The nature of these injuries and the prophylactic measures which may be employed to prevent them are discussed in another section of this book entitled Prognosis of Epilepsy (Chapter 17).

The most serious hazard of this form of epilepsy is not the seizures themselves but the associated mental retardation. Mental retardation of some degree is almost a constant finding in patients with minor motor epilepsy. Evidence of mental retardation may be apparent at the time of the onset of the seizures and then, on the other hand, signs of mental retardation may not become manifest until after the child has had seizures for a period of time. The degree of mental retardation found in association with minor motor epilepsy varies from mild to severe. In most instances, however, it is severe.

It is important that the parents of children with minor motor epilepsy be told about the most likely outcome of the condition, so that they can prepare themselves for the future and also make suitable arrangements for the care of the child. In many instances, institutional care is the only logical recourse.

OTHER TYPES OF EPILEPTIC SEIZURES

Since the introduction of electroencephalography, many other symptoms have been classified as manifestations of epilepsy. Some of these disturbances are: recurrent attacks of abdominal pain, headaches, attacks of dizziness, periodic vomiting, inappropriate laughing spells, emotional instability and fainting spells. These disorders, if thought to be of epileptic origin, are designated by various terms such as "diencephalic epilepsy," "autonomic epilepsy," "thalamic epilepsy," "hypothalamic epilepsy," "epileptic equivalent," "epileptic variant" and "non-convulsive epilepsy." The term "abdominal epilepsy" is assigned to those patients who suffer with recurrent attacks of abdominal pain thought to be epileptic in origin.

Since symptoms such as abdominal pain and headaches, for example, are among the most common complaints a physician is called upon to interpret and may be symptoms of many disorders, it is obvious that each patient must be investigated for all known causes of these symptoms before a diagnosis of an epileptic disorder should be made. As in the case of psychomotor epilepsy, it may be necessary for the physician to perform many brain wave tests and also to give the patient a trial on some of the drugs used to treat epilepsy before he can come to a definite conclusion in regard to the proper diagnosis.

Focal seizures are attacks which involve one part of the body. These seizures may appear as pure motor seizures such as jerking of one arm, or as sensory seizures such as numbness or tingling of some part of the body. A focal seizure is the one type of epileptic seizure which frequently occurs without associated loss of consciousness.

A typical so-called Jacksonian seizure is one which initially manifests itself by clonic movements of one part of the body (for example, the hand) which rapidly spread to involve the entire one side of the body. The clonic movements then spread in a similar fashion on the other side of the body and finally terminate in a generalized convulsion of the grand mal type. During the interval that the convulsive movements are spreading over the body the patient usually maintains consciousness. However, when the seizure becomes generalized, the patient falls into a state of unconsciousness just as with other types of grand mal convulsions.

AURA

An aura, or period of warning, is a disturbance which precedes an epileptic seizure. In other words, it is a premonitory sensation which indicates that the patient may have a seizure. Actually, an aura is an integral part of the attack.

It is exceedingly important that the physician study the seizure pattern of each patient for the occurrence of an aura. This information is of value to the neurosurgeon since it may give a clue as to the site of origin of an epileptic seizure.

TABLE 2

Sensations (Auras) Described by Some Epileptic Patients

A peculiar sensation which starts in the abdomen and then goes up to the chest and then to the head

I just feel funny all over my body

I feel different, but just can't describe the sensation

Abdominal pain or abdominal distress

Tingling, numbness or pain in various parts of the body

Headaches

A sensation of movements of the extremities which cannot be seen by the observer

Spots before the eyes

Various colors before the eyes

Impaired vision

A humming sensation

A buzzing sensation

Sounds of different types of music

Dizziness or unsteadiness

Peculiar or disagreeable tastes or odors.

The physician should always explain to the patient that an aura is a warning of an impending seizure. Therefore, if the aura is of long duration, the patient can utilize this interval of time to protect himself from injury if he should happen to be in a precarious position at the time of its occurrence. Table 2 gives a list of some of the sensations (auras) which regularly occurred before the seizures in some of my patients.

Auras occur mostly in patients who have grand mal seizures and to a lesser degree, in patients with psychomotor seizures. Patients with petit mal spells usually do not experience auras. The incidence of auras in minor motor epilepsy is impossible to determine because these spells occur almost entirely in the very young child. It is obvious that these young children would be unable to give a description of such an episode.

Chapter 5

FACTORS WHICH PRECIPITATE
EPILEPTIC SEIZURES

THERE is no doubt that epileptic seizures are produced by disturbances of nerve cell function of the brain. Although the specific cause of this cerebral dysfunction is not known, there are certain factors which are, on occasion, associated with the occurrence of epileptic seizures. In other words, in some patients the epileptic seizures occur spontaneously on some occasions and at other times they occur in association with these factors. Therefore, these factors cannot be considered the basic cause of their epileptic disorder, but merely the precipitating factors of some of the epileptic seizures.

EMOTIONAL DISTURBANCES

Emotional disturbances such as marked excitement, fear, frustration, tension and anxiety, are one of the most common, if not the most common, of the precipitating factors of epileptic seizures. This is particularly true in the case of the teenager and the younger adult. Emotional disturbances may increase the frequency of all types of epileptic seizures.

The nature and management of the emotional disorders encountered in epilepsy are discussed in detail in another section of this book entitled Behavior and Personality of the Epileptic (Chapter 13).

SLEEP

Many patients only have their seizures in association with sleep. Epileptic seizures may occur at any time during the sleep cycle, but they occur most frequently at two specific times (1) within the first or second hour after falling asleep, and (2) one to two hours before the usual time of awakening.

42

The fundamental changes which take place during sleep and which precipitate epileptic seizures are not known. Several investigators have determined the depth of normal sleep by various methods and concluded that, as a rule, the maximum depth of sleep is reached approximately one to two hours after falling asleep and again sometime near the usual time of awakening. These findings suggest that there may be some relationship between the depth of sleep and the occurrence of epileptic seizures.

Sleep, either natural or drug produced, is the most common means of evoking abnormal cerebral electrical activity. In some patients abnormal brain waves can only be elicited during certain stages of sleep and it may be necessary that the physician obtain an electroencephalogram under such circumstances in order to make the proper diagnosis.

If an individual is destined to have seizures, certainly the best time for them to occur is during sleep. People who have their seizures only in association with sleep experience less inconvenience and require fewer restrictions in their daily activities than those whose seizures occur during the daytime.

The patient who is subject to sleep seizures should be instructed against taking daily afternoon naps unless it is absolutely necessary. Such patients also should be definitely warned against the possibility of dozing off while operating an automobile. They should be told not to drive for prolonged periods of time particularly on super-highways or turnpikes, which are known to be conducive to dozing off or falling asleep. The rules and regulations concerning the operation of a motor vehicle are discussed in another section of this book entitled Socio-Economic Aspects of Epilepsy (Chapter 15).

The drug therapy for patients who suffer with seizures only in association with sleep differs from that which is prescribed for patients whose seizures occur during the daytime. Generally, for sleep seizures, either all or at least the greater part of the daily dosage is prescribed during the evening hours or at bedtime. A more detailed discussion of the treatment of sleep seizures is presented in another section of this book entitled Medical Treatment of Epilepsy (Chapter 8).

A question which is very frequently asked by the parents of an epileptic child who has sleep seizures is as follows: "Should such a child sleep in a room by himself or should someone sleep in the same bed with him or at least in the same room, so that he could be helped if he had a seizure?" I cite the case of a three year old girl who periodically had grand mal seizures about three or four o'clock in the morning while asleep. The mother informed me that she had been sleeping in her child's room every night since the seizures first occurred. Her husband became quite disturbed about this separation from his wife. The situation became so disturbing that he considered a divorce. The mother stated that she could not allow her child to sleep alone at night for fear that the child might have a convulsion, fall out of bed and hurt herself.

Generally, the policy of protecting a child by sleeping in the same room can do more harm psychologically, both to the patient himself and to the parent or guardian, than the calculated risk of accident to the child as a result of the seizure. The best policy to follow is to let nature take its course and allow the child to sleep unattended. Statistics show that only rarely does anything of a serious nature happen to an individual who has seizures during sleep. In practically all instances, the individual will have the spell and then go back to sleep. It is possible, however, to have protective sides installed on the beds of those patients who are known to have frequently fallen out of bed as a result of a seizure during sleep. This should not be done unless absolutely necessary, particularly in the case of older children since it could cause the patient considerable psychological harm.

MENSTRUATION

It has long been known that there is a direct relationship between epileptic seizures and menstruation. The physiological change or changes which occur during the menstrual cycle, and which are responsible for the precipitation of epileptic seizures, are not clearly understood and remain a highly controversial subject.

The retention of body fluids which occurs in association with the menstrual period is thought by some investigators to be the precipitant of seizures in some epileptic patients. Other physicians believe that it is possible that the complex hormonal changes which produce menstruation may play a prominent part in the precipitation of seizures.

Epileptic seizures may occur or become more frequent at any time during the menstrual cycle. However, the greatest tendency to seizures is observed during the first several days preceding the onset of the menstrual flow. In addition to the fact that the menstrual cycle is associated with an increase in the frequency of seizures in some epileptic patients, it is important to note that many females have their first epileptic seizure between the ages of eleven and thirteen. This is the period of life during which the onset of menses generally appears.

Some females have epileptic seizures only in association with their menstrual periods and not at any other time. If the seizures occur or become more severe only in association with the menstrual period, the physician should increase the dosage of the patient's regular medication for a few days before and during the menstrual cycle. A reduction of fluid intake and/or the administration of diuretics at this time is also helpful in some patients.

In spite of all types of therapy some patients continue to have seizures at the time of their menstrual periods and the patient must learn to accept the fact that she may experience a seizure during this period. If their employment permits, it may be advisable to forego work at this particular time.

Some of my patients who experienced seizures only in relation to their menses did not have a recurrence of these seizures after they passed through menopause. This finding suggests that the induction of artificial menopause should be seriously considered in those individuals who suffer with severe and incapacitating epileptic seizures in association with their menstrual periods.

In my experience pregnancy, per se, has no specific effect on the course of epilepsy. This subject is discussed in detail in the section of this book entitled Socio-Economic Aspects of Epilepsy (Chapter 15).

WITHDRAWAL OF ANTIEPILEPTIC DRUGS

The sudden withdrawal of antiepileptic medication is a very common cause of an increase in the frequency of a patient's seizures. It is also a very common cause for a return of seizures in a patient who has been taking medication for a prolonged period of time and who has been free of seizures for this period.

Particularly affected are those patients who have grand mal seizures and are taking barbiturate drugs such as phenobarbital, Mebaral and Gemonil.

In some instances a sudden withdrawal of antiepileptic drugs can cause status epilepticus, a condition which can be serious. This disturbance is described in detail in another section of this book entitled General Management of the Epileptic Patient (Chapter 7).

I have seen many patients who had been taking medication regularly experience an increase in the frequency of seizures or a precipitation of a seizure following the omission of one or two doses of medication. The patient and his parents should, therefore, always realize the importance of taking medication regularly and, particularly, of not discontinuing the medication, except upon the advice of his physician. I have seen many patients who, having been free of seizures for a prolonged period of time discontinued their medication of their own accord and soon thereafter began having seizures again.

For reasons which I cannot explain, in many patients it is more difficult to control a recurrence of seizures with the same medication which they had been taking successfully before.

I cannot emphasize too strongly that there is always a great possibility of recurrence of seizures associated with a sudden withdrawal of medication. The patient must fully appreciate the significance of this phenomenon. If the physician should inadvertently advise the patient to stop all of his medication abruptly, he should direct the doctor's attention to the fact that he has been taking antiepileptic medication for a long time.

I have also seen some patients who, having been free of seizures for a prolonged period of time, went of their own accord to a private electroencephalographic laboratory to check personally upon their medical progress by having a brain wave test performed. There they were told by the electroencephalographic technician to discontinue all medication so that a better reading might be obtained. This is a dangerous procedure and should be strictly avoided unless specifically authorized by a physician.

It is also important that the patient call attention to the fact that he has been taking antiepileptic medication when he is to be admitted to a hospital for diagnostic or surgical procedures. The busy physician or the busy hospital house-officer may overlook the fact that the patient has been taking antiepileptic medication and leave orders for the patient to receive nothing except specific medications prescribed for the specific disorder for which he was admitted to the hospital.

Occasionally, a patient may develop some unrelated intestinal disorder which is accompanied by vomiting. In such instances, the patient may be unable to swallow or retain his medication and it may be necessary, therefore, to administer the drugs by rectum or by hypodermic injection. There are also certain instances when all antiepileptic medication may have to be withdrawn. The responsibility for these decisions rests with the attending physician.

HYPERVENTILATION

It is well known that deep breathing will produce epileptic seizures in some patients. The primary importance of this procedure is that it provides a quick and simple means of activating seizures for diagnostic purposes.

In some instances, however, forced deep breathing will not precipitate a clinical spell in the patient, but will produce changes in the brain wave pattern which are of diagnostic significance to the physician. Hyperventilation is also employed as a routine part of an electroencephalographic examination.

This procedure appears to be almost specific for petit mal spells. Hyperventilation will precipitate a petit mal seizure in practically all cases. On the other hand, it has been my experience that forced deep breathing rarely, if ever, causes other types of epileptic seizures. I have had some patients who experienced other types of seizures, such as grand mal or psychomotor seizures, during the process of the hyperventilation test. However, these spells occurred so rarely with hyperventilation that I believe their occurrence was merely coincidental.

Hyperventilation is carried out by having the patient breathe deeply for a period of four to five minutes. If a seizure should occur while the test is being conducted, the patient will stop the hyperventilation of his own accord and it will not be necessary to continue it further.

When asked to continue forced breathing for this period of time, many patients will complain of sensations such as dizziness, light headedness or tingling of the hands and feet. These disturbances are not dangerous and may be considered as normal harmless reactions that also occur in many people who do not have seizures.

It is only natural for the parents to ask the following question: "Since it is medically known that deep breathing precipitates petit mal spells, should patients with these spells perform activities which bring about deep breathing such as running, bicycle riding and swimming?" I tell the parents that ordinary exercise is nearly always harmless and generally does not precipitate petit mal spells. The general activities which are recommended for an individual with epilepsy are discussed in detail in another section of this book entitled General Management of the Epileptic Patient (Chapter 7).

FEVER

(a) In Epileptic Patients

The effect of fever in individuals who suffer with epilepsy varies from patient to patient. In some instances, the frequency of seizures is increased, while in others it is lessened and in still others it remains unchanged.

The physician should make every attempt to remove all possible foci of infection in epileptic patients as soon as feasible, particularly in those who have experienced increased frequency or severity of seizures during acute infections.

(b) In Otherwise Normal Children

Convulsions or seizures are encountered very frequently in young children under three or four years of age in association with an elevation of temperature. The seizure usually occurs soon after the onset of the fever. In most instances, the convulsions which occur in young children with fever and extracranial infections are relatively innocuous. They are classified as simple febrile convulsions and are discussed in more detail in another section of this book entitled Disorders Simulating Epilepsy (Chapter 6).

ENVIRONMENT

A change of environment very frequently favorably affects the course of epileptic seizures, particularly in the case of children. I have seen many patients who experienced a marked decrease in the frequency and even a complete disappearance of seizures upon removal from their homes to other environments such as hospitals, camps, foster homes and special resident or hospital schools. They continued to do well throughout their entire stay in this new environment. However, when these children returned to their homes, the seizures reappeared with the same frequency which existed prior to the change of environment. The fact that these children took the same medication both at home and during the interval of their change of environment indicates very strongly that this latter factor was responsible for the temporary improvement in these patients.

It has been my experience that it is often difficult to get parents to agree to change their child's environment. Many will state: "I cannot see how removing my child to another environment could do him any good whatsoever. I treat him well and he seems to enjoy his existence at home." Nevertheless, there are many factors in a patient's environment which may adversely affect the course of his epileptic disorder. And, the one factor which I believe is by far the most significant is improper management of the child by his parents or guardian. CASE HISTORY NUMBER 6 illustrates the effect of environment on the course of an epileptic disorder.

Case History Number 6

H.M. is a nineteen year old white male whose birth and childhood development were essentially normal. There was no history of significant head injuries or of illness adversely affecting the brain prior to the onset of seizures.

He had his first convulsion when he was nine years old. This was a generalized major motor seizure lasting ten to fifteen minutes. Physical and neurological examinations revealed normal findings at that time. Laboratory studies, including x-ray of the skull, complete blood count and blood chemistries revealed normal findings. An electroencephalogram, however, showed abnormalities.

The patient continued to have similar major seizures once or twice a week in spite of treatment with many anticonvulsive drugs. Most of his spells occurred in the early morning hours just before the usual time of awakening and, therefore, he was able to attend school.

The mother was exceedingly over-solicitous and apparently was unable to cope with the problem. She watched "every movement" the patient would make and even resorted to sleeping in the same room with him. She would also walk him to school daily and call for him. She would not allow him to participate in physical or social scholastic activities. The patient showed evidence of marked resentment of his mother's attitude and often stated that she "treated him like a baby."

When the child was eleven years old he was admitted to the hospital for general observation and further investigation. He remained in the hospital for about one month. During this month's stay in the hospital, he had no seizures in spite of the fact that he took the same anticonvulsant medication which he had been taking previously. On two other occasions, when he was twelve and thirteen years of age, respectively, the mother was persuaded to allow the patient to attend a resident summer camp for a period of six weeks on each occasion. During both of these intervals, the patient remained completely free of seizures even though he received the same medication which he had been taking at home without benefit.

While away from home for prolonged periods, such as during his hospital admission and the two periods at the resident camp, the patient, in addition to remaining free from seizures, also behaved in an essentially normal fashion. However, at home he presented many emotional problems. He was constantly hostile, belligerent, resentful and showed evidence of marked insecurity and feelings of inferiority. He frequently stated that he loved his mother but resented the way she treated him. He said she would not allow him to act like a normal child and also that she watched every movement he made.

The mother's attention was called to the great disparity in her son's behavior while at home and when away from home. She was told that this finding indicated that environmental factors adversely affected the child's emotional state and that this, in turn, triggered off some of his epileptic seizures. It was suggested that improper parental management might possibly be one of the environmental factors causing the disturbances. At first the mother became exceedingly belligerent and stated that she loved her child very much and certainly would not do anything to cause him harm.

Subsequently, the mother was seen at regular intervals and given guidance in regard to the management of her child's disorder. She was gradually made to understand that she must learn to live with the situation and realize that her child must be given a chance to live as normal a life as possible, within the limits of his medical disorder. After a period of time, she became less over-protective and actually encouraged her son to participate in scholastic activities. She no longer treated him as a baby and, concurrent with the mother's more sensible approach to the problem, the patient's seizures gradually diminished and his behavior at home improved considerably.

When last seen, the patient was nineteen years of age. He was performing very well in every respect. When asked about his mother, he stated: "My mother finally learned to treat me like a boy my age should be treated, and because of this I now feel better and do not get as nervous as I did before." At this time he was having only an occasional seizure in association with sleep.

In addition to being responsible for improvement of seizures, change of environment also provides the physician with an opportunity to elicit important diagnostic information in some patients (Case History Number 7).

Case History Number 7

This case concerns an eight year old child who lived at home with her mother, grandfather and grandmother. Her father had divorced his wife because of incompatibilities. The child's seizures did not respond to the usual forms of therapy, and she was admitted to the hospital for further investigation. Shortly after admission, the seizures stopped and the child continued free of seizures during the entire stay in the hospital. When asked if she liked staying at the hospital she said: "Yes, I like it here." When asked whether she liked it better at home or at the hospital she stated: "I like it better at the hospital." However, when she was asked these same questions in the presence of her mother she did not give the same answers. She said that she liked it better at home.

The child was studied by a psychiatrist while at the hospital, and it was established that she had a deep-seated antagonistic feeling towards her mother. This was apparently the reason she liked it better at the hospital than she did at home. She was sent to a private resident school where, without medication, she remained free of seizures. Her relationship with her mother was finally brought to normal by psychiatric treatment, both of mother and of patient.

I have seen many patients in whom a change of environment was the only known factor which could have been responsible for a complete control of seizures. However, it is important to note that, in some instances, a reduction in the frequency of seizures may not occur until several weeks following the change of environment. In addition, those patients who respond to a change of environment would be well advised to remain in their new environment for a prolonged period of time before returning to their homes.

Change of environment can be brought about by removal to a foster home, private hospital school or state institution. The book entitled Directory for Exceptional Children supplies state-by-state listing and descriptions of educational and training facilities offered by many schools, homes, clinics, hospitals and services throughout the country for the epileptic. Unfortunately, most of the private hospital schools are exceedingly costly and are above the price range of most individuals.

Change of environment should be an important consideration for all patients who have not responded to the usual forms of anticonvulsive therapy. It has been my experience that this aspect of the treatment of epilepsy has been very much neglected. Physicians would do well to heed the advice of Hippocrates who, in the 5th Century B.C., stated that "Epilepsy in young perons is most frequently removed by changes of air, of country, and of modes of life."

PHOTIC STIMULATION

The earliest recorded evidence of the precipitation of epileptic seizures by photic stimulation is credited to Apuleius, a Roman contemporary of Galen, who mentioned in his Apologia that a seizure might be provoked when a potter's wheel was rotated before the eyes of a slave. Defending himself in the second century against charges of having practiced magic, Apuleius said: ".......... the spinning of the potter's wheel will easily infect a man suffering from this disease with its own giddiness; for the sight of its rotations weakens his already feeble mind, and the potter is more effective than the magician for casting epileptics into convulsions."

The first scientific evidence of the precipitation of epileptic seizures by stimulation with light was presented by Gowers in 1881. Early in the study of the electrical activities of the brain, Hans Berger noted that a photic stimulus to the retina of the eye altered the brain wave pattern.

Photic stimulation is employed as a diagnostic procedure in the investigation of patients with epilepsy in two ways: first, to determine if a clinical seizure can be precipitated with this procedure; and second, to determine if exposure to light will cause electroencephalographic abnormalities of the type which are observed in epileptic patients.

After the routine part of the electroencephalographic examination has been completed, the photic driving test is performed. An electroencephalographic tracing is obtained while a flickering light is shined in the region of the patient's eyes.

I have seen many epileptic patients in whom it was demonstrated that their seizures were precipitated by exposure to light. I can mention one child, a nine year old girl who for a period of several years had "passing out spells" in the mornings just as she left her house for school. The first reaction of the parents was that the child was "faking" and merely did not want to go to school. Later, attention was called to the fact that this child experienced these "passing out spells" on sunny days only and never on cloudy or sunless days. Diagnostic investigation revealed that these "passing out spells" were actually epileptic seizures which were triggered off by sudden exposure to direct sunlight when the child stepped out of her house in the mornings. She was fitted with appropriate sunglasses and has subsequently remained free of seizures.

In 1952, I reported the cases of three children who repeatedly experienced seizures while watching television. At first it was thought that the seizures had been precipitated by the excitement or tension caused by the television show. Later, however, it was learned that these children were sensitive to flickering lights. It was postulated that their seizures were triggered off by the television sets, which were known to have been defective and to have flickered very frequently. Similar instances of the precipitation of initial epileptic seizures by the flickering light of television screens were reported in 1961 by Mawdsley and also by Pallis and Louis.

In 1962, Bower and co-workers reported on fourteen children who had experienced epileptic attacks while viewing television. This group, comprised of six boys and eight girls, ages eight to fourteen, fell into two separate categories: six very sensitive to intermittent photic stimulation, liable to convulse while viewing television under normal conditions, and those less sensitive, tending to have a seizure when sitting very near to the screen (within two feet) or standing close to adjust the set. These physicians recommend that susceptible children should sit at least five feet from the screen; if the picture is faulty, the child should not try to adjust the set, but should look away and keep his eyes open. It is estimated that the flicker threshold for the American television system is five times greater than for the British system, probably explaining why television-induced convulsions are rare in America.

I have another patient whose case history is as follows: A white farmer, aged thirty-one, since the age of ten years had suffered from major convulsive seizures; these had gradually increased in severity and frequency until they numbered ten to twelve a year. The patient had noted no aura or warning while he was conscious.

The attacks, all preceded by exposure to bright or flickering light, consisted of a sudden loss of consciousness without warning, falling to the ground, and rolling up of the eyes, followed by generalized tonic and clonic convulsions. The average duration of such a seizure was fifteen to twenty minutes. During seizures the patient had bitten his tongue, injured his lips, and fractured his jaw. Occasionally, at the beginning of a seizure, he would involuntarily bring his left hand before his eyes, a movement which he was able to control, at times with great effort. The patient had learned that whenever he was exhausted, tense, or nervous he was more likely to have an attack.

No abnormalities were found on physical, ophthalmological, or neurological examination except for scars on the chin and tongue. The results of urinalysis and blood examinations were reported as normal. The photogenic attacks were studied in detail by Doctors Curtic Marshall and A. Earl Walker with a view to determining the parameters of excitation.

The patient was tested in the electroencephalographic laboratory with flickering red, blue and green lights and it was demonstrated that he was extremely sensitive to light toward the red end of the spectrum. As a result of these observations, he was fitted with eye glasses which filtered out red light and was instructed to wear these glasses whenever he was exposed to bright light. This patient experienced no recurrence of seizures when he wore his glasses in spite of the fact that he was repeatedly exposed to bright lights.

Patients who suffer from seizures while exposed to light are sometimes classified as having photogenic epilepsy. Patients in whom so-called photogenic epilepsy is suspected should have an electroencephalographic examination with photic stimulation by white and colored lights so that relevant sensitivity may be determined. Suitable colored eye glasses can then be prescribed if necessary.

DRUGS AND CHEMICALS

There are certain drugs and chemicals, such as Metrazol and strychnine, which are used in some patients to precipitate clinical epileptic seizures and/or electroencephalographic abnormalities for diagnostic purposes.

When taken in excess, many of the commonly used drugs will cause convulsions in most individuals. This applies to the epileptic as well as to the normal person.

There are also some individuals who have experienced convulsive seizures in association with the administration of the usual amounts of certain drugs, particularly the tranquilizing drugs. It is speculated that the convulsive reaction in these individuals was due to some type of hypersensitivity to the drug. It has been my experience, however, that such reactions are no more prevalent among epileptics than among non-epileptic patients receiving the usual therapeutic dosages of tranquilizing drugs, such as the phenothiazine derivatives. I have prescribed these tranquilizers to many of my epileptic patients and have not observed an incidence of convulsions greater than that which would be expected in the non-epileptic population.

In the past the ingestion of lead was one of the most common causes of convulsions in children. However, since manufacturers of children's toys and furniture no longer use paint containing lead,

lead poisoning in children today is generally the result of the ingestion of plaster and paint from the walls and window sills of old houses in which lead paint had been used. This can be exceedingly dangerous and a physician should be consulted immediately if lead ingestion is suspected.

Acute lead intoxication is not only associated with convulsions but can also cause irreversible brain damage. The residual brain damage caused by the lead can predispose an individual to recurrent seizures.

ALLERGY

Spangler and Dees and Lowenbach and several other investigators have reported a relationship between allergy and recurrent convulsive seizures. However, a study carried out in our clinic failed to reveal a specific relationship between allergy and epilepsy. This investigation was under the direction of Dr. Leslie N. Gay, Associate Professor Emeritus of Medicine of Johns Hopkins University School of Medicine and former Director of the Allergy Clinic of The Johns Hopkins Hospital.

ALCOHOL

The ingestion of alcoholic beverages can cause convulsions in any individual. However, in my experience, these convulsions almost always occur in association with an excessive consumption of alcoholic beverages. They generally occur either during the acute stages of alcoholic intoxication or immediately following an alcoholic debauch.

The problem of alcohol consumption for epileptic patients is discussed in detail in another section of this book entitled General Management of the Epileptic Patient (Chapter 7).

FLUID INTAKE

Investigations have shown that the ingestion and retention of large amounts of water may, in some epileptic patients, disturb cerebral function and cause convulsions. For these studies the retention of the water was effected by the administration of certain drugs such as Pitressin. This method of producing convulsions is the so-called Water-Pitressin Test for epilepsy. To my knowledge, this test has rarely been employed since the advent of electro-encephalography.

Many physicians in the past, and even some today, advise that the epileptic patient be placed on a restricted daily fluid intake. I do not believe that the ingestion of a normal amount of fluid by patients who have normal excretory functions has an adverse effect on the course of pre-existing epilepsy. I do not restrict the daily intake of fluids except in those patients whose seizures occur in association with the menstrual cycle, and in those patients who are receiving the ketogenic diet for their epilepsy.

ANESTHETICS

It is generally known that an occasional individual may experience a convulsion in association with the administration of an anesthetic. These seizures are usually designated as anesthetic convulsions.

I do not believe that anesthetic convulsions are more common among epileptics than among individuals who do not suffer with an epileptic disorder. It has been my experience that anesthetics generally do not adversely affect epilepsy. Hundreds of my patients have been exposed to anesthetics of all types without experiencing an increase in the frequency of their seizures.

MISCELLANEOUS

There are isolated instances where certain situations will precipitate or increase the frequency of epileptic seizures in some patients.

Keith and co-workers reported a patient in whom electroencephalographic changes and clinical seizures were precipitated by visual stimulation produced by *fine mesh patterns*.

There are instances of patients having had seizures which were thought to have been precipitated by certain types of *music*. This has been classified as musicogenic epilepsy. Critchley, in 1937, reported several instances of this disorder. In 1962, Joynt and co-workers reported another case of so-called musicogenic epilepsy and also reviewed the literature on this subject.

In 1956, Bickford and co-workers reported clinical and electro-encephalographic evidence of a new syndrome which was classified as *"reading epilepsy"* (epileptic seizures precipitated by reading). In 1961, Forstner and co-workers reviewed the literature on this subject and also reported the nineteenth case of so-called "reading epilepsy."

I have seen many instances where epileptic seizures were pre-cipitated by sudden noises or other *startling sensations*. These episodes are classified as reflex or startle epilepsy.

Some patients report an increase in frequency of seizures at certain seasons of the year and others report more numerous seizures over the weekends. In some instances, one is able to dis-cover a possible explanation for an increase in frequency of seizures at such times. For example, an exacerbation of seizures during Fall may be associated with the starting of school and an increase in the frequency of seizures over the weekend may be related to increased excitement at that time.

Some patients have reported numerous, vague, ill-defined situations which they said caused them to experience more seizures, such as "with the change of the moon," "only during certain seasons of the year," "only on rainy days" or "when it snows." I do not believe that the increase in the frequency of seizures in these patients was due directly to an external stimulus such as, for example, change of the moon, but rather to an emotional disturb-ance engendered by the specific situation. However, it is important for the physician to investigate the patient's complaints and observations regardless of their vagueness, since they may provide him with valuable leads in the treatment of the specific case.

Many epileptic patients report that their seizures occur or increase in frequency only when they become *fatigued*. As a result, epileptics are often advised to take frequent rest periods.

I have found it very difficult to evaluate the significance of fatigue as a precipitating factor of seizures in epilepsy. However, I believe that the general attitude of treating an individual with epilepsy as if he had tuberculosis or rheumatic fever and consequently encouraging or forcing him to take frequent rest periods should be discouraged. I believe that, if possible, the patient should be instructed and encouraged to conduct himself in the same manner as his normal associates.

The required amount of rest and physical activity suggested for the epileptic are discussed in the section of this book entitled General Management of the Epileptic Patient (Chapter 7).

Many parents have reported that their children have had their seizures only when they became constipated and others have stated that protracted convulsions have been terminated by an enema. I have also seen many adult patients who have related similar experiences.

In some of the older literature and textbooks, it is stated that *constipation* is a cause of recurrent convulsions. However, considering the prevalence of constipation among the non-epileptic population, one would hesitate to ascribe it as a primary cause or even as a significant precipitating factor of epileptic seizures.

It is true that constipation is a very common finding among epileptic patients and it probably occurs more frequently in this group than in the so-called normal population. The reasons for the high incidence of constipation in epileptic patients are that many of them lead a very sedentary life and that many of the commonly prescribed anticonvulsant drugs cause constipation.

BIBLIOGRAPHY

Apuleius: *Apulei Apologia*, with introduction and commentary by H. E. Butler and A. S. Owen. Oxford, Clarendon Press, 1914.

Bickford, R. G., Whelan, J. L., Klass, D. W., and Corbin, R. B.: Reading Epilepsy: Clinical and Electroencephalographic Studies of a New Syndrome. *Tr. Am. Neurol. A.*, 81st meeting, pages 100-102, 1956.

Bower, B. D., Pantelakis, S., and Jones, D.: *Convulsions and Television Viewing*. Program and Abstracts, The Society for Pediatric Research, Thirty-second Annual Meeting, May 8-10, 1962, page 6.

Critchley, M.: Musicogenic Epilepsy. *Brain*, *60*:13-27 (March) 1937.

Dees, S. C., and Lowenbach, H.: Allergic Epilepsy. *Ann. Allergy*, *9*:446-458, July-August, 1951.

Directory for Exceptional Children, Third Edition, 1958, Porter Sargent, Publisher, 11 Beacon St., Boston 8, Mass.

Forstner, G., Ferguson, R., and Jones, D. P.: Reading Epilepsy. *Canad. M. A. J.*, *85*:608, 1961.

Joynt, R. J., Green, D., and Green, R.: Musicogenic Epilepsy. *J.A.M.A.*, *179*:501-504, February 17, 1962.

Keith, M. H., Aldrich, R. A., Daly, D., Bickford, R. G., and Kennedy, R. L. J.: A Study of Light-induced Epilepsy in Children. *Am. J. Dis. Child.*, *83:*408-409 (March), 1952.

Livingston, S.: Comments on a Study of Light-induced Epilepsy in Children. *Am. J. Dis. Child.*, *83:*409, 1952.

Marshall, C., Walker, A. E., and Livingston, S.: Photogenic Epilepsy: Parameters of Activation. *A.M.A. Arch. Neurol. & Psychiat.*, *69:*760, 1953.

Mawdsley, C.: Epilepsy and Television. *The Lancet*, Jan. 28, 1961, pp. 190-191.

Pallis, C., and Louis, S.: Television-induced Seizures. *The Lancet*, Jan. 28, 1961, pp. 188-190.

Spangler, R. H.: Alergic findings in epileptic patients and ancestors. *Ann. Allergy*, *7:*91-114, September-October, 1943.

Chapter 6

DISORDERS SIMULATING EPILEPSY

THERE are many disorders which are associated with seizures or spells of various types; these disorders are listed in Chapter 2 (Table 1). This section is devoted to a discussion of some of the medical disturbances which should be considered in those patients who have had recurrent seizures or other epileptic-like attacks.

BRAIN TUMORS

A diagnosis of a brain tumor should be considered in every patient who suffers with a seizure. This is particularly true in the case of those individuals in whom the onset of seizures makes its appearance during adult life. The occurrence of seizures in association with a brain tumor is also observed in children but not nearly as frequently as in adults. Most of the brain tumors in children occur in areas of the brain (posterior fossa) which are not generally associated with seizures.

When I first started working in the field of convulsive disorders some twenty-five years ago, my interpretation of the prevailing medical opinion was that an individual who presented a seizure, especially a grand mal convulsion, most likely had a brain tumor. Consequently, I made great efforts at that time to submit each of my patients with seizures to very expensive investigative procedures which required hospitalization, such as pneumoencephalography. From the experience which I gained with the passage of time, I still believe that an individual with a seizure, particularly an adult, should be considered as a potential brain tumor patient. However, I now feel that investigative measures such as pneumoencephalography and cerebral arteriography should be considered only when the patient presents indications of a brain tumor, such as focal clinical seizures; or neurological abnormalities of cerebral origin other than those known to be due to previous trauma to the brain such as hemiplegia caused by a cerebral birth injury; or localized abnormalities in the electroencephalogram.

One could logically ask me the following question: How can you be sure that the first convulsion is not a manifestation of a brain tumor unless you investigate the patient extensively with studies such as pneumoencephalography and/or cerebral arteriography? My answer is as follows. I do not believe that any physician can be completely dogmatic about any given case. It has been my experience, however, that when a convulsion is a manifestation of a brain tumor, other signs or symptoms indicative of a brain tumor will generally be present at the time of the convulsion or will become apparent shortly thereafter. I base this statement on my experiences gained from following thousands of patients for a period of many years, many of whom consulted me after the occurrence of their first seizure. Many of these patients continued to have seizures without manifesting specific signs or symptoms indicative of a brain tumor. I submitted many of them to pneumoencephalographic and cerebral arteriographic examinations to investigate the possibility of a brain tumor and the findings were negative.

I would like to emphasize, however, that it is the responsibility of the physician to establish or rule out the presence of a brain tumor in each individual with seizures. I would also like to call attention to the fact that the absence of signs or symptoms indicative of a brain tumor in a patient in association with the first seizure should not be considered as positive evidence against a diagnosis of a brain tumor.

HYPOGLYCEMIC CONVULSIONS

Many patients with convulsions have been referred to me with a diagnosis of a hypoglycemic convulsive disorder. In some of these patients this diagnosis had been made merely on the basis that their seizures occurred during the latter part of the night or in the early morning, that is, after they had not eaten any food for a prolonged period of time; in others, because the patients had stated that their seizures were aborted by eating large amounts of carbohydrate-containing foods; and in still others, because their blood sugar levels were found on one or two occasions to be a little lower than that considered normal.

Some of these patients were instructed to eat large amounts of carbohydrate food in the evening before going to bed and in the morning as soon as they awakened; others were placed on special diets such as are employed in the treatment of hypoglycemia. In other words, these patients were treated medically as if the convulsions were related to an abnormally low blood sugar. After thorough study with appropriate laboratory investigations, however, it was established that these patients suffered with epileptic seizures and not hypoglycemic convulsions.

As far as the time of occurrence of epileptic seizures is concerned, it is well known that they very frequently occur in association with sleep, especially during the early morning hours just before the usual time of awakening. We investigated the fasting blood sugar values of hundreds of our epileptic patients who suffered with early morning convulsions and found normal values in practically all instances.

Many patients were referred to me with a diagnosis of hypoglycemic convulsions because they had presented blood sugar levels which were somewhat lower than that considered normal. Blood sugar levels vary from patient to patient and findings between 70 to 120 mg. per cent are generally designated as representing normal blood sugar values. However, I do not believe that a blood sugar level lower than that considered normal is in itself sufficient evidence to warrant a specific diagnosis of a hypoglycemic convulsion.

I can cite four of my patients who revealed exceedingly low blood sugar levels after prolonged periods of fasting, varying from two to four days. These patients were being starved prior to the institution of the ketogenic diet for their epilepsy. They received nothing but a restricted amount of water during this period. The blood sugar values in these patients were 8 mg. per cent, 14 mg. per cent, 18 mg. per cent and 24 mg. per cent, respectively. These patients did not have seizures at the times of these exceedingly low blood sugar values. In each instance the blood sugar concentration returned to normal upon institution of the ketogenic diet. Blood sugar determinations were also obtained on these hospitalized patients at the times they did have seizures, and the blood sugar values were found to be within normal limits.

One could definitely state that these patients presented laboratory evidence of hypoglycemia, but that there was no specific evidence that they suffered with hypoglycemic convulsions. The fact that all individuals who present laboratory evidence of low blood sugar levels, *including those with exceedingly low blood sugar values*, do not have convulsions indicates that factors other than the abnormally low blood sugar itself must be involved in the production of a so-called "hypoglycemic convulsion."

The differentiation between epileptic seizures and convulsive episodes associated with a low blood sugar should never be made merely on the basis of the time of occurrence of the seizures or on the finding of a blood sugar value considered to be lower than normal, but only after appropriate studies of carbohydrate metabolism have been carried out and it can be demonstrated that the blood sugar was abnormally low at the time of the occurrence of the seizure.

SIMPLE FEBRILE CONVULSIONS

Convulsions occur very frequently in association with an elevation of temperature, particularly in young children. The most common of the medical disorders which are associated with convulsions and fever are:

(1) Infections of the brain such as meningitis and encephalitis;
(2) Epileptic seizures triggered off by fever (fever caused by any intercurrent infectious illness); and
(3) Simple febrile convulsions. (These convulsions occur almost entirely in young children and are generally associated with extracranial infections such as tonsillitis and otitis media.)

It is obvious that the physician who sees an individual with a febrile convulsion will first rule out a cerebral infection such as meningitis or encephalitis since these diseases always require immediate definitive treatment. If there is no evidence of such disorders, the most likely diagnosis will be either simple febrile convulsions or epilepsy.

TABLE 3

FEATURES WHICH HELP TO DIFFERENTIATE SIMPLE FEBRILE CONVULSIONS
FROM EPILEPTIC CONVULSIONS PRECIPITATED BY FEVER

	Simple Febrile Convulsions	*Epilepsy*
Age of onset of seizures	under 6 years	any age
Duration of seizures	always very short	minutes to hours
Character of seizures	always generalized	focal or generalized
EEG	normal	abnormal in most cases
Relation of seizures to fever	occurs soon after onset of fever	anytime during febrile episodes
Frequency of seizures	1 to 4 per year	daily to yearly

Table 3 summarizes the clinical and laboratory features which assist the physician in distinguishing between a simple febrile convulsion and epilepsy triggered off by fever.

The physician should consider a diagnosis of simple febrile convulsions in those infants and pre-school children who suffer with fever and a generalized seizure of short duration (several minutes or so) in whom he is unable to elicit evidence of an infection of the brain such as meningitis or encephalitis.

The most common age of onset of simple febrile convulsions is between nine and fifteen months of age. They seldom appear in patients under six months of age and rarely, if ever, make their initial appearance or recur after five or six years of age.

Simple febrile convulsions generally appear soon after a sudden rise in temperature, usually within three or six hours after the onset of the fever. It is very rare for the convulsion to occur later than twelve or eighteen hours after the initial appearance of the elevation of temperature.

The electroencephalograms of patients who suffer with simple febrile convulsions are always normal when obtained at times other than those immediately following the occurrence of the seizure or at a time when the patient still has an elevation of temperature. Therefore, electroencephalographic studies of those children suspected of having simple febrile convulsions should be obtained at a time when the patient has been afebrile for at least two weeks. We obtained electroencephalograms of a group of children who had fever associated with disorders such as tonsillitis and otitis media but who did not have seizures, and observed electroencephalographic abnormalities which persisted in some instances for several weeks after defervescence.

A diagnosis of epilepsy should be assigned to those patients with febrile convulsions who present one or more of the following findings:

(a) Prolonged seizures;

(b) Focal convulsions of any duration;

(c) Convulsions associated with fever in children over the age of six years;

(d) Abnormalities in the electroencephalogram after the patient has been afebrile for at least two weeks.

The treatment of an isolated simple febrile convulsion does not require special consideration since the duration of the seizure is so brief that it would be terminated before any therapeutic measures could be instituted. These seizures are almost always associated with an extracranial infection such as tonsillitis or otitis media. It has been my experience that the administration of daily anticonvulsant medication is generally ineffective in preventing the recurrence of simple febrile convulsions. However, phenobarbital and aspirin may be prescribed at the first signs of an infection and continued for at least twenty-four hours thereafter. This type of therapy is generally of no avail since the convulsion is frequently one of the first manifestations of the febrile disorder. In other words, I have been told by many parents that they did not know that their child had a febrile disorder until the occurrence of the convulsion.

My experience based on the results of two independent studies carried out in our clinic over the past twenty-five years has taught me that the general outlook for patients who suffer with the disturbance which I classify as a simple febrile convulsive disorder is excellent. Most of the patients had one to four convulsions per year during the first four or five years of their lives. Simple febrile convulsions did not recur in any of these patients after six years of age.

To date, non-febrile seizures had developed in only a very small number of these patients, a percentage not much greater than is seen in the general population. There is no clinical evidence which suggests that the simple febrile convulsions caused brain damage in any of these patients.

Because of these findings, I believe that when the physician is confronted with a child who has experienced his first simple febrile convulsion, he should advise the parents of the good prognosis. However, I do not believe that he can be completely dogmatic and tell the parents that there is absolutely no chance of their child's developing epilepsy later in life. I feel it is important that these patients be observed periodically by the physician. If the patient should have a recurrence of seizures other than that typical of simple febrile convulsions or if the convulsions should recur more frequently than four times a year or after six years of age, the physician should then change the diagnosis to that of an epileptic disorder and treat the patient accordingly.

The treatment and outcome of patients who suffer with epileptic seizures triggered off by fever are essentially the same as that of other types of epilepsy.

BIBLIOGRAPHY

Fowler, M.: Brain Damage After Febrile Convulsions. *Arch. Dis. Child.*, *32:*67, 1957.

Friderichsen, C., and Melchior, J.: Febrile convulsions in children, their frequency and prognosis. *Acta paediat. Supp.*, *100:*307, 1954.

Livingston, S., and Kajdi, L.: Importance of Heredity in the Prognosis of Febrile Convulsions. *Am. J. Dis. Child.*, *69:*324, 1945.

Livingston, S., Bridge, E. M., and Kajdi, L.: Febrile convulsions: A clinical study with special reference to heredity and prognosis. *J. Pediat.*, *31:*509, 1947.

Livingston, S.: Comments on Febrile Convulsions, in *Year Book of Pediatrics.* Chicago, The Year Book Publishers, 1953-1954, page 371.

Livingston, S : Febrile Convulsions, in *The Diagnosis and Treatment of Convulsive Disorders in Children.* Springfield, Ill., Thomas, 1954, page 75.

Livingston, S.: Comments on Brain Damage after Febrile Convulsions, in *Year Book of Pediatrics.* Chicago, The Year Book Publishers, 1957-1958, page 372.

Livingston, S.: Febrile Convulsions, in *Advances in Pediatrics.* Chicago, The Year Book Publishers, Inc., 1958, page 113.

Livingston, S.: Comments on Critical Evaluation of Therapy of Febrile Seizures, in *Year Book of Pediatrics.* Chicago, The Year Book Publishers, 1960-1961, page 380.

Livingston, S.: Febrile Convulsions in Children: Simple or Epileptic? *Consultant*, March 1962, page 34.

Millichap, J. G., Aledort, L. M., and Madsen, J. A.: Critical Evaluation of Therapy of Febrile Seizures. *J. Pediat.*, *56:*364, 1960.

Peterman, M. G.: Febrile Convulsions. *J. Pediat.*, *41*:536, 1952.
Prichard, J. S., and McGreal, D.: The EEG in Febrile Convulsions. *Electroencephalog. & Clin. Neurophysiol.*, *9*:166, 1957.

BREATH-HOLDING SPELLS

Holding of the breath during the course of crying is observed very frequently in young children. A typical simple breath-holding spell is easily recognized and usually follows a more or less constant pattern. After some event as a result of which the child has become angry, afraid or has injured himself even slightly, he starts crying. As the crying increases in intensity, the child appears to be in a rage, begins holding his breath and becomes slightly cyanotic around the lips. The entire episode may be over in a minute or so. Generally, such spells are of little significance and should cause little concern either to the parents or to the physician. In other instances, however, the breath-holding episodes are of a more violent nature and may be associated with unconsciousness and/or frank convulsive movements (Case History Number 8).

It is of interest to note that Mark Twain in his book *Pudd'nhead Wilson* describes an instance which sounds very much like a typical breath-holding spell:

" 'Tom' was a bad baby from the very beginning of his usurpation. He would cry for nothing; he would burst into storms of devilish temper without notice, and let go scream after scream and squall after squall, then climax the thing with 'holding his breath'—that frightful specialty of the teething nursling, in the throes of which the creature exhausts its lungs, then is convulsed with noiseless squirmings and twistings and kickings in the effort to get its breath, while the lips turn blue and the mouth stands wide and rigid, offering for inspection one wee tooth set in the lower rim of a hoop of red gums; and when the appalling stillness has endured until one is sure the lost breath will never return, a nurse comes flying, and dashes water in the child's face, and—presto! the lungs fill, and instantly discharge a shriek, or a yell, or a howl which bursts the listening ear and surprises the owner of it into saying words which would not go well with a halo if he had one. The baby Tom would claw anybody who came within reach of his nails, and pound anybody he could reach with his rattle. He would scream for water until he got it, and then throw cup and all on the floor and scream for more. He was indulged in all his caprices, howsoever troublesome and exasperating they might be; he was allowed to eat anything he wanted, particularly things that would give him the stomach-ache."

The convulsive movements observed in some patients with breath-holding spells look quite similar to those seen in some patients with epilepsy and because of this, the patient may be erroneously diagnosed as having epilepsy and treated accordingly. I have seen many young children who were treated for epilepsy, when actually they suffered with breath-holding spells. Case History Number 9 is an example of a patient with breath-holding spells who was mis-diagnosed as having epilepsy.

Breath-holding episodes are usually fairly easy to recognize since they present a relatively consistent stereotyped pattern. Firstly, there is a precipitating factor such as a slight injury or some other minor provocative incident which creates an acute emotional upset in the child (Table 4); and secondly, the child starts to cry, holds his breath and becomes cyanotic around the lips. This is then followed by a short period of unconsciousness and/or convulsive movements which usually lasts two or three minutes or so.

TABLE 4

LIST OF INCIDENTS WHICH PARENTS CONSIDERED AS CAUSES
OF BREATH-HOLDING SPELLS

When he bumps his head	When he is examined by a doctor
When he is frightened	When he is forced to do something
When he is angry	he does not want to do
To get attention	When his playmates take something
When he is displeased	he wants
When he hurts himself	When he gets a spanking

Table 5 lists some of the features which assist in differentiation between convulsions associated with breath-holding spells and epileptic convulsions. Breath-holding convulsions are almost always preceded by an obvious precipitating factor, whereas in most instances epileptic seizures occur spontaneously without any apparent preceding disturbing factor; breath-holding episodes are always preceded by crying and holding of the breath, whereas

TABLE 5

FEATURES WHICH HELP TO DIFFERENTIATE CONVULSIONS ASSOCIATED WITH
BREATH-HOLDNG SPELLS FROM EPILEPTIC CONVULSIONS

	Convulsions Associated with Breath-holding Spells	Epileptic Convulsions
Precipitating factor	Always present	Usually not apparent in young children
Crying	Always present before onset of convulsion	Not usually present
Cyanosis	Always occurs before onset of convulsion	When present, occasionally occurs at onset of convulsion, but usually after convulsion has been in progress (prolonged convulsion)
Opisthotonus	Usually present	Rarely occurs
EEG	Always normal	Usually abnormal, but may be normal

young children with epilepsy rarely cry before an attack; cyanosis appears with the crying and precedes the convulsions of breath-holding spells, whereas in epilepsy the cyanosis usually appears after the onset of the convulsive movements; opisthotonus almost always occurs in association with breath-holding spells, whereas it rarely occurs with epileptic seizures; and the electroencephalogram is always normal in patients with breath-holding spells, whereas it is abnormal in most patients with epilepsy.

Breath-holding spells most often appear during the first two years of life, but rarely before six months of age. The average age of onset in my group of patients was twelve months of age.

The frequency of spells varies considerably. Some of my patients had one spell every several months or so, while others had as many as five to ten a day. Generally, breath-holding spells recur infrequently at the onset of the disorder. However, in many instances, the frequency of spells gradually increases as the child becomes older. In my group of patients the frequency reached a peak between the ages of two and three years. Breath-holding spells tend to disappear spontaneously after three or four years of age and rarely recur after six years of age.

The convulsive movements associated with breath-holding episodes are always very short and innocuous and require no immediate care. The administration of antiepileptic therapy, in my experience, is of no value in the prevention of the recurrence of breath-holding spells. I have also had similar experience with the use of the tranquilizing drugs.

The treatment of breath-holding spells consists primarily of parent-child guidance and reassurance. I inform the parents of the harmlessness of the individual attacks, reassure them that their child does not have epilepsy and direct my treatment toward a solution of a parent-child conflict, if such a situation is apparent.

The general outlook for children with breath-holding spells is excellent. Follow-up studies made on hundreds of my patients with breath-holding spells over a period of many years revealed an incidence of epilepsy no greater than that which exists in the general population.

However, it is noteworthy that many of my patients with breath-holding episodes manifested behavioral disturbances, such as enuresis, head-banging and temper tantrums. In some instances, these latter disturbances appeared during early years of life concurrent with the breath-holding spells. However, in many cases behavioral disturbances did not become apparent until after the child had "out-grown" the breath-holding spells. Dr. Leo Kanner studied a group of children with breath-holding spells and observed similar behavioral disturbances.

The frequent occurence of behavioral disturbances in patients with breath-holding spells is, in my opinion, evidence that the breath-holding spell itself is also most likely a manifestation of an emotional disturbance of some type.

I have been impressed with the fact that breath-holding spells are observed almost entirely in children with normal intelligence. Only rarely have I encountered a typical breath-holding spell in a brain damaged child. Long-term follow-up studies made on my group of patients did not present the slightest indication that the occurrence of convulsions associated with breath-holding spells, regardless of their frequency, caused demonstrable evidence of brain damage.

BIBLIOGRAPHY

Bridge, E. M., Livingston, S., and Tietze, C.: Breath-holding Spells. *J. Pediat.*, *23:* 539, 1943.

Hinman, A., and Dickey, L. B.: Breath-holding spells: Review of Literature and Eleven Additional Cases. *A.M.A. Am. J. Dis. Child.*, *91:*23, 1956.

Kanner, Leo: *Child Psychiatry*, 2nd edition. Springfield, Ill , Thomas, 1949.

Livingston, S.: Breath-holding Spells, in *The Diagnosis and Treatment of Convulsive Disorders in Children.* Springfield, Ill., Thomas, 1954, page 71.

Livingston, S.: Breath-holding Spells, in *Advances in Pediatrics.* Chicago, The Year Book Publishers, Inc., 1958, page 119.

Low, N. L., Gibbs, E. L., and Gibbs, F. A.: Electroencephalographic Findings in Breath-holding Spells. *Pediatrics*, *15:*595, 1955.

TETANY

Tetany is a condition characterized by convulsions and other spasmodic manifestations which are dependent upon a state of increased excitability of the nervous system. Tetanic symptoms may appear during the course of any disturbance associated with hypocalcemia or alkalosis.

It is important that the physician rule out the possibility of tetany in the diagnosis of any case of convulsions, particularly in infants.

NARCOLEPSY AND CATAPLEXY

Narcolepsy is a condition characterized by paroxysmal and recurrent diurnal attacks of irrepressible sleep. Patients with narcoplesy may go to sleep at inappropriate times and in unsuitable places, such as while standing or walking, during conversation, and while sitting at the dinner table. I can mention one of my patients, a boy nine years of age, who, during the course of a baseball game in which he was participating, left the field of play for no apparent reason, sat beside a tree and fell asleep.

The narcoleptic "sleep" is generally very shallow and the patient can usually be easily aroused. The patient almost always exhibits mental alertness after being aroused or awakening spontaneously.

Narcolepsy is also sometimes associated with sudden attacks of loss of muscular tone and weakness, the so-called cataplectic attacks. These attacks last a few seconds or so. Patients frequently fall to the floor utterly powerless to speak, but consciousness is maintained throughout the entire spell. These cataplectic attacks are frequently induced by an abrupt emotional disturbance, such as being startled or frightened and are also frequently precipitated by violent laughter.

A narcoleptic attack may simulate some aspects of an epileptic seizure because of its paroxysmal and recurrent nature.

Narcolepsy differs from epilepsy in the following respects. The narcoleptic sleep is usually shallow and the patient can be easily aroused, whereas the patient cannot usually be aroused from the unconsciousness associated with an epileptic spell; there is mental alertness following recovery from a narcoleptic attack, whereas the epileptic attack is generally followed by a post-convulsive period of disorientation and drowsiness; and patients with narcolepsy present normal electroencephalograms, whereas in epilepsy the electroencephalogram reveals abnormalities in most patients.

The cataplectic attack may simulate the akinetic or "drop" epileptic seizure in the brevity and general appearance of the spell. The cataplectic spell differs from the epileptic seizure in the following respects. Firstly, the cataplectic attack is almost always precipitated by some emotional disturbance, whereas the akinetic or "drop" epileptic seizure generally occurs spontaneously. Secondly, consciousness is maintained throughout the cataplectic attack, whereas there is at least a momentary disturbance of consciousness associated with the epileptic spell.

EMOTIONAL (FUNCTIONAL) DISTURBANCES

There are many paroxysmal and recurrent disturbances which require considerable evaluation and diagnostic investigation before the physician can decide whether these disturbances are emotional (functional) in origin or symptoms of an epileptic disorder. Examples of such disturbances are fainting or syncopal attacks, recurrent headaches, recurrent attacks of abdominal pain, recurrent vomiting spells, and tics.

I have encountered many patients whose symptoms of recurrent headaches or recurrent attacks of abdominal pain were first thought to be on a functional basis, but were subsequently placed into the epileptic category because of abnormal electroencephalographic findings and/or favorable response to antiepileptic drugs.

I have also seen many infants who were considered as having colic by their parents and also by their physicians because they frequently issued a sharp cry, suddenly pulled their thighs up towards their abdomen and appeared as if they were in pain. Actually these infants suffered with what is known as minor motor epilepsy, a disturbance which frequently manifests itself in such a manner. A detailed description of minor motor epilepsy is presented in another section of this book entitled Classification of Epileptic Seizures (Chapter 4).

Electroencephalography provides the physician with considerable help in differentiating between an emotional disturbance and epilepsy. When this examination reveals abnormal findings, the physician has no alternative but to consider that the disturbance is most likely a manifestation of epilepsy. In those instances where the electroencephalogram reveals normal findings, it is my general policy to treat the patient with antiepileptic drugs; a satisfactory response to this therapy would favor a diagnosis of an epileptic disorder. It is obvious that in some instances psychiatric investigations may reveal the proper diagnosis. I would like to note that I have seen many patients in whom I could not be certain of the diagnosis in spite of all of the diagnostic techniques currently available.

One of the most frequent problems with which I am confronted is to decide whether a given patient suffers from psychomotor epilepsy or whether his symptoms are best classified as an emotional or psychiatric disorder. This problem is discussed in more detail in another section of this book entitled Classification of Epileptic Seizures (Chapter 4).

I frequently have been confronted with the dilemma of deciding whether a grand mal seizure was epileptic in origin or related to an emotional disturbance (hysterical convulsion).

Hysterical convulsions are observed most frequently in older individuals, but they also occur in children. In some instances the appearance of a hysterical convulsion is exceedingly difficult to differentiate from a true epileptic seizure. However, in most instances the differentiation does not present too much of a problem.

Hysterical convulsions are not usually associated with biting of the tongue and there is usually no urinary or fecal incontinence. The onset of the hysterical convulsion is generally less sudden than that of true epilepsy, and in most instances bodily injury from this spell does not occur. The hysterical patient does not pass into a true stupor at the end of a convulsion as the epileptic usually does. The brain wave pattern of a patient with hysterical convulsions is normal, whereas the electroencephalographic examination reveals abnormalities in most patients with epilepsy.

CONGENITAL AND DEGENERATIVE DISEASES OF THE BRAIN

There are certain congenital and degenerative diseases of the brain which are associated with recurrent epileptic-like seizures and, therefore, may be confused with true epilepsy.

Generally, some of these disorders can be differentiated easily from true epilepsy because they manifest characteristic findings on physical and roentgenological examination. For example, the condition known as tuberous sclerosis shows typical acne-like lesions on the nose, cheeks and chin which are knows as adenoma sebaceum and also reveals areas of calcification in the brain substance demonstrable by routine x-ray of the skull. Also, the typical case of the Sturge-Weber syndrome can be diagnosed by the presence of a characteristic skin lesion on one side of the face (nevus vasculosis) and intracranial calcification visible by routine x-ray of the skull.

There are many other congenital and degenerative diseases of the brain which are associated with recurrent seizures. The reader may refer to the standard textbooks on neurology for a discussion of these disorders.

Case History Number 8
Breath-holding Spells of the Convulsive Type of the Usual Pattern

K.E.: Birth and development were normal. The mother stated that following a spanking given the patient at twenty months of age, he began to cry, became blue in the face and went into a generalized convulsion which lasted about a minute. During the course of the subsequent months he had several other convulsions which were precipitated by spanking, fright or minor injury. He was admitted to the hospital for study at the age of twenty-four months. While hospitalized, he had numerous short convulsions which were precipitated by being forced to do things which he resented. One typical spell occurred during the preparations for a lumbar puncture. Physical and laboratory examinations were negative. An EEG revealed normal findings. He continued to have frequent attacks for another year, after which time they gradually decreased in frequency. At five years of age he was attending kindergarten and had had no attacks for the preceding six months. He was seen again at seven years of age and again at eleven years of age. There had been no recurrence of spells whatsoever.

Case History Number 9

Breath-holding Spells Previously Mis-diagnosed as Epilepsy

R.N. At the age of ten months the patient developed spells consisting of breath-holding and cyanosis which were followed by generalized convulsions lasting for five minutes. He was sleepy and drowsy after the spells. They were always precipitated by temper or minor injuries. At first the attacks recurred infrequently, but during the course of the subsequent six months they recurred on the average of once or twice a day. When he was one year of age he was examined by his family physician and a diagnosis of grand mal epilepsy was made. Antiepileptic medication was prescribed. He continued, however, to have frequent spells in spite of the antiepileptic medication. At sixteen months of age he was referred to our clinic with a diagnosis of epilepsy. After a thorough evaluation, it was decided that he had breath-holding spells and not epilepsy. The antiepileptic medication was discontinued and the spells continued as before. When he was four years old, he was sent to a private boarding home for children where he remained for about one year. During the first two or three weeks, he had several breath-holding spells, after which time they completely disappeared. He continued to do well upon returning home and when last seen at the age of eleven years had had no recurrence of spells.

Chapter 7

GENERAL MANAGEMENT OF THE EPILEPTIC PATIENT

THE PATIENT SHOULD REALIZE THAT EPILEPSY MAY CAUSE A HANDICAP

THE EPILEPTIC patient must realize that he does have a handicap and that he must adjust his life accordingly. In many instances this applies also to the patient who has been free of seizures for many years.

The controlled epileptic must learn to cope with the many unwarranted adverse attitudes which the public at large has toward epilepsy. The patient who is still having seizures has what may be called a two-fold handicap. First, he has the same handicap as that of the controlled epileptic, that is, he must learn to cope with the many misconceptions which the public has concerning epilepsy; and second, he must realize that because of his seizures, he may have to live with some restrictions as far as his physical activities and employment are concerned, although, in many instances, these restrictions may be minimal.

There is no doubt that most epileptic patients with infrequent seizures can be rehabilitated to the extent that they can live essentially normal lives. The patient should be told that this can usually be accomplished by learning "to live with his seizures." He should be encouraged to disregard the layman's adverse attitude toward epilepsy. He should realize that he, himself, cannot correct the ignorance and prejudices of the general public which undoubtedly stem from a misunderstanding of the disorder. This advice is exceedingly important. Many of my patients became pathologically restless, belligerent and antagonistic after having made many fruitless attempts to convince certain individuals that they were not "different people" or "second rate citizens."

77

The patient should be emphatically told that there is no reason why epilepsy should carry a stigma, and that it is a disorder which should differ in no way in its social implications from rheumatic fever, tuberculosis, heart disease or diabetes. He also should be told that the misunderstandings concerning epilepsy undoubtedly will gradually disappear as the public becomes more and more aware of the real nature of the disorder.

The epileptic patient must realize that he does have a disorder which because of its tendency to manifest itself periodically does justify some restrictions, such as automobile driving and certain types of employment. It is true that in those instances where patients have been free of seizures for many years, the application of many of the restrictive measures is completely unwarranted. However, the seizure-free patient must understand that such is the case at the present time and he must acclimate himself to these unwarranted restrictions.

The patient must attempt to deal as effectively as possible with the emotional problems which may be associated with his illness. It is true that many epileptic patients develop emotional disturbances which are moreorless related to their disorder. These emotional problems stem mostly from two sources: first, from the public's attitude toward the disorder of epilepsy; and second, from the patient's fear or anxiety of having a recurrence of his seizures. Emotional shocks themselves, in all probability, never cause seizures if the potential cerebral disorder is not already present, but they certainly can act as a factor in the precipitation of seizures in many epileptic patients. Therefore, if the patient can readjust his way of thinking and learn to "live with his epilepsy," the frequency of the seizures may decrease.

The patient must be taught that he may have to accept certain limitations in living that are imposed by the epileptic disorder. The patient must realize that in spite of the fact that he does have a handicap, he should endeavor to maintain the highest degree of normal activity as possible. The epileptic patient will have to face much prejudice and ignorance on the part of society, but he should realize that great progress is being made toward breaking down these barriers.

IMMEDIATE CARE OF THE PATIENT AT THE TIME OF AN EPILEPTIC SEIZURE

This section is written primarily to provide the parents and guardians of epileptic patients with some instructions relative to the general management of the patient at the time of the occurrence of a seizure. This information will also be of value to individuals such as nurses, school teachers and others who have occasion to witness epileptic seizures.

Generally, most epileptic seizures are of short duration and do not require immediate specific care. This is particularly true in the case of petit mal and minor motor seizures, since these spells seldom last longer than fifteen to twenty seconds. In fact, most epileptic seizures are terminated before any assistance could be rendered. The physician should emphasize to the patient and/or his parents or guardian that the occurrence of epileptic seizures of short duration is no cause for undue alarm and also that these attacks do not damage the brain.

In the case of those seizures of prolonged duration, the patient should be allowed to remain, if possible, at the place where the seizure occurred until the active portion of the spell has subsided. Of course, it is obvious that a patient must be moved, regardless of the convulsive movements, if he happens to fall on a busy street or in any other precarious place.

The patient should be placed in such a position that he cannot hurt himself by knocking his body against hard objects. One of my patients, for example, broke his arm by striking it against a metal bedpost during a severe seizure.

Tight clothing, especially around the neck, should be loosened or removed.

If the seizure occurs while the patient is in bed, he should be observed so that he does not fall to the floor. Such falls can be prevented either by observation or by placing protective guard-rails or boards on the sides of the bed. All pillows should be removed from the bed. The patient should not be allowed to lie on his abdomen since respiratory difficulties may result from pressing the face into the mattress or other soft bed clothing.

If possible, the patient should be kept on his side so that mucus and saliva will flow more freely from the mouth. Since patients are unable to swallow during convulsive episodes, mucus and/or saliva may flow down into the lungs and cause respiratory distress; therefore, the patient should not be placed or be permitted to lie flat on his back for any length of time. Another reason why it is important to keep the patient on his side rather than on his back is that vomiting sometimes occurs during a seizure; it is obvious that if a patient were on his side, the vomitus would more likely be expelled from the mouth than flow back down into the lungs.

In the older writings on epilepsy it is routinely stated that some object should always be inserted between the teeth of a patient having an epileptic seizure. I would like to emphasize the fact that in most instances this is an unnecessary procedure and sometimes can do more harm than good. However, this procedure should be carried out in those patients who bite their tongue or cheeks or show marked evidence of respiratory difficulty during a convulsive episode. Any firm, blunt, non-damaging object of the right size and not too hard, such as a padded tongue depressor, a folded leather belt or a leather glove can be inserted between the patient's teeth. This object should be placed on one side of the mouth, between the back teeth for the following two reasons: (1) it is easier to insert an object in this area; and (2) the front teeth are more easily broken. Extreme care should be taken when any object is inserted into the mouth of an individual with carious teeth, because such teeth are easily broken and can cause respiratory difficulties if aspirated. False teeth should be removed for the same reason.

No effort should be made to stop the muscular contractions by forceful means such as holding down the patient's arms and/or legs. It is also not advisable to lift the patient, or carry him from place to place while he is in the active stages of the convulsion, unless absolutely necessary.

No special efforts such as shaking the patient, applying cold applications to the face or pinching should be made as an endeavor to terminate the unconsciousness associated with an epileptic seizure as they are of no avail and consciousness will automatically return of its own accord. In most instances the unconsciousness associated with an epileptic seizure is of relatively short duration, generally lasting not longer than five to ten minutes. In the case of patients who manifest prolonged unconsciousness, a physician should be consulted immediately.

The practice of placing a child with a convulsion in a tub of hot water or in the so-called mustard bath is not only a worthless procedure but can cause harm in some patients.

I also question the value of mouth-to-mouth breathing which is practiced so frequently in patients with epileptic seizures. I believe that this procedure causes more anxiety to the bystanders and to the individual performing the mouth-to-mouth breathing than the good it does the patient.

Most epileptic seizures are of short duration and rarely endanger the life of the patient directly. In the case of the known epileptic it is generally not necessary to consult a physician for immediate treatment of the convulsive episode itself. The physician should subsequently be informed of the seizure so that he can make appropriate adjustments, if necessary, in the patient's regular antiepileptic regimen.

In the case of the known epileptic there are several exceptions to the general rule of letting a seizure run its course without medical advice. These are: (1) when the seizure lasts much longer than previous ones; (2) when the seizure is different in character from previous ones; (3) when the seizure occurs in association with circumstances different from previous ones; and, (4) when a patient experiences one seizure after another without regaining consciousness. This latter condition is known as status epilepticus and is discussed in another section of this book entitled Classification of Epileptic Seizures (Chapter 4). Each of these exceptions should be considered as an emergency and a physician should be consulted or the patient should be immediately taken to the nearest hospital.

A fallacy which has been carried down from generation to generation and which is prevalent even today is that extreme vigilance should be exercised during an epileptic seizure to prevent the patient from swallowing his tongue and choking to death. This is one of the most common fears of the patient, his parents and individuals witnessing an attack. I would like to emphasize the fact that this fear should be completely dispelled, since it would be utterly impossible for an epileptic to die in this manner. If he were to swallow his tongue, which I think is mechanically impossible, it would go down into the esophagus which leads to the stomach, and obviously, one could not block off the air passage in this manner. In order to block off the air passage, it would be necessary for the tongue to go down into the trachea. I cannot imagine a circumstance in which the tongue could go down into the trachea in such a manner as to completely obstruct the air from flowing in and out of the lungs. It is true that in some instances patients present indications of breathing difficulties during convulsions. However, these difficulties are usually due to one or more of the following situations: excessive accumulation of mucus in the trachea, swelling at the base of the tongue or a temporary disturbance of the part of the brain which controls breathing.

It is not unusual for a patient recovering from a grand mal attack to manifest bizarre activities such as talking incoherently, extreme restlessness, and conducting himself in a generally confused state. Due to a lack of knowledge and understanding of seizures by the general public, the epileptic patient is frequently subjected to considerable ridicule and mockery by the individuals who witnessed the episode. In some instances, the patient is aware of and sensitive to the reactions of the bystanders. The patient's embarassment can be greatly intensified and aggravated by expressions of shock and horror by individuals witnessing the attack. Individuals witnessing an epileptic seizure can greatly lessen a patient's embarrassment and feelings of shame by displaying nonchalance and casualness for the episode. Perhaps the most valuable service which a bystander can render to a patient recovering from a seizure is an expression of encouragement, understanding and a desire to lend assistance.

Because grand mal seizures generally follow a moreorless stereotyped pattern, the specific instructions heretofore stated can be given to the parents or guardians of patients who suffer with such seizures. However, since psychomotor seizures vary considerably from patient to patient, the instructions relative to the general management of patients with psychomotor epilepsy will necessarily have to parallel the specific type of seizure. A description of psychomotor epilepsy is given in another section of this book entitled Classification of Epileptic Seizures (Chapter 4).

Sometimes a patient with psychomotor seizures can cause himself bodily injury and also cause harm to other individuals and/or their property. Therefore, the most valuable help the bystander can render is to attempt to prevent the patient from performing any of these activities. Frequently, the patient having a psychomotor seizure requires constant supervision and the attendant may have to follow the patient from place to place until the seizure has terminated. In some instances it may be necessary that the patient be completely restrained or immediately removed to a hospital.

It is obvious, in many instances, that patients with prolonged seizures and unconsciousness and those with status epilepticus should be seen by a physician or immediately taken to a hospital so that appropriate therapeutic measures can be instituted to terminate the seizure. Some of the many drugs currently employed to terminate prolonged seizures and status epilepticus are phenobarbital, Seconal, Dilantin, paraldehyde, chloral hydrate and Amytal. The reader may refer to the various textbooks on epilepsy and neurology for specific instructions in regard to dosage and administration of these agents.

PHYSICAL ACTIVITY FOR THE EPILEPTIC

The attitude that physical activities should be curtailed in epileptic patients still exists to a great extent among the parents and guardians of many epileptics and also to some degree among physicians. Many of these parents expressed the belief that physical activity itself may precipitate seizures and also that there is a great chance that the epileptic may injure his head during the course of physical activity and thereby make his epilepsy "worse." My experience has taught me that these attitudes are unwarranted and definitely should be discouraged.

I have seen many epileptic patients who were living a very sedentary existence when they first consulted me. In some instances this inactivity was so complete that the patients were conducting themselves as invalids. When asked why they were conducting themselves in such a fashion, some patients stated that they were instructed to do so by their physicians. Also, many parents were under the impression that epilepsy was a disease comparable to rheumatic heart disease and tuberculosis, and that rest was beneficial for the disorder. They believed that epileptics should get "plenty of rest" and, in many instances, should take naps during the afternoon. These attitudes definitely are unsound and frequently can do the patient much more harm than good. It should be noted that today most physicians believe that the importance of rest is overemphasized, even in patients who suffer with disorders such as rheumatic heart disease and tuberculosis. The current medical attitude is that patients suffering with these disorders should be allowed more physical activity than was previously permitted.

The amount of rest needed by most epileptics is only that which is sufficient for any healthy child or adult; over-fatigue, obviously, should be avoided by all individuals, whether they have epilepsy or not.

Lennox appropriately states, "Physical and mental activity seems to be an antagonist of seizures. Enemy Epilepsy prefers to attack when the patient is off guard, sleeping, resting, or idling."

The fact that epileptic seizures very frequently occur in association with sleep tends to refute the belief that rest exerts a beneficial effect on epilepsy. In fact, many epileptic patients only have their seizures in association with sleep. These patients should be instructed not to take afternoon naps unless absolutely necessary. It is also of interest to note that electroencephalographic abnormalities can only be elicited in some patients when they are dozing or asleep; these abnormalities may not appear when they are awake. This is another factor which indicates that it is better for most epileptics to be physically and mentally active rather than to get more than the usual amounts of rest and sleep.

It is definitely known that fresh air, sunshine and exercise generally exert a favorable effect on the course of epilepsy. By and large, the epileptic, if physically capable, should be encouraged to participate in most physical activities. Many epileptic patients experience fewer seizures when engaged in such activities as compared to when they are idle or at rest. The vast majority of epileptics can engage in all physical activities, the performance of which would not be associated with a significant risk of injury to himself or to others.

It is obvious that the epileptic who is still having seizures should not perform activities such as riding horseback or climbing to high altitudes. By "high altitudes" I do not mean to infer that a change in atmospheric pressure is likely to precipitate an epileptic seizure. I do not believe that such is the case. A considerable number of my patients have traveled into areas of exceedingly high altitude and did not experience an increase in frequency of seizures. By "high altitude" I refer to situations such as tree climbing, mountain climbing and working on ladders.

I allow my patients to go swimming if they care to do so, but only under supervised circumstances such as in the presence of a life guard or a competent swimming companion. However, I advise my patients against diving or jumping into deep water.

A question which I have been asked very frequently by parents is, "What about bicycle riding?" Generally, I answer this question in the following manner. I call attention to the fact that bicycle riding carries with it a calculated risk of injury for every child, epileptic and non-epileptic, and that, by and large, this risk is primarily related to traffic. For the epileptic who has never ridden or expressed a desire to ride a bicycle, it is probably best not to encourage him to ride a bicycle. Also, it is obvious that those individuals who have very frequent seizures (daily or weekly) should be prohibited from riding a bicycle. However, in those patients with infrequent seizures who have already established the practice of bicycle riding, the problem consists essentially of weighing the risk of injury associated with bicycle riding against the risk of causing emotional harm or making the child feel "different" if he is prohibited from riding a bike. I usually present this dilemma to the parents and let them help me make the decision. I do, however, tell them that my patients have not experienced significant injuries in association with bicycle riding as a result of their epileptic disorder. Therefore, I generally advise that the child be allowed to ride a bicycle. Obviously, he should be instructed not to ride a bicycle in heavy traffic.

Many parents prohibit their children from engaging in physical activities because of the fear that overbreathing may precipitate petit mal spells. It is true that overbreathing does precipitate petit mal spells in some patients; however, it has been my experience that the usual physical activities do not cause an individual to hyperventilate to a degree which would bring about a seizure.

Many of my patients had been advised against participating in body contact sports such as boxing, wrestling and football. The performance of these sports is associated with a calculated risk of injury which is the same for all individuals, epileptic and non-epileptic. A common attitude which exists among the parents of epileptics and also among some physicians is that epileptics should not be allowed to participate in body contact sports, particularly football and boxing, because of the possibility of injury to the head which would "make the epilepsy worse."

It is true that individuals who sustain penetrating injuries to the head are probably made more susceptible to epilepsy. However, there is no conclusive evidence, to my knowledge, that closed head injuries resulting from the performance of body contact sports either aggravate a pre-existing epileptic disorder or "cause" an epileptic disorder. I base this statement on my experience with more than 15,000 epileptic patients. Many of these patients are currently participating or have indulged in body contact sports and I know of no adverse consequences relative to their pre-existing epileptic disorders.

I believe that the relationship of the adverse effect of head injuries per se on the course of pre-existing epilepsy has been completely exaggerated and probably does not exist. A highly significant point which argues against the effect of non-penetrating injuries to the head as a factor in aggravating or increasing the frequency of epileptic seizures is found in minor motor epilepsy. Of the various forms of epilepsy, minor motor epilepsy is the one type associated with frequent injuries to the head. Many of my patients with minor motor seizures have fallen and injured their heads very frequently; many have sustained lacerations to the head on the average of two or three times a week. I do not know of any instance where these injuries to the head have increased the incidence of the patient's seizures. I believe that this finding is almost conclusive evidence that closed head injuries of the type which consists of hard bumps to the head sustained in falls to the floor or ground do not adversely affect the course of epileptic seizures, at least those associated with minor motor epilepsy.

In his book published in 1962, Jennett presented evidence that closed head injuries increase the possibility of the development of epilepsy above that which exists in the general population. Silverman and others have reported that electroencephalographic abnormalities, consisting primarily of abnormally slow waves, occur in patients shortly after closed head injuries. However, I am not convinced that these findings represent conclusive evidence that closed head injuries play a great part in the causation of epilepsy. I believe that significant evidence in favor of my conviction is that almost every child sustains some type of closed head injury during the period of growing up, and if this type of injury were a major factor in the causation of epilepsy, the incidence of this disorder would approach 100 per cent of the general population.

Some patients who are prohibited from participating in sports can be caused great harm emotionally. I do not believe the calculated risk of sustaining brain damage of the type which would aggravate a pre-existing epileptic condition outweighs the chances of causing serious emotional disturbances in some individuals. I cite the following case as an example.

The parents of an eighteen year old student recently consulted me in regard to the feasibility of their son's playing football. This young man was an excellent football player on a college freshman team and the expectation of his playing on the varsity squad was very great. He loved to play football and, in fact, stated that he would not continue at college unless he could play football. He had two short grand mal convulsions six months apart and was diagnosed as having epilepsy. Both of these seizures occurred in the early morning hours while at home. His parents were very fearful of allowing him to continue playing football because of the impression that he might sustain a head injury of some type which would aggravate his epileptic disorder. They had been instructed by their personal physician to prohibit their son from participating in this sport. This young man subsequently developed serious psychological disturbances because he was not allowed to play football and he withdrew from college. His psychological difficulties cleared up soon after I recommended that he be allowed to resume his football career.

SHOULD AN EPILEPTIC CARRY OR
WEAR AN IDENTIFICATION BADGE?

In certain illnesses, particularly diabetes, it is sometimes advisable for the patient to carry some type of identification badge so that if he should become ill while away from home, the badge would identify the illness to the passerby. If a diabetic should be found unconscious on the outside, the passerby could, because of the identification badge, ascertain the nature of the illness and notify the patient's immediate relative or a physician or have the patient removed to a hospital. Most individuals with diabetes do not object in any manner whatsoever to wearing or carrying an identification badge.

However, the vast majority of my epileptic patients expressed considerable reluctance to wearing any form of identification or even carrying a card indicating that they are epileptic.

I have asked many of my epileptic patients if they would desire to carry an identification badge of some type. Only the occasional patient stated that he would like to wear an identification badge, because it may give him a feeling of some security. The vast majority of my patients stated that they definitely would not carry or wear an identification badge because of two major reasons: (1) they feared that it may unnecessarily expose their condition to the public; and (2) it would keep them "constantly conscious" of their illness. They considered this latter reason as very important, since they were making every effort to forget about their illness. They stated that an identification emblem would serve as a "constant reminder" of their epileptic disorder and would, therefore, seriously impede their efforts to live as normal a life as possible. They also expressed the fear that such identification badges might also serve as "constant reminders" to their relatives, close associates and fellow-employees and thereby engender attitudes which might intensify their feelings of being "different."

It is my belief that the decision as to whether or not an epileptic should wear an identification badge should be left entirely up to the individual patient, except in certain specific instances. For example, I think the physician should recommend the wearing or carrying of some type of identification badge in (1) those patients who have psychomotor seizures which consist of prolonged periods of amnesia or aphasia or prolonged states of confusion; (2) those patients who experience frequent or prolonged grand mal seizures; and (3) those patients who are receiving dosages of anticonvulsive medication which may cause reactions such as marked drowsiness or ataxia.

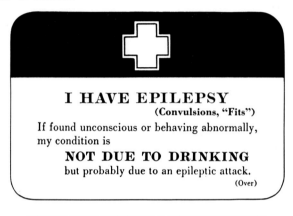

Figure 5. This photograph shows both sides of an identification card which can be obtained by physicians from Ayerst Laboratories, Medical Department, 22 E. 40th Street, New York 16, New York.

I can cite several instances in which identification badges were of considerable help. One such instance was that of a 12 year old girl who had frequent episodes during which she would awaken from her sleep, leave her home and roam the streets at night in a confused state. On all occasions she was returned home by the

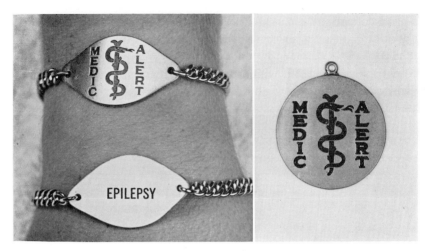

Figure 6. Photograph shows both sides of an identification bracelet and one side of an emblem. The reverse side of the emblem is not shown, but it identifies the disorder. This emblem can be worn on a charm bracelet or on a necklace. I recommend that the patient's name and address be engraved on the reverse side of these identification badges. These photographs were supplied by Medic-Alert Foundation, Turlock, California.

police or a passerby, since her disorder and identity were designated on her identification bracelet.

Several of my patients have been arrested by the police and accused of being "drunk." One of these patients manifested the bizarre behavior which is so commonly observed following a grand mal convulsion. The arresting officer assumed that the patient's abnormal behavior was the result of alcoholic intoxication. A routine search of the patient at the police station revealed his identification card which designated the patient's illness and it was subsequently established that the patient had been ill and not drunk.

Another of my patients suffered with ataxia caused by his anti-epileptic medication. This patient was stopped on the street by a policeman who thought that he was drunk. The patient produced his identification card which stated that he was an epileptic and the officer allowed him to "go on his way."

One of my patients experienced a seizure soon after leaving a restaurant in which he had eaten his dinner. He had consumed one bottle of beer during the course of the meal. He was found unconscious on the ground by a policeman, and because of the odor of alcohol on his breath, he was taken to the police station and arrested for being under the influence of alcohol. Upon examination of the patient's personal papers, the officer found an identification card which indicated that the individual was an epileptic patient. The patient, of course, was immediately released.

Identification badges are available in various forms, such as cards (Figure 5), bracelets and emblems (Figure 6).

In some instances it may be advisable for the patient to carry a card designating the names and dosages of his antiepileptic medications. This could be of considerable value in case the patient were brought into a hospital in an unconscious state, particularly during the late hours of the night.

THE USE OF ALCOHOL AND TOBACCO BY EPILEPTICS

It has been my experience that the ingestion of an occasional alcoholic drink is not harmful to most epileptics. In fact, I cannot recall more than an occasional patient who informed me that drinking made his seizures worse. It should be noted that Rodin and co-workers administered sufficient alcohol to produce obvious intoxication to twenty-five hospitalized epileptic patients and did not observe an increase in the frequency of seizures.

It is obvious that all individuals should refrain from the excessive use of alcohol and individuals who have learned that alcohol causes them difficulties or does not "agree" with them should abstain from the consumption of alcoholic beverages.

I allow my patients to take a "social highball" if they care to do so. The decision is entirely up to the individual patient. However, the epileptic patient who is taking large amounts of antiepileptic drugs should be definitely warned against the ingestion of excessive amounts of alcohol for two major reasons: first, it is known that alcohol may increase the sedative action of antiepileptic drugs, particularly the barbiturates; and, second, there is great likelihood that the patient may "forget" to take his antiepileptic medication regularly during periods of excessive alcohol consumption.

It is my belief that the danger of alcohol consumption is not its effect on the seizures themselves, but lies in the possibility of the patient's developing chronic alcoholism, as is the case with many individuals who suffer with disorders which have a tendency to be chronic. Therefore, the physician should definitely advise those individuals who have experienced an improvement in seizures during an alcoholic debauch that it is probably best that they not drink alcoholic beverages.

Some of my patients developed anti-social tendencies and feelings of marked inferiority because they were instructed by their physicians "never to drink an alcoholic beverage." They were told that epileptics should not consume alcoholic drinks and also that alcohol and antiepileptic medications "do not mix." Many of these patients subsequently refused to attend various social functions. They stated that it disturbed them considerably when they "couldn't join the crowd" in all of the activities of a party. They also said that the "forced" abstinence made them feel "different."

Several persons have asked me if the consumption of alcohol would increase the chances of epilepsy developing in their offspring, since mention is made of such a relationship in the medical literature. My observations are in complete agreement with those of Diethelm, who conducted an extensive study of the incidence of epilepsy in the relatives of chronic alcoholics and concluded that: "Idiopathic epilepsy does not occur in the relatives of alcoholics considered in the present study...........Our findings throw a new light on the frequent statements in the older literature that epilepsy and alcoholism arise from the same constitutional background or that alcoholism frequently causes epilepsy in the offspring. The very low incidence of epilepsy in the relatives of intelligent alcoholics argues against these assumptions."

Many of my patients were told that they should not use tobacco in any form. To my knowledge, there is no medical evidence which even suggests that tobacco adversely effects the course of epilepsy.

SHOULD RECORDS OF SEIZURES BE KEPT?

Generally, I advise my patients and their parents against keeping detailed written records of the frequency of spells. Many of them told me that they were informed by their previous physicians that it was absolutely necessary to keep a detailed written report of spells so that he could adequately evaluate the efficacy of their medication.

I have encountered instances where "complete bookkeeping systems" were set up relative to the patient's seizure disorder. The exact number of seizures, the precise minute of occurrence of each seizure, the exact duration of spells by the minute and second, and many other insignificant details were meticulously recorded in a ledger. All members of the family were instructed to immediately record every detail of each seizure in this ledger. At the end of each day or each week, the frequency of the spells and other details were tabulated. In other instances, the record of frequency and time of occurrence of seizures were recorded on a large calendar which hung in the most conspicuous place in the house.

I believe that such procedures may cause patients and their families much more harm emotionally than it could benefit the physician medically. I have found, in many instances, that it keeps both the patient and the family constantly aware of the illness. I stress the policy of "trying to forget about the seizures" and advise the patients and their families merely to keep a mental note of frequency of spells.

As far as the physician is concerned, I believe it is important that he know approximately how many spells the patient has had during intervals between visits, but not necessarily the exact number. In those patients who suffer with petit mal or minor motor epilepsy, for example, the physician could get, under normal circumstances, only an approximate idea of the frequency of spells, since many such spells go unobserved. I can cite several instances where parents, who were told by their physicians that they must have an accurate account of the spells, kept their children under constant vigilance, for fear that they might "miss a spell." It is obvious that such a situation could do harm both to the parents and also to the child.

I also believe that the family should be warned against constantly asking the afflicted individual, "Did you have any spells today?" The parents of many of my patients had made a routine practice of asking their child this question after he had been away from home for a period of time, such as attending school or some social function. This definitely is a harmful practice since it obviously keeps both the patient and his parents constantly conscious of the illness.

I advise the parents to assume the attitude: "What they don't know won't hurt them."

It is true that in certain instances it may be advisable for the parent, guardian or patient to keep a modest record of the approximate frequency of spells, the approximate time of occurrence, the approximate duration of the spells and other details concerning the illness which might be of value to the physician. However, I believe that the continued detailed recording of these episodes can definitely be harmful to many individuals.

ANESTHETICS FOR THE EPILEPTIC

I have frequently been asked the following questions by physicians:

(1) Is there any reason why an epileptic should not be given a general anesthetic?

(2) Are there any specific anesthetics which are best for epileptics?

(3) Are there any specific anesthetics which should not be administered to an epileptic?

(4) Do you have any specific recommendations in regard to the administration of an anesthetic to an epileptic?

(5) Are there any specific precautions which should be taken in association with the administration of an anesthetic to an epileptic?

My general answer to these questions is that I can see no reason why an epileptic patient cannot be given any type of anesthetic in the same manner as any other individual. This statement is based on the fact that I have not encountered any specific difficulties in the hundreds of my epileptic patients who have been exposed to general anesthetics of all types. I can definitely state that none of my patients experienced an increase in the frequency of their seizures in association with the administration of an anesthetic.

When an epileptic has to undergo a surgical procedure which requires an anesthetic, it is important that he remind his physician that he is taking anticonvulsant drugs, if such be the case. It is also important that he remind the surgeon of this fact so that the anticonvulsant medication will not be withdrawn while the patient is in the hospital, unless the surgeon specifically authorizes the discontinuance of the medication.

In those instances where it is impossible for the patient to take his medication by mouth, it should be administered parenterally. Both phenobarbital and Dilantin may be administered parenterally. However, if the patient's antiepileptic medication consists of drugs, such as Mysoline, which are not prepared for parenteral administration, the physician should prescribe another drug such as phenobarbital or Dilantin during the period which the patient is unable to take his regular medication orally.

It has been my experience that epileptics can receive any type of general anesthetic. However, I would like to call attention to the fact that in those instances where a barbiturate, such as Pentothal Sodium, is to be administered as an anesthetic to epileptic patients who had been taking a barbiturate for control of their seizures, the anesthetist should bear in mind that it may be necessary to administer lesser amounts of the barbiturate-anesthetic in order to produce the desired anesthetic state. It is also important for the physician to keep in mind the fact that epileptics receiving anticonvulsant medication may require a lesser dosage of drugs which are administered preparatory to a surgical procedure.

SHOULD CHILDREN WITH CONVULSIVE DISORDERS RECEIVE ROUTINE PROPHYLACTIC IMMUNIZATIONS?

The routine prophylactic immunizations employed in the United States today consist of the following: diphtheria, pertussis, poliomyelitis, smallpox and tetanus. It is known that some of these immunizations, particularly pertussis, have caused neurological reactions with resultant brain damage which, in turn, predisposed some individuals to recurrent convulsions later in life. Therefore, it is only natural for the physician and also the parent who is cognizant of this reaction to ask the following question: "Should a patient who suffers or has suffered with convulsions receive routine prophylactic immunizations?"

I have not observed that pertussis immunizations adversely affect the brains of epileptic patients to any greater degree than would be expected in non-epileptic individuals. Several of my patients did develop "encephalopathies" in association with pertussis immunizations. Also, a few of my epileptic patients had seizures in association with these immunizations and some of my patients who suffered with simple febrile convulsions also experienced seizures. I attributed these seizures to an elevation of temperature in both groups of patients.

On the other hand it is known that whooping cough itself adversely affects the central nervous system of children with especial severity and also is responsible for bronchiectasis in some patients. I believe that the chances of a child's developing these complications of whooping cough are much greater than the chances of his being adversely affected by the immunization itself. Therefore, it is my general policy to recommend that all of my patients be routinely immunized against pertussis. Similar attitudes have been expressed by Byers, Melin and Peterman.

I presented a detailed discussion in regard to the administration of prophylactic pertussis immunizations to children with convulsive disorders in an editorial (*J. Pediat.*, *43*:746-750, 1953) which also contains the attitudes of other physicians including Byers, Lennox and Peterman.

On the other hand, recommendations against the use of pertussis immunizations in children with a personal and/or family history of convulsions or epilepsy have been made by Cockburn, Köng and others.

In 1960, Ström reported that the incidence of neurological complications of pertussis vaccine was exceedingly high in Sweden and he raised the question as to whether immunizations against pertussis should be continued in that country. He stated that the incidence of neurologic reactions following pertussis vaccination was approximately four times greater than the incidence of neurologic complications following whooping cough. Ström's findings appear comparable to the more frequent occurrence of post-vaccinal encephalitis in the Netherlands than in other countries and suggest an increased host susceptibility rather than a faulty vaccine.

I have not experienced significant neurological difficulties in my group of epileptic patients in association with smallpox immunizations. It is my understanding that the concensus of opinion is that there is a low incidence of neurological complications associated with this immunization. However, it is of interest to note that Hoefnagel, in 1962, reported four young children who developed acute transient encephalopathy following smallpox vaccination.

I am not cognizant of significant neurologic reactions occurring in association with the other routine prophylactic immunizations, such as diphtheria, poliomyelitis and tetanus.

BIBLIOGRAPHY

Cockburn, W. C : Whooping-cough Immunization. *The Practitioner*, *167:*232, 1951.

Diethelm, O. (Editor): *Etiology of Chronic Alcoholism*. Springfield, Ill., Thomas, 1955.

Hoefnagel, D.: Acute, Transient Encephalopathy in Young Children Following Smallpox Vaccination. *J.A.M.A.*, *180:*525, 1962.

Jennett, W. B.: *Epilepsy After Blunt Head Injuries*. Springfield, Ill., Thomas, 1962.

Köng, E.: Pertussis Immunization and Its Contraindications. *Helvet. paediat. acta*, *8:* 90, 1953.

Lennox, W. G.: *Science and Seizures*. New York, Harper and Bros., 1941, p. 134.

Melin, K-A.: Pertussis Immunization in Children with Convulsive Disorders. *J. Pediat.*, *43:*652, 1953.

Rodin, E. A., Frohman, C. E., and Gottlieb, J. S.: Effect of Acute Alcohol Intoxication on Epileptic Patients: A Clinical Experimental Study. *AMA Arch. Neurol.* *4:*103-106, 1961.

Silverman, D.: Electroencephalographic Study of Acute Head Injury in Children. *Neurology*, *12:*273, 1962.

Ström, J.: Is Universal Vaccination against Pertussis Always Justified? *Brit. M. J.*, *5207:*1184, 1960.

Chapter 8

MEDICAL TREATMENT OF EPILEPSY

GENERAL PRINCIPLES OF DRUG THERAPY

ALTHOUGH epilepsy has been known as far back as Hippocrates, few major advances in the treatment of this disorder had been made until recent years. Within the past several decades new therapeutic measures, both medical and surgical, have been developed and have proved to be effective in the treatment of epilepsy. The advent of electroencephalography has further stimulated interest and research in the field of convulsive disorders.

The ideal objective in the treatment of epilepsy is complete control of seizures and provision for normal physical, mental and social development. The degree of success in attaining this goal depends upon many factors such as the type of epilepsy, the duration of the illness, the absence or presence of brain damage and the cooperation of the patient and his parents. This last factor, the cooperation of patient and parents, is extremely important. It has been my experience that in order to obtain good results, the patient and his parents must have confidence in the attending physician and follow his instructions "to the letter."

One must realize that there are some patients whose seizures cannot be satisfactorily controlled with the available medical therapy. However, this group of so-called refractory epileptics is becoming progressively smaller with the passage of time. This is due to a better understanding by physicians of the disorder of epilepsy and to many new therapeutic procedures which are being developed.

For many years the bromides and phenobarbital were essentially the only two anticonvulsant drugs employed in the treatment of epilepsy. Bromide was first employed for the treatment of epilepsy by Sir Charles Locock in 1853 and it continued to be essentially the only valuable drug used for the control of epileptic seizures until the introduction of phenobarbital by Dr. A. Hauptmann in 1912. No significant further advances in drug therapy were made until 1938 when Drs. H. H. Merritt and T. J. Putnam introduced Dilantin as a treatment for epilepsy. Since that time other new drugs have been developed and successfully employed in the control of epileptic seizures. All of the anticonvulsant drugs which were being used for the control of epileptic seizures at the time of this writing are discussed in the section of this chapter entitled Antiepileptic Drugs.

The following general principles have been found to be exceedingly helpful in the medical management of the epileptic patient and are generally employed in the Epilepsy Clinic of The Johns Hopkins Hospital.

1. Patient and parental cooperation is very important. Therefore, the physician should explain to the patient and/or his parents the methods and goal of treatment of epilepsy

Obviously the ultimate goal in every case of epilepsy is to completely control or at least reduce the frequency of seizures to the extent that they do not interfere with the patient's general wellbeing.

It is exceedingly important that the patient and/or his parents clearly understand the methods which the physician uses to treat the disorder of epilepsy. He should be told that in some patients the desired goal may be attained after a short trial on one particular drug, and then again, in other patients it may be necessary to try several drugs or a combination of drugs before a satisfactory result is reached. I tell my patients and/or their parents that there are no "wonder drugs" for epilepsy and also that in order to obtain good results, the treatment must be carried out in a systematic manner.

I frequently use the disorder of diabetes as an analogy in explaining the systematic manner of treatment. I tell them that in the case of diabetes the physician initially prescribes the average amount of insulin for the patient in question and subsequently, at regular intervals, he prescribes either more or less insulin, depending upon the patient's needs. In some instances the physician may administer more insulin than the patient requires, causing the patient to have an insulin reaction. In the case of diabetes, the physician utilizes the patient's symptoms and blood and urine sugar determinations to establish the daily maintenance dosage of insulin required for the case in question. I explain to the patient and/or his parents that in order to get a satisfactory result in epilepsy, a similar systematic method of treatment must be employed. Each dosage of anticonvulsant medication must be given a satisfactory trial. Changes in dosages are made, if necessary, at regular intervals, according to the frequency of the seizures and the patient's tolerance to the medication. In this manner the physician is able to establish the daily maintenance dosage of medication necessary for the individual case of epilepsy.

I have found that when the general plan of therapy is explained in detail to the patient and/or his parents, the physician gains their confidence and they will then co-operate to the best of their abilities. The physician will also relieve himself of many "annoying" telephone calls, such as "Doctor, the medicine which you prescribed for my child the other day has not yet stopped his seizures. I think you ought to try another drug, don't you?" etc.

2. Treatment should be instituted as soon as the diagnosis has been established

This is a most important aspect of the treatment of epilepsy for the following reasons. First, in most cases, the degree of success in the control of seizures bears a direct relationship to the duration of the epilepsy: the longer the duration, the less likely a satisfactory result will be obtained, regardless of the type of therapy employed. Second, it is exceedingly important to institute measures to prevent a recurrence of seizures, not only because of the seizures themselves, but also because of injuries, brain damage and emotional disorders which are sometimes associated with the occurrence of seizures.

I have been frequently asked, "Should a child with one convulsion be treated with regular daily anticonvulsant medication over a prolonged period of time?" My answer is, "It depends upon the diagnosis that the physician assigns to the individual case in question." Every patient with a convulsion should be investigated for diseases known to be associated with seizures such as hypoglycemia, hypocalcemia and brain tumor. I make a diagnosis of epilepsy in each case of convulsions where no definite disease can be demonstrated, regardless of whether the patient has had only one seizure or many. Actually the term epilepsy is a so-called "wastebasket diagnosis" and is assigned to all patients who suffer with seizure disorders of undetermined etiology.

I believe, however, that much harm may be done to some patients and also to their parents if treatment is not instituted immediately after the occurrence of the first epileptic seizure. I prescribe regular daily anticonvulsant medication to those patients who have had only one convulsion of undetermined etiology (epilepsy). My general policy is that these patients be treated in essentially the same manner as those patients who have had more than one seizure. In the past, I did not routinely prescribe regular daily anticonvulsant medication to patients after the occurrence of their first epileptic seizure. However, I did have the opportunity to follow most of these patients and observed that approximately 80 per cent of them had a recurrence of a similar seizure. However, since I instituted the policy of treating patients immediately after their first epileptic seizure, I have observed a marked reduction in the number of patients who had a recurrence of epileptic seizures.

Emotional disturbances constitute a major problem in most epileptic patients and their parents, and in some instances, these disorders are a greater problem than the seizures per se. A marked reduction has been observed in emotional disorders in my patients and their parents since this plan of therapy was instituted. I would like to emphasize that this plan of therapy is unwarranted in children with simple febrile convulsions and convulsions associated with breath-holding spells.

3. The selection of the drug of first choice for the treatment of any case of epilepsy depends upon: the type of seizure, the toxicity of the drug and the cost of the drug

a. *Type of Seizure*

Table 6 gives a list of the useful drugs for the control of various forms of epilepsy which were available at the time of this writing.

TABLE 6

UsEFUL DRUGS FOR CONTROL OF VARIOUS FORMS OF EPILEPSY*

Major Motor	Petit Mal	Minor Motor**	Psychomotor
Phenobarbital	Benzedrine or	Phenobarbital	Dilantin
Dilantin	Dexedrine Sulfate	Mebaral	Phenobarbital
Mysoline	Zarontin	Miltown or Equanil	Benzedrine or
Peganone	Tridione	Bromides	Dexedrine Sulfate
Mebaral	Paradione	Benzedrine or	Mysoline
Gemonil	Diamox	Dexedrine Sulfate	Peganone
Bromides	Atabrine	Celontin	Celontin
Elipten		Milontin	Mebaral
Diamox		Gemonil	Elipten
Mesantoin		ACTH and Steroids	Tridione
		Diamox	Mesantoin
			Phenurone

*Arranged in order of preference, based on relative effectiveness, toxicity and cost of drugs.

**Minor motor seizures are exceedingly difficult to control with any of the available anticonvulsant drugs. Occasional good results are obtained with the drugs listed in this table. The ketogenic diet is the only effective form of therapy for minor motor seizures.

Some antiepileptic drugs are more effective in controlling certain types of seizures and, on the other hand, some drugs often increase the frequency of certain types of seizures. Therefore, it is important that each drug be prescribed in the type of epilepsy in which it is most likely to be effective.

For example, phenobarbital and Dilantin are particularly effective in the control of major motor seizures but sometimes accentuate petit mal spells. Tridione is an effective agent for petit mal spells but sometimes precipitates major seizures or increases the frequency of pre-existing major motor seizures.

It is important that all patients with petit mal epilepsy be given a drug such as phenobarbital, Dilantin or Mysoline in addition to the drug prescribed for control of the petit mal spells. The reason for the combined therapy is that other types of seizures are prone to develop in patients with petit mal epilepsy, particularly those treated with Tridione. Before this combined therapy was instituted, I observed that a very high percentage (approximately 60%) of patients with pure petit mal epilepsy developed other types of seizures, especially major motor seizures. The latter spells appeared at different periods of life after the onset of petit mal, but the most frequent time was at puberty.

We are in the process of analyzing the results of those patients with petit mal epilepsy who were treated with combined therapy and, although we had not completed our investigation at the time of this writing, it appears that the number of patients who developed major seizures has been reduced considerably.

My method of treatment for patients with pure petit mal epilepsy is as follows. I prescribe phenobarbital alone for the first month of treatment to determine the patient's tolerance to this drug and also to ascertain whether it causes an increase in the frequency of the petit mal spells. In some patients, both phenobarbital and Dilantin increase the frequency of these spells. Patients who react adversely to phenobarbital should be given Dilantin or Mysoline and the patient's tolerance to these drugs should be determined in the same manner as for the phenobarbital. A drug to treat the petit mal spells (Table 6) should be added to the therapeutic regimen after the tolerated "prophylactic" major motor anticonvulsant (phenobarbital, Dilantin or Mysoline) has been selected.

b. *Toxicity of Drugs*

Treatment should be started with the drug which is known to be the least toxic. In the event that the patient fails to respond to the essentially non-toxic drugs, such as phenobarbital, Dilantin and Mysoline, the physician has no alternative except to treat the patient with other drugs which may have more severe side effects in some patients. For example, Phenurone is an effective anticonvulsant for psychomotor epileptic seizures. However, since this drug is known to be exceedingly toxic, it should not be used until after an attempt has been made to control the patient's seizures with all of the other antiepileptic agents recommended in Table 6 for this form of epilepsy.

Periodic physical examinations and at least monthly blood, urine and liver function tests should be performed on all patients receiving certain drugs which are known to have adversely affected the hemapoietic, genitourinary or hepatic systems, such as Mesantoin, Tridione, Paradione, Celontin and Phenurone.

Complete blood counts should be made on all patients receiving such drugs before the institution of therapy and at least at monthly intervals thereafter. If no abnormalities occur within twelve months, the interval between counts may be extended. It is my policy to discontinue the use of the drug in patients in whom the total white count drops below 3,500, or in whom there is a marked percentage reduction in the neutrophils, or in whom the platelet count drops to below 125,000. The drug may be readministered when the blood count returns to normal. In such cases, however, blood counts should be made twice a week for a month or so thereafter. The parents or the patient should be instructed to report immediately any sign or symptom of possible damage to the hemapoietic system, such as fever, sore throat, easy bruising, petechiae, ecchymosis or epistaxis.

Periodic urine examinations should be performed on patients receiving drugs which are known to have adversely affected the genitourinary system, such as Tridione, Paradione and Milontin.

Liver function tests should be performed on patients receiving drugs such as Phenurone before the institution of therapy and at regular intervals thereafter. The parents or the patient should be advised to report immediately to the physician the appearance of jaundice, dark urine, general malaise, fever, gastrointestinal upset or any other disturbance which may be indicative of a hepatitis. Drugs such as Phenurone should be employed with caution in any individual with a history of previous liver damage.

A drug should be discontinued immediately at the first appearance of any type of cutaneous reaction. It is important that the patient be protected with some other type of drug when this is done, as sudden withdrawal may precipitate a recurrence of seizures or status epilepticus. If the rash is of the milder type, such as a morbilliform, scarlatiniform or urticarial rash, therapy with the same drug may be started after the rash has completely disappeared. Continued use of the drug in patients with purpuric rashes, exfoliative dermatitis, or other serious skin reactions is inadvisable. A recurrence of the rash is also a contraindication to continued use of the drug. Approximately 25 per cent of my patients had a recurrence of rash when the same drug was readministered. In eash instance treatment was started with smaller dosages than previously.

TABLE 7

Cost of Antiepileptic Medication

Name of Drug	Dosage	Cost for Year*
Phenobarbital	32 mg. (½ gr.) 3 times daily	$3.50–$6.00
Dilantin	100 mg. (1½ gr.) 3 times daily	15.00–20.00
Mysoline	250 mg. (3¾ gr.) 3 times daily	62.00–75.00
Tridione	300 mg. (4½ gr.) 3 times daily	30.00–35.00

*Based on average cost of 1000 capsules or tablets purchased from local drug store. These prices were obtained from questionnaires received from sixty-five drug stores located in Baltimore City.

c. *Cost of Antiepileptic Medication*

The cost of the drug therapy for epilepsy varies from patient to patient and depends upon the dosage and the number of drugs required for any individual case. The cost of a year's supply of anticonvulsant medication may range from $3.50 to as high as several hundred dollars.

Table 7 gives the approximate cost for a year's supply of some of the more commonly used antiepileptic drugs, at an average dosage.

The patient can save considerable money if he purchases his antiepileptic medication in large quantities. For example, the average price range for a one month's supply (100 tablets) of 32 mg. phenobarbital tablets purchased from the local drug store is $1.00 to $2.00, while the price range for one year's supply (1000 tablets) of the same medication is but $3.50 to $6.00 The advantage of purchasing this medication in large quantities is quite obvious. Similar monetary savings can be realized with the purchase of other anticonvulsant drugs in large quantities.

I initially prescribe a small supply of medication until I determine the appropriate therapy for the individual case. After this has been determined, I then prescribe a sufficient quantity of medicine to last six months or one year.

I have observed that many physicians prescribe phenobarbital in a liquid form (Phenobarbital Elixir), particularly for younger children. The cost of medication is increased considerably when phenobarbital is prescribed in this form. The average cost for a one year's supply of liquid phenobarbital (Phenobarbital Elixir) is

$60.00, as compared with $5.00, which is the approximate average cost of a one year's supply of the same dosage of phenobarbital when it is prescribed in tablet form.

I have found liquid phenobarbital (Phenobarbital Elixir) to be a very unsatisfactory medication for prolonged usage for many reasons. Many patients have expressed a frank dislike for the taste of the liquid preparation. Many children refuse to take Phenobarbital Elixir after a period of time, probably because of the sameness of its taste, and also because of its alcoholic content, 13 to 15 per cent. Since tablets of phenobarbital are tasteless, their usage can eliminate these objections and may result in the patient's adhering to his dosage schedule more faithfully. Phenobarbital tablets can readily be administered to young children if they are crushed into small particles and suspended in a teaspoonful of fluid, such as orange juice, milk or water, or mixed with substances such as apple sauce or preserves.

When liquid phenobarbital is prescribed, one cannot be certain of the exactness of the dosage, since the patient frequently does not use a standard 5 cc. measuring spoon. The capacity of various household teaspoons has been found to vary from slightly less than 4 cc. to slightly more than 6 cc. This difference in the size of teaspoons can be responsible for the patient's receiving different quantities of phenobarbital from time to time. Also, varying amounts of liquid medication may be wasted when it is administered, particularly to the younger child, resulting in a reduced dosage of the drug and an increase in the cost of therapy.

When phenobarbital tablets are used in place of the liquid form, the patient cannot inadvertently alter the dosage and an exact amount of the medication can be administered repeatedly. Also, waste and loss resulting from the spillage and breakage are reduced to a minimum with the use of the tablet form of phenobarbital.

When phenobarbital is prescribed in liquid form, it causes the patient considerable inconvenience in those instances where the physician desires to supply the patient with sufficient medication to last for a prolonged period of time. As an example, liquid medications are usually prescribed in 4 oz., 6 oz. and 8 oz. bottles and occasionally in 16 oz. and 32 oz. bottles. A 32 oz. bottle of liquid phenobarbital would last a patient receiving the average dosage of phenobarbital just about one month. Therefore, it would be necessary to have the medication renewed at frequent intervals. This inconvenience could be easily eliminated if the medication were prescribed in tablet form.

The patient would be further inconvenienced in the handling and transportation of large volumes of liquid phenobarbital such as while traveling on vacation. Whereas a one or two month's supply of phenobarbital tablets can easily be carried in the pocket of a shirt or dress, a comparable quantity of Phenobarbital Elixir will not fit into an ordinary shoe box and would weigh approximately seven pounds.

The same increased costs of therapy, inaccuracies of dosage and inconveniences also apply to the other liquid forms of antiepileptic drugs. Of course, it is true that in some instances, the liquid anticonvulsive medication may be the only form which the patient will take or tolerate.

In May, 1960, The National Epilepsy League, 203 Wabash Avenue, Chicago 1, Illinois, organized a central pharmacy which provides antiepileptic drugs to its members at wholesale prices. It is necessary for the patient to submit his physician's prescription before medication can be obtained from this source. I do not completely approve of this method of obtaining antiepileptic medication. I believe that it may be of value for patients residing in close proximity to Chicago. However, in the case of those individuals living outside of the Chicago area, I believe that this mail order method of obtaining medication can create some difficult situations.

I have encountered some instances where a patient who did not know the nature of his medicine, misplaced or lost his medication at a time when I was out of town. If the medication had been obtained from Chicago, it is obvious that the patient would be unable to receive an additional supply in ample time, whereas had the prescription been filled at a local pharmacy, the patient could very quickly obtain an additional supply of medication.

Also, there is a natural tendency for many patients to wait until they are "down to their last few pills" before obtaining an additional quantity of medication. Obviously, in the time required for the transportation of mail to and from Chicago, the patient's small supply of medication may be exhausted, resulting in an unfavorable situation. In most instances, however, medication can be obtained from a local pharmacy in a matter of minutes.

An exceedingly major problem would arise if a patient were to attempt suicide by ingesting all of his medication at a time when his personal physician was unavailable. If the patient is taken to a hospital in an unconscious state and the nature of his medication is unknown to anyone else, definitive treatment might be dangerously delayed. I do not know if the central pharmacy in Chicago designates the nature of the drug on the container, but even so, it is quite possible that the container would not be available to the hospital physicians, having been destroyed or misplaced by the patient. It is reasonable to assume that if the antiepileptic medication had been obtained from a local pharmacy, the nature or ingredients of the medication could be ascertained almost immediately.

4. Treatment should begin with one drug. Other drugs should be prescribed, if necessary, only after it has been determined that the maximal tolerated dosage of the starting drug failed to produce a satisfactory clinical response

The major reasons for instituting treatment of an epileptic patient with one drug are as follows: (a) Since there are only three or four "really good" drugs available for the control of seizures and since it is known that the dosage necessary to control epileptic seizures varies from patient to patient, the physician should give each drug a thorough trial before resorting to another drug. I have found that this is a very satisfactory method of titrating the dosage of drug therapy for any individual case. (b) If two drugs of completely different chemical structure were initially prescribed and the patient were to manifest some type of untoward reaction such as marked drowsiness or a cutaneous eruption, it is quite obvious that the physician may have considerable difficulty in determining which of the two drugs was responsible for the unfavorable reaction.

In those patients who suffer with relatively infrequent seizures (monthly or less often) the conventional starting dosage (Table 8) should be prescribed initially. The dosage should then be increased if necessary until a satisfactory control of seizures is attained or

TABLE 8

AVERAGE STARTING AND AVERAGE MAXIMUM DOSAGES* OF ANTIEPILEPTIC DRUGS
EMPLOYED AT THE EPILEPSY CLINIC OF THE JOHNS HOPKINS HOSPITAL

		Starting Dosage‡			Maximum Dosage‡		
Drug	Age, Yr.	Mg.	Grains	Times/Day	Mg.	Grains	Times/Day
Bromides	Under 6	320	5	2	640	10	3
	Over 6	320	5	3	1000	15	3
Phenobarbital	Under 6	16	¼	3	65	1	3
	Over 6	32	½	3	100	1½	3
Mebaral	Under 6	32	½	3	130	2	3
	Over 6	65	1	3	200	3	3
Gemonil	Under 6	50	¾	3	100	1½	3
	Over 6	100	1½	3	200	3	3
Mysoline	Under 6	62.5	1	2	250	3¾	4
	Over 6	250	3¾	2	500	7½	3
Dilantin	Under 6	32	½	3	100	1½	3
	Over 6	100	1½	2	200	3	3
Mesantoin	Under 6	50	¾	3	200	3	3
	Over 6	100	1½	3	400	6	3
Peganone	Under 6	250	3¾	3	750	11¼	4
	Over 6	500	7½	3	1000	15	4
Benzedrine	Under 6	2.5	1/24	2	5	1/12	3
Sulfate	Over 6	5	1/12	2	15	¼	3
Dexedrine	Under 6	2.5	1/24	1	2.5	1/24	3
Sulfate	Over 6	2.5	1/24	2	7.5	⅛	3
Paradione	Under 6	150	2¼	2	300	4½	3
	Over 6	300	4½	2	600	9	3
Tridione	Under 6	150	2¼	2	300	4½	3
	Over 6	300	4½	2	600	9	3
Milontin	Under 6	250	3¾	2	500	7½	3
	Over 6	500	7½	2	1000	15	4
Celontin	Under 6	150	2¼	3	300	4½	4
	Over 6	300	4½	2	600	9	4
Zarontin	Under 6	250	3¾	2	250	3¾	4
	Over 6	250	3¾	3	500	7½	4
Diamox	Under 6	125	2	3	250	3¾	3
	Over 6	250	3¾	2	250	3¾	4
Equanil	Under 6	200	3	3	400	6	3
Miltown	Over 6	400	6	2	400	6	4
Phenurone	Under 6	250	3¾	3	1000	15	3
	Over 6	500	7½	3	2000	30	3
Elipten	Under 6	125	2	2	250	3¾	3
	Over 6	250	3¾	2	250	3¾	4

*The conversion of the metric system of weights to the apothecary system is approximate.

‡The starting and maximum dosages listed in this table are for patients under six years of age and for those over six years of age. This latter group also includes adults. Older children can tolerate as much antiepileptic medication as adults and in most instances it is necessary to prescribe these higher dosages in order to obtain satisfactory results.

until the limit of tolerance for the drug has been reached. In some cases, it may be necessary to prescribe a second drug, but this should not be done until after it has been determined that the maximal tolerated dosage of the first drug failed to produce a satisfactory clinical response. If the maximal tolerated dosage of the first drug fails to give satisfactory control of seizures, but does reduce their frequency or severity to some extent, it should be continued at that same dosage and a second drug should be added to the therapeutic regimen. The dosage of the second drug should be increased, as needed, to tolerance. However, if the maximal tolerated dosage of the first drug fails to help the patient in any manner, it should be gradually withdrawn simultaneously with the administration of the second drug. If during the process of withdrawal of the first drug and the addition of the second drug a satisfactory combination of dosages of both drugs is found, then the patient should continue with both drugs. Occasionally, it may be necessary to prescribe the maximal tolerated dosage of more than two drugs in order to obtain a good control of seizures.

For patients who suffer with relatively frequent (daily, weekly) seizures, the average maximum dosage should be prescribed initially (Table 8). This dosage should be decreased or increased, if necessary, depending upon the patient's tolerance and the occurrence of the seizures. Other drugs should be added to the therapeutic regimen, if necessary, as previously described.

5. The medication should be taken daily, at times of the day, such as with meals, upon returning home from school and at bedtime, which do not interfere with the patient's routine activities

It is important that patients and their parents realize that it is not necessary for the medication to be taken at the same minute of each day. I have had many patients who were forced to interrupt some recreational activity, such as baseball, because it was "time for them to take their medicine." This procedure is not only unnecessary, but can cause some patients considerable emotional distress.

Generally, I advise that the medication not be administered to children, particularly the young child, at school because it may unnecessarily expose a child's illness to his classmates. It is true that I stress the fact that one should not deliberately conceal a diagnosis of epilepsy. However, I believe that nothing is gained when it is unnecessarily exposed. A suggested dosage schedule for the epileptic patient who attends school is as follows: the first dose, with breakfast; the second, when he returns home from school; and the other dosage, either with the evening meal or at bedtime, or at both times, depending upon the case in question.

It has been suggested by several investigators that the total daily dosage of antiepileptic drugs such as phenobarbital and Dilantin be administered at bedtime. I do not believe that sufficient clinical studies have been carried out which prove that the administration of the total daily amount of anticonvulsant medication given in one dosage at bedtime is superior or even as effective as when it is given in divided dosages throughout the day. We are currently in the process of evaluating the clinical effectiveness of these two methods of administering anticonvulsant medication.

The physician should emphasize to the patient the importance of taking the medication exactly as prescribed. I have seen many patients who were instructed to take their antiepileptic medication three times daily and who on numerous occasions either neglected or forgot to take one of the dosages of medication. These omissions were shortly followed by a seizure. The occurrence of seizures in association with the omission of daily medication may occur with any of the antiepileptic drugs, but in my experience, it is most commonly observed with phenobarbital.

Many parents have asked the following question: "What should I do in the case where a dose of medication was administered to my child and for some reason or other it was vomited up?" I advise the parents that the patient should be given another dosage of medication in the following situations: (1) if it is thought that all of the medication was vomited up and they were able to see the drug; or (2) if the vomiting occurred within fifteen minutes after the administration of the medication.

Also, in many instances, patients have told me that on certain occasions they were not absolutely sure that they had taken one of the dosages of their medication and they were quire concerned as to whether or not they should take another dosage. I advise my patients that if they are not certain that they have taken a dosage of medication, they should then take another dosage. This will alleviate any anxiety on the part of the patient in regard to his having a seizure because of the omitted dosage of medication. Even if the patient had taken the medication and would take another dose, the only inconvenience which he would be liable to suffer would be a transient reaction such as drowsiness.

I have seen many patients who were taking their medication every four hours around the clock, that is, the individual was awakened during the middle of the night to be given his dosage of medication. I asked the patients or the parents why the medication was being administered in this manner. I was told that the medication was started in this manner while the individual was a patient in the hospital and that no one had instructed them to administer the medication differently when the patient was discharged. Hospital routine is generally such that it is necessary for the medication to be prescribed at certain times of the day. However, I do not advise that medication be taken in that manner when the patient is at home.

At the present, I recommend that the antiepileptic medication be taken in equal amounts throughout the day. However, in the treatment of seizures which occur in association with sleep or with the menses, it is frequently of value to vary this regimen, as follows:

(a) Early nocturnal seizures (those which occur soon after falling asleep).

Let us suppose that we have to prescribe for a seven year old child with major motor seizures which occur only at night shortly after falling asleep. Such a patient initially should be given 32 mg. of phenobarbital, three times a day. The first dose should be given with lunch, the second dose with supper and the third dose at bedtime. If the seizures should recur, the second dose should be increased to 64 mg., the first and third doses remaining at 32 mg. The second dose should be increased still higher, if necessary, until a satisfactory control of seizures is attained or until the limit of tolerance for the drug has been reached.

(b) Late nocturnal or early morning seizures (those which occur shortly before the usual time of awakening).

Patients who suffer with such seizures should be treated initially with the appropriate dosage of phenobarbital, three times a day. The first dose should be given with lunch, the second dose with supper and the third dose at bedtime. If the seizures should recur, the third (bedtime) dosage of the drug should gradually be increased until a satisfactory control of seizures is attained or until the limit of tolerance for the drug has been reached.

(c) Epileptic seizures which occur in association with the menses.

Epileptic seizures which occur in association with the menses are generally difficult to control. I have found the following plan to be of value in those patients whose menstrual periods recur at regular intervals. For example, a fourteen year old girl who has major motor seizures in association with her menstrual periods, initially should be given 96 mg. of phenobarbital daily in three equal doses. If there should be a recurrence of seizures at the time of menstruation, the dosage of phenobarbital should be increased to 128 mg. daily. This increased dosage should be given for approximately three days before the expected date of menstruation, throughout the menstrual period and for about three days thereafter. During the remainder of the month, the patient should be given the initial maintenance dosage (96 mg. daily). The dosage of phenobarbital should be further increased, if necessary, during the menstrual cycle until the seizures are controlled or the maximal tolerated dosage has been reached.

Limitation of total daily fluid intake and reduction of salt intake for a few days preceding and during the menstrual period is of benefit in some cases. Several workers have observed some good results with Diamox when given premenstrually. However, we have observed no significant benefit in any of our patients treated with this drug.

I have followed a few patients who, during their early years, had epileptic seizures only in association with their menstrual periods. These seizures were uncontrollable with antiepileptic drugs. However, when these patients passed into natural menopause, the seizures no longer recurred and they remained free of seizures without anticonvulsant medication. This observation certainly indicates that one might consider the induction of menopause, either surgically or by x-ray, in those patients who suffer with severe and incapacitating seizures in association with their menstrual cycles.

6. The dosage of anticonvulsant medication varies from patient to patient

The proper dosage of antiepileptic medication for any given patient is that which controls his seizures without producing untoward reactions which interfere with his general well-being. Obviously, the ideal goal in the treatment of epilepsy is to attain a complete control of seizures. However, the drug dosage necessary for a complete control of seizures may in some patients, produce unpleasant reactions, such as drowsiness, which are more of a handicap to the patient than the seizures themselves.

Some patients may be better off leading a normal life between occasional seizures than living seizure-free in a perpetual state of drug-induced drowsiness and confusion. I can mention one of my patients, a very important business executive, who has infrequent short epileptic seizures. In many instances I prescribed a dosage of anticonvulsant medication which rendered him completely seizure-free, but this amount of medication, so the patient told me, made him drowsy to the point where he could neither think as clearly nor perform as acutely as when he took smaller amounts of medication. This lower dosage reduced the frequency of the seizures but did not stop them completely. This individual has repeatedly stated that he would much prefer to have an occasional seizure and the "clearer mind" than to be "made dull" by the amount of medication required to completely control his seizures.

In many instances, reactions such as drowsiness can be alleviated somewhat by the daily administration of stimulating drugs, such as Benzedrine or Dexedrine Sulfate or Ritalin.

The average daily starting and maximum dosages of the anticonvulsants which are employed in the Epilepsy Clinic of The Johns Hopkins Hospital are given in Table 8.

7. The medication should be taken for a prolonged period of time

It has been my experience that the longer anticonvulsant medication is continued in any epileptic patient, the less likely it is that he will have a recurrence of seizures after his therapy is stopped. It is my general policy to continue the antiepileptic medication in full dosage in children for at least four years after the last seizure, and in adults for the rest of their lives. I do make exceptions to this general plan of duration of therapy, some of which are discussed below.

The onset of puberty, especially in females, is a time of life when epilepsy frequently makes its initial appearance and also when a previously controlled epileptic has a recurrence of seizures. Therefore, if the four year period of freedom from seizures should coincide with the onset of puberty, I continue the medication in full dosage throughout the adolescent period. This is particularly important in the case of females.

In some instances, I discontinue the medication sooner than four years after the patient's last seizure. For example, one should consider discontinuing the medication in those patients where there is evidence that the taking of the medication per se is causing significant psychological difficulties. This is particularly true in the case of the teen-ager. I have observed many teen agers in whom I believed that the continued use of anticonvulsant medication was at least partially responsible for psychological disturbances. These patients objected to taking medication every day because of reasons such as "it makes them feel different from other people, they just don't want to be bothered, and they feel it is a nuisance to take the medicine."

When I am confronted with such problems, I study each patient individually and make the decision to withdraw the medication in those cases where it appears that the psychological difficulties caused by the taking of the medication markedly outweigh the calculated risk of a recurrence of seizures which may be associated with withdrawal of the medication. I also consider the withdrawal of medication in those patients who "refuse" to take their medication regularly. I would like to emphasize the fact that it is better to start a withdrawal of medication in a systematic manner than to have the patient take the medication irregularly.

It is needless to say that the medication should be discontinued immediately in patients when there is evidence that it is causing them organic damage.

I only recommend that adults continue taking medication for the rest of their lives when they are receiving drugs such as phenobarbital or Dilantin, which are known to be essentially free of side effects and which are also known to have been taken successfully by many patients for long periods of time. Many of my patients have taken phenobarbital or Dilantin or a combination of both daily for twenty to twenty-five years without manifesting evidence that these drugs disturbed their general well-being in any manner whatsoever.

8. **The medication should be discontinued very gradually**

A sudden withdrawal of anticonvulsant medication is a frequent cause of a recurrence of seizures or status epilepticus. It has been my experience that this is particularly true in the case of phenobarbital. Therefore, when the physician decides to withdraw anticonvulsant medication in a patient who has been seizure free for a period of time, he should reduce the dosage gradually over an interval of time. This interval of time is governed by the amount and type of medication which the patient had been taking. Generally, I withdraw the medication by gradually reducing the dosage over a period of one to two years in those patients who had been taking the average amount of anticonvulsant medication. For example, if the patient had been taking four dosages of medication daily, I advise that for a period of six months the medication be reduced to three dosages daily, during the next six months to two dosages daily, during the next six months to one dosage daily and then no medication thereafter. In those patients who had been receiving considerably more than the average dosage of antiepileptic drugs, it is usually advisable to extend the period of withdrawal to longer intervals of time.

The dosage of medication should be increased immediately to the original level if there should be a recurrence of seizures during the period of reduction.

I have observed that some physicians use the EEG to determine whether a patient's epileptic disorder has improved and whether or not the anticonvulsant therapy should be continued. In such instances, the patient is instructed to discontinue all medication for several days before the test is performed. It is my definite belief that the information thus obtained is of insufficient value to out-weigh the likelihood of precipitating status epilepticus or of causing a recurrence of seizures by the sudden withdrawal of medication. I emphatically advise against such a procedure.

9. Regular medical care (routine follow-up visits) is one of the most important aspects in the medical management of the epileptic patient

The physician should see the epileptic patient at regular inter-vals to regulate the dosage of his medication, to examine him for untoward drug reactions and to discuss social problems, if present. I generally instruct the patient to return within two to three weeks after the initial administration of his anticonvulsant medication, primarily to determine his tolerance to the prescribed dosage. The frequency of the patient's return visits is governed by the magnitude of his medical and social problems. It is my routine policy to see all patients at least once every six months during the entire time they are receiving treatment, including those who have been rendered free of spells.

It is true that many physicians are exceedingly busy and may not have sufficient time to see each patient often enough to ade-quately discuss all of his problems, particularly the socio-economic problems. In such instances, the physician should refer the patient to one of the national lay epilepsy organizations or a local affiliate if available in his community. The names of the national organi-zations are given in another section of this book entitled Services Available for the Epileptic Patient (Chapter 11).

BIBLIOGRAPHY

Livingston, S.: Management of the Child with One Epileptic Seizure. *J.A.M.A., 174:* 135, 1960.
Gellis, S. S. (Editor): *Yearbook of Pediatrics.* Chicago, Year Book Medical Publishers, Series 1961-1962, p. 383.

ANTIEPILEPTIC DRUGS

The indications for usage (Table 6), the recommended dosages (Table 8), the untoward reactions and dosage forms (how supplied) of each of the drugs which were being used at the time of this writing for the treatment of epilepsy are presented in this section.

Since the number of papers which has been written on these drugs is so vast, it did not seem advisable for the purpose of this book to make mention of each of these articles. Instead, at the end of this section, there is a short bibliography which is divided into two sections: (1) general bibliography which includes a review article and several textbooks; these writings contain a list of most of the references to the antiepileptic drugs and (2) specific bibliography which gives pertinent references to each antiepileptic drug.

The interested reader may also refer to the other textbooks on epilepsy or to the general medical literature for additional bibliography.

Bromides

Untoward Reactions

Drowsiness, acne-like rashes, psychoses and neurologic manifestations are the most significant side reactions encountered with bromide therapy.

Drowsiness is an indication of overdosage. It is more likely to occur during hot weather, when perspiration is marked. Reducing the dosage of bromide or giving additional salt and a generous intake of fluid will usually bring about improvement of mild drowsiness within five to ten days.

The acne-like rashes rarely occur in infants and young children, but are frequently observed in adolescent children and adults. Pre-existing acne is generally made much worse by bromides.

It has been my experience that psychoses and neurologic abnormalities are observed most frequently in adults.

How Supplied

Bromide is most often prescribed in liquid form. However, it is also supplied in tablet form by numerous manufacturers in a wide range of doses.

The technique of administration of bromide is not as simple as that of most of the other antiepileptic drugs. An increase in the intake of salt decreases the accumulation of bromide, the bromide ion being replaced by chloride. The effectiveness of bromide therapy, therefore, necessitates a lowered, but fairly constant intake of salt. Epileptic patients given bromides should be instructed to cook foods without adding salt and not to eat foods of high salt content. When there is unusual salt loss, as from vomiting or excessive perspiration, the bromide intake should be reduced or temporarily discontinued.

Phenobarbital

Untoward Reactions

Drowsiness and hyperactivity are frequent untoward reactions observed with phenobarbital therapy.

Drowsiness is generally a symptom of overdosage and can usually be alleviated by reducing the dosage of the drug.

Although phenobarbital is generally considered a sedative drug, it causes hyperactivity in many patients, particularly children. Many of my young epileptic patients became so restless, irritable and "mean" following the institution of phenobarbital therapy that it was necessary to discontinue the drug, in spite of the fact that it had proved to be very helpful in controlling the seizures. Hyperactivity is an indication of an idiosyncrasy to the drug and is not related to the dosage.

Phenobarbital only rarely causes skin rashes. Thousands of my patients have received this drug some time during the course of their illness and in only a few instances did a skin rash occur which was attributable to the phenobarbital.

How Supplied

Phenobarbital Tablets—16 mg.
Phenobarbital Tablets—32 mg.
Phenobarbital Tablets—65 mg.
Phenobarbital Tablets—100 mg.
Phenobarbital Elixir, U.S.P.—20 mg. per 5 cc. (teaspoonful)
Phenobarbital Sodium Sterile Powder—Ampoule—120 mg.
Phenobarbital Sodium Solution—1 cc. Ampoules—120 mg. in propylene glycol
Eskabarb Spansule Capsules—65 mg. phenobarbital
Eskabarb Spansule Capsules—97 mg. phenobarbital
Luminal Elixir—20 mg. phenobarbital per 5 cc. (teaspoonful)
Luminal Ovoids—16 mg. phenobarbital—yellow
Luminal Ovoids—32 mg. phenobarbital—light green

Luminal Ovoids—100 mg. phenobarbital—dark green

Luminal Sodium Hypodermic Tablets—60 mg. phenobarbital sodium

Luminal Sodium Ampuls—Powder—130 mg.

Luminal Sodium Ampuls—Powder—320 mg.

Luminal Sodium Solution for Injection—1 cc. Ampuls—130 mg. —in a special vehicle

Luminal Sodium Solution for Injection—2 cc. Ampuls—320 mg. —in a special vehicle

Luminal Sodium Solution for Injection—10 cc. Vials—160 mg. per cc.—in a special vehicle

Mebaral (Mephobarbital)

Untoward Reactions

The side reactions of Mebaral are similar to those of phenobarbital, but do not occur as frequently.

How Supplied

Mebaral Tablets—32 mg.—white tablet

Mebaral Tablets—50 mg.—white tablet

Mebaral Tablets—100 mg.—white tablet

Mebaral Tablets—200 mg.—white tablet

Mebroin Tablets—a combination of Mebaral 90 mg. and diphenylhydantoin 60 mg.; peach colored tablet

Gemonil (Metharbital)

Untoward Reactions

Gemonil is relatively free of toxic effects. Drowsiness and rashes were the only significant untoward reactions observed in our patients.

Drowsiness is related to the dosage of the drug and can generally be alleviated by reducing the dosage of the drug.

How Supplied

Gemonil Tablets—100 mg.—white tablet

Dilantin Sodium (Diphenylhydantoin Sodium)

This drug is known by a variety of trade names: in Brazil, as Epelin; in Uruguay, as Epanutin; in other Latin American countries, as Epamin; and in the British Commonwealth, as Epanutin.

TABLE 9

UNTOWARD REACTIONS OF DILANTIN THERAPY

Definite*	Questionable**
Disturbed equilibrium	Toxic amblyopia
Diplopia	Agranulocytosis
Nystagmus	Thrombocytopenia
Dysarthria	Pancytopenia
Skin rashes	Megaloblastic anemia
(measles-like and scarlatiniform	Aplastic anemia
frequently associated with	Alopecia
lymphadenopathy and a leukopenia)	Myocardial damage
Hyperplasia of gums	Systemic lupus erythematosus
Hypertrichosis	Polyarthropathy
Constipation	Hematuria
Nausea	Albuminuria
Vomiting	Periarteritis nodosa
Drowsiness	Pulmonary abnormalities
Behavioral disturbances	Hepatitis
Headaches	Exfoliative dermatitis
Tremors	Erythema bullosum malignans
Lymphadenopathy	Hemorrhagic erythema multiforme
(clinically and pathologically	
simulating malignant lymphomas)	

*Definite—those reactions which have been observed very frequently; those reactions which have been observed infrequently but have been reproduced with readministration of the drug.

**Questionable—those reactions in which a definite relationship with the drug has not been conclusively established.

Untoward Reactions

A comprehensive list of the untoward reactions which have been encountered in patients receiving Dilantin is shown in Table 9.

Serious disorders such as hepatitis, exfoliative dermatitis, aplastic anemia, periarteritis nodosa and systemic lupus erythematosus are included because their occurrence has been reported in association with Dilantin therapy. However, I do not believe that a specific relationship between these disorders and Dilantin has been definitely established. At least 50 per cent of my 15,000 patients have taken Dilantin some time during the course of their illness and hundreds of them have taken Dilantin continuously for more than twenty years. In my experience, serious toxic reactions to Dilantin were very rare, and I have not encountered a single instance where the reaction was not reversible.

Disturbance of equilibrium is the most frequent side reaction encountered with Dilantin therapy. This disturbance is due to overdosage, and almost always disappears within one to two weeks after the dosage has been reduced to the tolerated level.

In some instances, unsteadiness is so severe that the patient may give the impression of being "drunk from alcohol." I can mention the case of one of my patients who was so unsteady that he fell on the street. He was picked up by a police officer and accused of being under "the influence of alcohol."

Diplopia is frequently encountered and is generally related to the dosage of the drug.

Nystagmus, dysarthria and drowsiness are other side effects related to overdosage and usually disappear soon after the dosage is reduced to the tolerated level. Drowsiness is less common with Dilantin than with most other antiepileptic drugs.

Skin rashes are frequently encountered, a measles-like eruption being the most common. This cutaneous reaction usually appears ten to fourteen days after the start of therapy and is frequently associated with fever and occasionally with lymphadenopathy and a leukopenia. The rash sometimes involves the mouth and throat. It is of interest to note that this rash simulates that of measles so precisely (Figure 7) that many of my patients were diagnosed as having measles, when actually they were manifesting a reaction to the Dilantin therapy. These measles-like rashes probably represent a drug sensitivity, since they develop irrespective of the dosage prescribed.

There is no doubt that measles-like and scarlatiniform rashes are caused by Dilantin, as they are observed so frequently and can be reproduced in many patients with readministration of the drug. However, the etiology of some of the other skin lesions which have been reported in association with Dilantin therapy, such as exfoliative dermatitis is not so clear.

Gingival hyperplasia may be observed in patients receiving Dilantin. Hyperplastic gums are usually quite firm and faintly pink in color. Some of my patients complained of bleeding occurring either spontaneously or when the teeth were brushed. In a few instances, the hyperplastic tissue was so extensive that it covered the cutting edges of the teeth. Among my adult epileptic

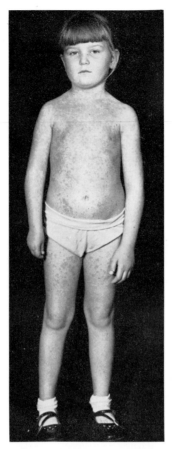

Figure 7. Photograph shows measles-like rash which appeared twelve days after the onset of Dilantin therapy.

patients with marked gingival hyperplasia, two of their own accord, had all their teeth extracted; they continued to take Dilantin for many years thereafter, but the hyperplasia receded spontaneously and has not recurred. This suggests the possibility that hyperplasia of the gums does not occur in the absence of teeth.

The occurrence or degree of gingival hyperplasia is not related to the dosage, and probably represents a specific drug sensitivity reaction. In most cases, the gums return to normal within a year after the drug has been withdrawn. The occurence of hyperplasia is in itself not an indication for discontinuing therapy. In some cases, however, it may be necessary to withdraw the drug because the hyperplastic tissue does not respond to corrective measures and becomes so marked that it interferes with chewing or is disfiguring.

Gingival hyperplasia can be reduced somewhat by strict oral hygiene and daily vigorous massaging of the gums. Repeated excision of excessive hyperplastic tissue is helpful in some instances. The daily administration of chlorpheniramine (Chlor-Trimeton, Teldrin) reduced the degree of gingival hyperplasia in several of our patients.

Figure 8 shows the gums of a sixteen year old girl who had been receiving a total of 700 mg. of Dilantin daily for about five years. The Dilantin was withdrawn gradually over a period of two months, starting at the time this photograph was taken. Phenobarbital was substituted for the Dilantin. Figure 9 shows this patient's gums one year later (she had been receiving no Dilantin for ten months).

Hypertrichosis is observed in some patients in association with the administration of Dilantin. In my group of patients who presented this reaction, the hair growth was related neither to the dosage, nor to the type of epilepsy, nor was there evidence of any endocrine abnormality.

Gastrointestinal disturbances, such as a "heavy feeling in the stomach," nausea or vomiting, also occur in some patients, but they are in general relatively minor. Frequently, such reactions can be prevented or minimized if the patient takes the drug only with or immediately after meals, or by using a gelatin capsule containing a suspension of Dilantin in vegetable oil.

Obstinate constipation is observed very frequently in patients who have been receiving Dilantin for prolonged periods of time.

Lymphadenopathies of great magnitude which simulated malignant lymphomas both clinically and pathologically have been observed with Dilantin therapy.

Behavioral disturbances have also been encountered in association with Dilantin therapy. In some instances, it was quite evident that Dilantin was the causative factor; in other instances, the relationship between the Dilantin and the behavioral disturbances

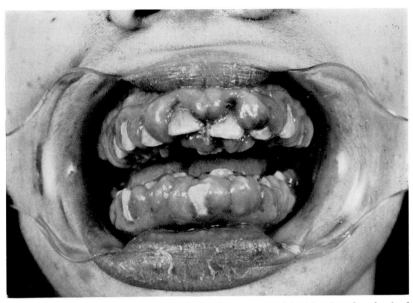

Figure 8. Severe gingival hyperplasia in sixteen year old white female who had been receiving Dilantin for about five years.

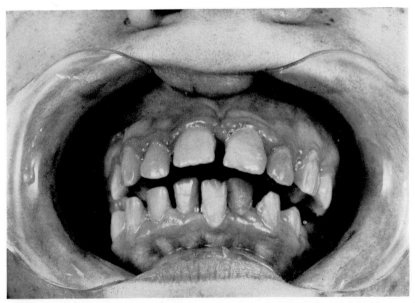

Figure 9. Gums of the patient in Figure 8 one year later. She had not received any Dilantin for approximately ten months.

was not clear. However, it is important that the physician keep in mind the possibility of these disturbances.

Other untoward reactions, such as periarteritis nodosa, toxic amblyopia, systemic lupus erythematosus, hepatitis, genitourinary and cardiovascular disturbances have been observed in association with Dilantin therapy. I do not believe that one can be completely certain that Dilantin was the cause of these disturbances, since they have been observed so infrequently and, to my knowledge, have not been reproduced in the same patient.

In 1959, Moore reported a high incidence of pulmonary changes in a group of his patients who had been taking Dilantin for prolonged periods of time. This finding was not confirmed by a study carried out in our clinic, nor by a similar investigation by Low and Yahr.

How Supplied

Dilantin Sodium Kapseals—30 mg.—hard capsule with pink band

Dilantin Sodium Kapseals—100 mg.—hard capsule with orange band

Dilantin Sodium Steri-Vials—250 mg. with 5 cc. ampoule of special solvent (40% Propylene Glycol and 10% Alcohol in Water for Injection) adjusted with sodium hydroxide to pH 12

Dilantin D. A. Kapseals—100 mg.—hard special capsule formulated to delay absorption; orange opaque band

Dilantin Infatabs—50 mg.—triangular, grooved, cream colored, palatably flavored tablets

Dilantin in Oil Capsules—100 mg.—in a vegetable oil; soluble gelatin capsule

Dilantin Suspension—100 mg. per 4 cc.—flavored—orange color

Dilantin Sodium with Phenobarbital Kapseals—100 mg. with Phenobarbital 16 mg.—hard capsule with garnet band

Dilantin Sodium with Phenobarbital Kapseals—100 mg. with Phenobarbital 32 mg.—hard capsule with black band

Phelantin Kapseals—Dilantin Sodium 100 mg. with Phenobarbital 30 mg. and Desoxyephedrine Hydrochloride 25. mg.—hard yellow capsule with transparent orange band

Mesantoin (Methylphenylethylhydantoin)

Untoward Reactions

A comprehensive list of the untoward reactions which have been encountered in patients receiving Mesantoin are shown in Table 10.

TABLE 10

UNTOWARD REACTIONS OF MESANTOIN THERAPY

Definite*	*Questionable***
Leukopenia	Hepatitis
Thrombocytopenia	Psychoses
Agranulocytosis	Periarteritis nodosa
Pancytopenia	Systemic lupus erythematosus
Aplastic anemia	Exfoliative dermatitis
Skin rashes	
(Measles-like and scarlatiniform)	
Purpuric rashes	
(associated with thrombocytopenia)	
Marked drowsiness	
Ataxia	
Diplopia	
Nystagmus	
Lymphadenopathy	
(clinically and pathologically	
simulating malignant lymphomas)	

*Definite—those reactions which have been observed very frequently; those reactions which have been observed infrequently but have been reproduced with readministration of the drug.

**Questionable—those reactions in which a definite relationship with the drug has not been conclusively established.

The most significant and alarming toxic effect of Mesantoin is hemapoietic. We experienced no fatalities, but a significant number of deaths from hematologic disturbances has been reported. Since the physician cannot predict which patient may be affected in this manner, it is advisable that patients have periodic blood examinations during the period of treatment with this drug.

Deaths due to hepatitis, periarteritis nodosa and severe dermatological disturbances have also been reported. Systemic lupus erythematosus has also been mentioned as a toxic reaction of Mesantoin. I do not believe that it has definitely been proved that Mesantoin was the causative factor in these cases.

Drowsiness is a common side reaction and its appearance indicates that the maximal tolerated dosage has been exceeded. This effect can usually be alleviated by reducing the dosage.

Mesantoin causes measles-like and scarlatiniform skin rashes resembling those observed with Dilantin. Purpuric rashes associated with abnormally low platelet counts were encountered in four of our patients.

Lymphadenopathies of great magnitude which simulated malignant lymphomas both clinically and pathologically have been observed with Mesantoin therapy.

Ataxia, diplopia and nystagmus are encountered in some patients. These reactions can be eliminated, or at least minimized, by a reduction in the dosage of the drug.

Hyperplasia of the gums, which is seen so frequently with Dilantin, was not encountered in any of our patients.

How Supplied
Mesantoin Tablets—100 mg.—pale pink color
Hydantal Tablets—a combination of Mesantoin 100 mg. and phenobarbital 20 mg.; glazed white tablet

Peganone (Ethotoin)
Untoward Reactions
Peganone appears to have fewer side effects than the other hydantoin derivatives which are currently being employed as anticonvulsants (Dilantin and Mesantoin).

The only significant untoward reaction observed in our clinic was a cutaneous eruption (measles-like) similar to that which is seen with other hydantoinates.

How Supplied
Peganone Tablets—250 mg.—white tablet
Peganone Tablets—500 mg.—white tablet

Mysoline (Primidone)
Untoward Reactions
A comprehensive list of the untoward reactions which have been encountered in patients receiving Mysoline are shown in Table 11.

TABLE 11

Untoward Reactions of Mysoline Therapy

Definite*	Questionable**
Marked drowsiness	Alopecia
Skin rashes (morbilliform)	Psychoses
Megaloblastic anemia	Edema of the eyelids
Dizziness	Painful gums
Ataxia	Nystagmus
Diplopia	Polyuria
Personality changes	Sexual impotence
Nausea	Headaches
Vomiting	Leukopenia
	Systemic lupus erythematosus

*Definite—those reactions which have been observed very frequently; those reactions which have been observed infrequently but have been reproduced with readministration of the drug.
**Questionable—those reactions in which a definite relationship with the drug has not been conclusively established.

The most common side reaction of Mysoline is drowsiness, varying in degree from mild, transient sleepiness to severe lethargy. In the majority of cases the drowsiness appears within the first few days of the beginning of Mysoline therapy. In some cases it appears after the first few doses are taken. Several of my patients stated that they slept for approximately twenty-four hours after ingesting their first tablet of Mysoline.

The drowsiness disappears, in most instances, within several weeks after the initial administration of the drug. The initial drowsiness can be minimized, in most cases, if treatment is started by giving very small amounts (50 mg.) of the drug at bedtime for one week and then subsequently increasing the dosage at weekly intervals as indicated.

Dizziness and ataxia are encountered in some patients. In most instances, these reactions disappear with a reduction in dosage of the drug.

Skin rashes, usually of the morbilliform type, are occasionally observed in association with Mysoline therapy.

Diplopia, personality changes, nausea and vomiting are also occasionally observed.

No hematologic disturbances were encountered in any of our patients. However, since megaloblastic anemia occurring with Mysoline therapy has been reported by other physicians, it is advisable that patients receiving this drug have periodic blood examinations.

How Supplied
Mysoline Suspension—250 mg. per 5 cc. (teaspoonful)—white color
Mysoline Tablets—50 mg.—white tablet
Mysoline Tablets—250 mg.—white tablet

Tridione (Trimethadione)

Untoward Reactions
A comprehensive list of the untoward reactions which have been encountered in patients receiving Tridione are shown in Table 12.

TABLE 12

UNTOWARD REACTIONS OF TRIDIONE THERAPY

*Definite**	*Questionable***
Leukopenia	Alopecia
Agranulocytosis	Systemic lupus erythematosus
Thrombocytopenia	Hepatitis
Pancytopenia	Exfoliative dermatitis
Aplastic anemia	
Nephrosis	
Hematuria	
Photophobia	
Hiccoughs	
Drowsiness	
Headache	
Vertigo	
Diplopia	
Nausea	
Vomiting	
Abdominal pain	
Painful and swollen joints with fever	
Personality changes	
Behavioral disturbances	
Skin rashes (morbilliform and urticarial)	

*Definite—those reactions which have been observed very frequently; those reactions which have been observed infrequently but have been reproduced with readministration of the drug.

**Questionable—those reactions in which a definite relationship with the drug has not been conclusively established.

The most significant toxic reactions of Tridione are its adverse effects on the hemapoietic and genitourinary systems. We have had no fatalities from these disorders, but fatal cases have been reported by others. Therefore, it is important that patients have periodic blood and urine examinations during the course of Tridione therapy.

Photophobia is an exceedingly common side effect caused by Tridione. This reaction is not related to the dosage of Tridione and in all probability represents a sensitivity to the drug. Therefore, a reduction of dosage is generally of no avail in alleviating this disturbance. Many patients are helped by wearing dark glasses.

Diplopia, vertigo, increased irritability and drowsiness are encountered, usually when excessive amounts of the drug are taken. Headaches, insomnia, personality changes, and behavior difficulties have been seen occasionally.

Hiccoughs is seen quite frequently. This disturbance usually makes its appearance a week or two after the initial administration of the drug. It usually persists for two or three days and generally disappears spontaneously.

Skin rashes, usually of the morbilliform or urticarial type, are encountered occasionally.

Several of our patients developed swollen joints and fever which disappeared on withdrawal of Tridione and recurred when the drug was readministered.

Systemic lupus erythematosus, hepatitis, exfoliative dermatitis and alopecia have been mentioned as untoward reactions of Tridione. However, I do not believe that it has been definitely established that Tridione was the causative factor in these reactions.

How Supplied

Tridione Capsules—300 mg.—white capsule

Tridione Solution—150 mg. per fluid dram (3.7 cc.)—aqueous; flavored; light orange color

Tridione Dulcet Tablets—150 mg. with Magnesium Trisilicate 80 mg.—white, aromatic tablet

It is important that Tridione Capsules be kept in a cool place, since Tridione melts when exposed to excessive temperatures (when exposed to direct sunlight during the summer, if kept in the glove compartment of a car during the summer months, if stored in any place which is likely to be exposed to excessive heat, etc.). The official compendia, The Pharmacopeia of the United States and The National Formulary, both direct that Tridione preparations be stored at temperatures preferably not exceeding 86°F.

My attention was called to the fact that several of my patients had been taking Tridione Capsules which contained less than half the original contents. One of my patients, a young child, had been taking empty Tridione Capsules for a period of time before the parents became cognizant of the situation. In each instance the Tridione Capsules had been stored in an exceedingly hot place.

Paradione (Paramethadione)

Untoward Reactions

The untoward reactions of Paradione are similar to those of Tridione, but have been observed less frequently This finding may be explained by the fact that Paradione has not been used as extensively as Tridione.

How Supplied

Paradione Capsules—150 mg.—red color
Paradione Capsules—300 mg.—red color
Paradione Solution—300 mg. per cc. This preparation contains
65 per cent alcohol and must be diluted prior to administration; it may be mixed easily with orange juice or milk. It is available in bottles of 50 cc. with a graduated dropper, permitting the withdrawal and delivery of 0.5 or 1 cc. doses.

Benzedrine Sulfate (Amphetamine Sulfate)
Dexedrine Sulfate (Dextro-Amphetamine Sulfate)

Untoward Reactions

I have prescribed the amphetamines to hundreds of my patients and the only significant side reactions which I observed were insomnia, loss of weight, increased irritability and restlessness. These reactions can be alleviated, or at least minimized, in most patients by a reduction in the dosage of the drug.

How Supplied

Benzedrine Sulfate Ampul Solution—20 mg. per cc. in 1 cc. Ampuls

Benzedrine Sulfate Spansule Capsules—15 mg.

Benzedrine Sulfate Tablets—5 mg.

Benzedrine Sulfate Tablets—10 mg.

Dexedrine Sulfate Elixir—5 mg. per 5 cc. (teaspoonful)

Dexedrine Sulfate Spansule Capsules—5 mg.

Dexedrine Sulfate Spansule Capsules—10 mg.

Dexedrine Sulfate Spansule Capsules—15 mg.

Dexedrine Sulfate Tablets—5 mg.

Phenurone (Phenacemide)

Untoward Reactions

Phenurone is an exceedingly toxic drug and should be used only in those patients whose seizures are refractory to the other standard antiepileptic drugs.

Fatalities from hemapoietic, genitourinary and hepatic disturbances have been reported in association with Phenurone therapy. Therefore, it is imperative that blood, urine and liver function tests be performed periodically on patients during the course of treatment with Phenurone.

An exceedingly common untoward reaction caused by Phenurone is an adverse change in personality or behavior. Suicidal tendencies, paranoia and acute psychotic states have been observed in association with the administration of Phenurone.

Other relatively frequent side reactions include skin rashes of maculopapular or scarlatiniform type, severe headaches, anorexia, loss of weight, vomiting and vague abdominal pains.

How Supplied

Phenurone Tablets—500 mg.—white tablet

Milontin (Phensuximide)

Untoward Reactions

Milontin appears to be relatively free of significant side reactions. Disturbances such as nausea, vomiting, drowsiness and skin eruptions have been observed in association with Milontin therapy.

Microscopic hematuria has been reported by several physicians in patients receiving this drug.

How Supplied

Milontin Suspension—250 mg. per 4 cc.—Anise-pineapple flavored aqueous suspension—white color

Milontin Kapseals—500 mg.—hard, light orange capsule with orange band

Celontin (Methsuximide)

Untoward Reactions

Side reactions such as drowsiness, periorbital edema, dizziness, gastrointestinal disturbances and skin eruptions have been observed in association with Celontin therapy.

A fatal case of bone marrow aplasia which occurred in association with the administration of this drug was also reported. There is also suggestive evidence that Celontin adversely affected the kidney and liver in several patients. In view of these findings, patients receiving Celontin should have periodic blood, genitourinary and hepatic examinations during the course of its administration.

How Supplied

Celontin Kapseals—300 mg.—hard, yellow-tint capsule with orange band

Zarontin (Ethosuximide)

Untoward Reactions

Zarontin had not been used very extensively at the time of this writing. Untoward reactions such as nausea, gastric distress, drowsiness, dizziness, headache and skin rashes have been observed in association with its administration.

A report of fatal aplastic anemia in an eight and a half year old girl receiving Zarontin has been called to my attention. She had been given combined anticonvulsant medication consisting of Zarontin, Peganone, Diamox and Gemonil. The exact relationship of the part played by Zarontin in this case has not been established.

I recommend that periodic blood, urine and liver function tests be performed on patients receiving Zarontin until the toxicity of this drug has been definitely established.

How Supplied

Zarontin Capsules—250 mg.—soluble gelatin capsule—orange color

Elipten (Amino-Glutethimide)

Untoward Reactions

To my knowledge, no serious toxic reactions have been observed at the time of this writing with Elipten therapy. Skin rashes, pruritic dermatitis, marked drowsiness and transient leukopenia had been encountered in some patients.

How Supplied

Elipten Tablets—125 mg.—white tablet
Elipten Tablets—250 mg.—white tablet

Diamox (Acetazolamide)

Untoward Reactions

Undesirable side effects of Diamox therapy, though rather frequent, are usually not serious and are rapidly reversible. Drowsiness and paresthesias are the most commonly encountered side effects. Fatigue, excitement, gastrointestinal upset and polydipsia have been observed less frequently.

How Supplied

Diamox Tablets—250 mg.—white tablet

Miltown, Equanil (Meprobamate)

Untoward Reactions

This drug appears to be relatively free of serious side reactions. Drowsiness occurs in some patients; this reaction is related to the dosage in most instances and can usually be minimized by a reduction of dosage.

Among the common untoward reactions encountered with this drug are the hypersensitivity reactions which usually manifest themselves in pruritis and urticarial eruptions. Non-thrombocytopenic purpura has also been reported.

How Supplied

Meprospan Capsules—200 mg. Miltown—yellow-topped capsule

Meprospan Capsules—400 mg. Miltown—blue-topped capsule
Meprotabs—400 mg. Miltown—white coated tablet
Miltown Tablets—200 mg.; 400 mg.—white tablets
Equanil Suspension—200 mg. per 5 cc. (teaspoonful)—pink color
Equanil Tablets—200 mg.—white pentagonal tablet
Equanil Tablets—400 mg.—white tablet
Equanil Wyseals—400 mg.—especially coated yellow tablets
Equanil L-A (continuous release) Capsules—400 mg.—red-topped capsule

Additional Drugs

Other preparations which have been reported by some physicians to be effective in the treatment of epilepsy include ACTH and steroids, Atabrine, Pyridoxine and Librium. These preparations have not proved to be of significant value in the treatment of our patients.

BIBLIOGRAPHY

General Bibliography

Goodman, L. S., and Gilman, A.: *The Pharmacological Basis of Therapeutics*(2nd ed.). New York, Macmillan, 1955.

Lennox, W. G.: *Epilepsy and Related Disorders,* 2 vols., Boston, Little, Brown and Co., 1960.

Livingston, S.: *The Diagnosis and Treatment of Convulsive Disorders in Children.* Springfield, Ill., Thomas, 1954.

Livingston, S.: Drug Therapy for Childhood Epilepsy. *J. Chron. Dis.,* 6:46, 1957. (This article contains approximately 250 references relative to the use of antiepileptic drugs in children and adults.)

Livingston, S.: Convulsive Disorders in Infants and Children, in *Advances in Pediatrics.,* Chicago, The Year Book Publishers, Inc., 1958.

Specific Bibliography

Pertinent articles referrable to each antiepileptic drug which are either not included or not discussed in detail in the General Bibliography.

ACTH and Steroids

Pauli, L., O'Neil, R., Ybanez, M., and Livingston, S.: Minor Motor Epilepsy, Treatment with Corticotropin (ACTH) and Steroid Therapy. *J.A.M.A.,* 174:1408, 1960.

Atabrine

Livingston, S.: Drug Therapy for Childhood Epilepsy. *J. Chron. Dis.,* 6:73, 1957.

Sibley, W. A., Tucker, H. J., and Randt, C. T.: Quinacrine in the Treatment of Refractory Petit Mal. *New England J. Med.,* 267:332, 1962.

Benzedrine and Dexedrine Sulfates

Livingston, S., Kajdi, L., and Bridge, E. M.: The Use of Benzedrine and Dexedrine Sulfate in the Treatment of Epilepsy. *J. Pediat.*, *32:*490, 1948.

Bromides

Livingston, S., and Pearson, P. H.: Bromides in the Treatment of Epilepsy in Children. *A.M.A. Am. J. Dis. Child.*, *86:*717, 1953.

Celontin

Green, R. A., and Gilbert, N. G.: Fatal Bone Marrow Aplasia Associated with Celontin Therapy. *Minnesota Med.*, *42:*130, 1959.

Livingston, S., and Pauli, L.: Celontin (PM-396) in the Treatment of Epilepsy. *Pediatrics*, *19:*614, 1957.

Scholl, M. L., Abbott, J. A., and Schwab, R. S.: Celontin—A New Anticonvulsant. *Epilepsia*, *1:*105, 1959.

Diamox

Chao, D. H., and Plumb, R. L.: Diamox in Epilepsy: Critical Review of 178 Cases. *J. Pediat.*, *58:*211, 1961.

Livingston, S., Petersen, D., and Boks, L. L.: Ineffectiveness of Diamox in the Treatment of Childhood Epilepsy. *Pediatrics*, *17:*541, 1956.

Dilantin

Bray, P. F.: Diphenylhydantoin (Dilantin) After Twenty Years. A Review with Reemphasis by Treatment of Eighty-four Patients. *Pediatrics*, *23:*151, 1959.

Kurtzke, J F : Leukopenia with Diphenylhydantoin. *J. Nerv. Ment. Dis.*, *132:*339, 1961.

Livingston, S., Petersen, D., and Boks, L. L.: Hypertrichosis Occurring in Association with Dilantin Therapy. *J. Pediat.*, *47:*351, 1955.

Livingston, S.: Treatment of Epilepsy with Diphenylhydantoin Sodium (Dilantin Sodium). *Post Graduate Med.*, *20:*584, 1956.

Livingston, S., Whitehouse, D., and Pauli, L. L.: Study of the Effects of Diphenylhydantoin Sodium on the Lungs. *New England J. Med.*, *264:*648, 1961

Low, N. L , and Yahr, M. D.: The Lack of Pulmonary Fibrosis in Patients Receiving Diphenylhydantoin. *J.A.M.A.*, *174:*1201, 1960.

Lustberg, A., Goldman, D., and Dreskin, O. H.: Megaloblastic Anemia Due to Dilantin Therapy. *Ann. Intern. Med.*, *54:*153, 1961.

Moore, M. T.: Pulmonary Changes in Hydantoin Therapy. *J.A.M.A*, *171:*1328, 1959.

Rallison, M. L., Carlisle, J. W., Lee, R. E.. Jr., Vernier, R. L., and Good, R. A.: Lupus erythematosus and Stevens-Johnson Syndrome; Occurrences as reaction to anticonvulsant medication *Am. J. Dis. Child.*, *101:*725, 1961.

Rosenfeld, S., Swiller, A. I., Shenoy, Y. M., and Morrison, A. N.: Syndrome Simulating Lymphosarcoma Induced by Diphenylhydantoin Sodium. *J.A.M.A.*, *176:*491, 1961.

Weintraub, R. M., Pechet, L., and Alexander, B.: Rapid Diagnosis of Drug-induced Thrombocytopenic Purpura. *J.A.M.A.*, *180:*528, 1962.

Elipten

Bauer, R. B., and Meyer, J. S.: Clinical Evaluation of Elipten: A New Anticonvulsant Drug for Epilepsy. *J. Michigan M. Soc.*, *59:*1829, 1960.

Pearce, K. I.: Elipten: A Clinical Evaluation of a New Anticonvulsant. *Canad. M. A. J.*, *82:*953, 1960.

Gemonil

Perlstein, M. A.: Gemonil (5,5-diethyl l-methyl barbituric acid). New Drug for Convulsive and Related Disorders. *Pediatrics, 5:*448, 1950.

Librium

Kaim, S. C., and Rosenstein, I. N.: Anticonvulsant Properties of a New Psychotherapeutic Drug. *Dis. Nerv. Syst., 21*(3) Suppl: 46-8, 1960.

Livingston, S., Pauli, L., and Murphy, J. B.: Ineffectiveness of Chlordiazepoxide Hydrochloride in Epilepsy. *J.A.M.A., 177:*243, 1961.

Meprobamate

Livingston, S., and Pauli, L.: Meprobamate in the Treatment of Epilepsy of Children. *A.M.A. Arch. Dis. Child., 94:*277, 1957.

Mesantoin

Kozol, H. L.: Mesantoin in the Treatment of Epiepsy. *Arch. Neurol. & Psychiat., 63:* 235, 1950.

Saltzstein, S. L., and Ackerman, L. V.: Lymphadenopathy Induced by Anticonvulsant Drugs and Mimicking Clinically and Pathologically Malignant Lymphomas. *Cancer, 12:*164, 1959.

Milontin

Doyle, P. J., Livingston, S., and Pearson, P. H.: Use of Milontin in the Treatment of Petit Mal Epilepsy (Three per Second Spike and Wave Dysrhythmia). *J. Pediat., 43:*164, 1953.

Millichap, J. G.: Milontin: A New Drug in the Treatment of Petit Mal. *Lancet, 2:* 907, 1952.

Mysoline

Christenson, W. N., Ultmann, J. E., and Roseman, D. M.: Megaloblastic Anemia During Primidone (Mysoline) Therapy. *J.A.M.A., 163:*940, 1957.

Livingston, S., and Petersen, D.: Primidone (Mysoline) in the Treatment of Epilepsy. *New England J. Med., 254:*327, 1956.

Timberlake, W. H., Abbott, J. A., and Schwab, R. S.: Mysoline: Effective Anticonvulsant with Initial Problems of Adjustment. *New England J. Med., 252:*304, 1955.

Paradione

Livingston, S., and Boks, L. L.: Use of the Dione Drugs (Propazone, Tridione, Paradione, Dimedione and Malidone) in the Treatment of Epilepsy of Children. *New England J. Med., 253:*138, 1955.

Peganone

Livingston, S.: The Use of Peganone (AC 695) in the Treatment of Epilepsy. *J. Pediat., 49:*728, 1956.

Schwade, E. D., Richards, R. K., and Everett, G. M.: Peganone, A New Antiepileptic Drug. *Dis. Nerv. Syst., 17:*155, 1956.

Phenurone

Livingston, S., and Pauli, L. L.: Phenacemide in the Treatment of Epilepsy. *New England J. Med., 256:*588, 1957.

Pyridoxine

Ernsting, W., and Ferwerda, T. P.: Vitamin B$_6$ (pyridoxine, adermine) in therapy of epilepsy. Nederl. tijdschr. geneesk., *95:*3643, 1951 (Dutch).

Livingston, S., Hsu, J. M., and Petersen, D. C.: Ineffectiveness of Pyridoxine (Vitamin B$_6$) in the Treatment of Epilepsy. *Pediatrics, 16:*250, 1955.

Tridione

Benton, J. W., Tynes, B., Register, H. B., Alford, C., and Holley, H. L.: Systemic Lupus Erythematosus Occurring During Anticonvulsive Therapy. *J.A.M.A., 180:* 115, 1962.

Mustard, H. S., and Livingston, S.: Tridione Therapy in Epilepsy: Review of the Results in 156 Patients with Petit Mal Epilepsy with Special Reference to Side Reactions. *J. Pediat., 35:*540, 1949.

Zarontin

Goldensohn, E. S., Hardie, J., and Borea, E. D.: Ethosuximide in the Treatment of Epilepsy. *J.A.M.A., 180:*840, 1962.

Livingston, S., Pauli, L., and Najmabadi, A.: Ethosuximide in the Treatment of Epilepsy. *J.A.M.A., 180:*822, 1962.

ARE ANTIEPILEPTIC DRUGS HABIT FORMING?

Some of the medicines used in the treatment of epilepsy fall within the habit forming category, but virtually never lead to undue dependence or addiction when administered in connection with the treatment of epilepsy. Most of the anticonvulsive drugs have no habit forming capacity whatsoever and many are completely benign in their general effect.

My experience has been that drug addiction is not a problem in the treatment of epilepsy, particularly in the case of children. I have seen many patients who had taken drugs such as phenobarbital or Dilantin daily for five or six years or even longer in whom no significant difficulties were encountered after the medication was discontinued. Some of these patients did experience a recurrence of seizures, but I do not recall observing signs or symptoms of true drug addiction in any of these patients. It is true that some of them manifested anxieties during the interval of withdrawal of medication and also for a period of time after the medication had been completely withdrawn. However, these anxieties were related mostly to a fear of having a recurrence of epileptic seizures.

PATIENT SHOULD BE CAUTIONED AGAINST
UNETHICAL TREATMENTS

The physician should caution the patient against treating himself with proprietary medications which may be sold over the counter in drug stores and also against resorting to medications and treatments which are advertised as "sure cures for epilepsy" in some of the non-ethical advertising journals and lay magazines.

The discovery of an effective anticonvulsant or a "sure cure for epilepsy" by some obscure individual working in a make-shift laboratory is so remote a likelihood as to be almost inconceivable. The modern drugs of today are neither discovered by accident nor produced by a semi-scientific or hit-and-miss program of research. Rather, they are the results of highly specialized programs of discovery, development and evaluation conducted in medical schools and hospitals and by the ethical pharmaceutical manufacturers. The discovery, evaluation and production of new drugs involve chemical, pharmaceutical and medical procedures of a highly scientific and technically complex nature. The concerted efforts of experts in the fields of medicine, pharmacology, toxicology, pharmacy, engineering, statistics and chemistry must be reviewed, evaluated and coordinated. Each new drug is subjected to rigid chemical, biological and clinical controls, analyses and assays. New drugs must also withstand the inexorable scrutiny of the medical profession with respect to efficacy and relative safety. In addition, the amount of money required to support and operate the intensive programs of research and evaluation required in the production of a single drug may exceed several millions of dollars. It is quite obvious, therefore, that any progress made in the control of epileptic seizures will not result from the efforts of mail order houses and other firms whose advertising is restricted to non-ethical journals and magazines.

In the past, the "mail order" treatment of epilepsy was practiced very frequently and the perpetrators of these frauds reaped huge profits without having substantially benefited the epileptic patient. Today, however, because of more stringent regulations governing and restricting the sale of drugs and because of more efficient methods of enforcement by the postal authorities and by the Food and Drug Administration, the problem of misleading and false advertising of medications and treatments for epilepsy has been resolved to a large extent. The patient should rigidly adhere to the recommendations and suggestions of his physician in regard to treatment and medication and he should obtain his anticonvulsive medications only from recognized, legitimate and ethical sources.

In some instances, advertisements in non-ethical journals and magazines request that the patient send his medical history and state that after this has been studied, he will in turn receive medication which has proved to cure epilepsy in many patients. I would like to call attention to the fact that besides being worthless and extremely costly, such type of treatment can sometimes be very dangerous. The patient should also realize that it is virtually impossible for anyone to competently diagnose and treat convulsive disorders by mail.

I can mention two instances where patients of mine who suffered with seizures mailed their case histories to one of these mail order houses. They received medication at monthly intervals, predicated on their case histories of seizures. Because these patients were not examined by a physician associated with the mail order house, it was impossible for the mail order house to know that the seizures in one of these patients were associated with a brain tumor and in the other, with syphilis of the brain.

Although the "mail order" treatment for epilepsy has diminished considerably in recent years, it is still being currently practiced. I recently had one of my patients write to one of these mail order outfits in response to an advertisement which appeared in one of the "love and sex" magazines. The following is a copy of the letter which he received. The name and address of the company, the name of the medication and the name of the signer of the letter are deleted for obvious reasons.

"Dear Friend:

Thank you for writing. Enclosed you will find helpful information about (name of drug) treatment for epilepsy.

Why have you shown interest in this disease? Are you or one of your loved ones afflicted with epilepsy? If so, from our long experience we are aware of what you may have suffered. Furthermore, we feel that we can help you find relief from your suffering. Let us tell you about (name of drug).

For years, (name of drug) treatment, consisting of easy-to-take tablets, has provided effective relief from the symptoms of epilepsy. Our files are filled with cases where (name of drug) has checked attacks. It has made possible the joy of living without the fears and embarrassments of further attacks.

Read the enclosed leaflet, 'Words of Gratitude.' Although it contains only a few of hundreds of letters praising the splendid work of (name of drug), it will help you understand our faith in (name of drug) treatment.

So great is our faith that we now make this binding agreement on your first month's treatment. If for any reason you are not satisfied with the results, without question your money will be promptly and cheerfully refunded.

Perhaps you are disappointed because other medicines you tried have failed. Probably these medicines have cost you money that you could not afford to spend. Don't be discouraged. (Name of drug) has helped many others find relief from attacks—it might help you! With our money-back agreement you have nothing to lose. Send for (name of drug) today.

Fill out the Case History Chart. Mail it together with your check or money order. (Name of drug) will be sent C.O.D. on request. Your order will receive our personal attention. Please use caution to take the medicine only as directed.

Sincerely yours,"

Since my patient's original correspondence, he has been receiving periodic letters from this mail order outfit requesting that he send his case history together with the money for the tablets. The fifth letter stated that if he would send his case history immediately, he would be given a 40 per cent reduction in the price of the first month's supply of tablets.

Chapter 9

DIETARY TREATMENT FOR EPILEPSY

Many dietary "cures" for epilepsy have been practiced in the past. Almost every type of animal, vegetable and mineral substance has been recommended for the control of epileptic seizures.

Favorable results in the treatment of grand mal epilepsy with the dehydration regimen (marked reduction in the total daily fluid intake) were first reported by Dr. Fay of Philadelphia in 1930. I have not had sufficient experience with the dehydration procedure advocated by Dr. Fay to comment on the efficacy of such a form of treatment. To my knowledge, this type of therapy is not used to any great extent for the treatment of epilepsy at the present time.

The relation of seizures to food allergy is discussed in another section of this book entitled Factors Which Precipitate Epileptic Seizures (Chapter 5).

The only dietary regimen which I have found to be of value in the control of epileptic seizures is the ketogenic diet.

THE KETOGENIC DIET REGIMEN

The value of fasting in the control of epileptic seizures has been recognized for centuries. It is of interest to note that fasting is mentioned as a "cure" for seizures in the following quotation from the Bible (St. Mark 9:14-29):

"14 And when he came to his disciples, he saw a great multitude about them, and the scribes questioning with them.

15 And straightway all the people, when they beheld him, were greatly amazed, and running to him saluted him.

16 And he asked the scribe, What question ye with them?

17 And one of the multitude answered and said, Master, I have brought unto thee my son, which hath a dumb spirit;

143

18 And wheresoever he taketh him, he teareth him; and he foameth, and gnasheth with his teeth, and pineth away: and I spoke to thy disciples that they should cast him out; and they could not.

19 He answereth him, and said, O faithless generation, how long shall I be with you? how long shall I suffer you? bring him unto me.

20 And they brought him unto him: and when he saw him, straightway the spirit tare him; and he fell to the ground, and wallowed foaming.

21 And he asked his father. How long is it ago since this came unto him? and he said, Of a child.

22 And ofttimes it hath cast him into the fire, and into the water, to destroy him: but if thou canst do any thing, have compassion on us, and help us.

23 Jesus said unto him, If thou canst believe all things are possible to him that believeth.

24 And straightway the father of the child cried out, and said with tears, Lord, I believe; help thou mine unbelief.

25 When Jesus saw that the people came running together, he rebuked the foul spirit, saying unto him, Thou dumb and deaf spirit, I charge thee, come out of him, and enter no more into him.

26 And the spirit cried, and rent him sore, and came out of him: and he was as one dead; insomuch that many said, He is dead.

27 But Jesus took him by the hand, and lifted him up; and he arose.

28 And when he was come into the house, his disciples asked him privately, Why could not we cast him out?

29 AND HE SAID UNTO THEM, THIS KIND CAN COME FORTH BY NOTHING, BUT BY PRAYER AND FASTING."

(This sentence is capitalized for emphasis. It does not appear in the Bible in this form.)

To my knowledge, the first scientific report on the value of fasting in the control of epileptic seizures was presented in France by Guelpa and Marie in 1910. Subsequently, other investigators observed that abstinence from food for a few days or so resulted in temporary cessation of seizures and improvement in the mental activity in many patients with epilepsy, but that the beneficial effects did not extend beyond the starvation period.

The beneficial results of fasting in the control of epileptic seizures influenced Dr. R. M. Wilder of the Mayo Clinic to attempt to reproduce the ketosis caused by starvation by means of a special diet and in 1921 he introduced a high fat, low carbohydrate diet as a treatment for epilepsy. Because this diet causes a patient to remain in a constant state of ketosis, it became known as the "keto" or ketogenic diet.

HOW DOES THE KETOGENIC DIET CONTROL SEIZURES?

The specific mechanism or mechanisms by which the ketogenic diet controls epileptic seizures is not clearly understood and much work yet remains to be done to settle this problem. It is thought that the beneficial effect produced by the ketogenic diet is related in some manner to one or a combination of the physiologic effects of acidosis, ketosis and dehydration. Dr. James B. Sidbury is now conducting a series of metabolic studies which may throw some light on this subject.

Although the ketogenic diet is an excellent form of therapy for epileptic seizures, there are many factors which influence its effectiveness, such as, the age of the patient, the type of epilepsy and the willingness and capability of both the patient and the parents to cooperate satisfactorily.

AGE OF PATIENT

The ketogenic regimen is most effective in children between the ages of two and five years for the following reasons: (1) they usually maintain the desired level of ketosis with the diet; and, (2) children of this age can be closely and regularly supervised and, therefore, would be less likely to eat foods other than those prescribed in the diet. In selected cases, we have had good results in some children older than five years of age. Generally, however, the diet is not a suitable form of therapy for the older child and adult, due primarily to the fact that a palatable diet cannot be prepared with the ratio of fat, carbohydrate and protein necessary to produce ketosis. A diet for an older individual prepared in the proper proportions would contain so much fatty substance that it is unlikely that a patient would either eat it or tolerate it.

Generally, the ketogenic regimen is not helpful in very young children, particularly those under the age of one year, because they usually will not maintain the desired state of ketosis.

TYPE OF EPILEPSY

There is no specific relationship between the type of epilepsy and the likelihood of a satisfactory response to the ketogenic diet. However, we have had our best results in the treatment of major motor and minor motor epilepsy. This latter finding is of utmost importance since none of the antiepileptic drugs currently available are, in my experience, particularly effective in the treatment of minor motor epilepsy.

In addition to its excellent anticonvulsant value, the ketogenic diet also favorably affects the general well-being of many patients. It does not dull mental functioning, as anticonvulsant drugs so frequently do. It also acts as a tranquilizing agent for the increased restlessness and irritability (the hyperkinetic syndrome) which is seen so frequently in young children with epilepsy. Many of my patients were described by their parents, before the institution of the ketogenic diet, as "wild as a little Indian" and after the diet was started, as being as "calm as a lamb." It is of interest to note that several of the parents were reluctant to discontinue the diet, in spite of a poor control of seizures, because their children's behavior and disposition were so much better while on the ketogenic regimen than when they were being treated with antiepileptic drugs.

COOPERATION OF PARENTS AND PATIENT

The success of the ketogenic diet often is dependent upon the parents' willingness to cooperate and conscientiously adhere to the diet and rules as instructed. It is imperative to maintain the diet exactly as given. It is also important to make the meals as attractive and palatable as possible for the child. The parents should not make any changes in the diet unless specifically authorized by their physician.

The feasibility of prescribing the ketogenic diet in any given case is governed more by the circumstances within the home than by any other factor. To be effective, the ketogenic diet must be rigidly controlled. This regimen, therefore, should not be attempted unless both the parents and the patient are capable of cooperating satisfactorily. One must be dealing with parents who are at least moderately intelligent and who will appreciate the importance of maintaining and adhering strictly to the diet.

Once it is started, the diet must be followed closely or its entire beneficial effect is lost. All articles of food must be weighed carefully and the directions must be faithfully followed. Even a cookie or a small piece of candy contains enough carbohydrate to nullify the benefit temporarily.

Some children with strong dietary likes and dislikes may find it difficult to eat the large amounts of fatty foods contained in a ketogenic diet. The diet, therefore, should not be prescribed to those patients in whom feeding difficulties are anticipated.

Since the diet must be continued for at least two or three years, the financial status of the parents should be taken into consideration. The high content of fat makes the ketogenic diet somewhat more expensive than a normal diet. The cost of many anticonvulsants, however, is also considerable in many instances.

MANAGEMENT OF THE KETOGENIC REGIMEN

A starvation period of approximately five to seven days must be instituted prior to starting the ketogenic diet. Careful observation, preferably in a hospital, is mandatory during this interval of fasting. During this period of starvation, the patient receives nothing but a limited amount of water by mouth. A daily measured water intake of not less than 400 cc. (13 oz.) and not more than 800 cc. (26 oz.) is required to obtain the desired degree of dehydration. This starvation results in ketosis which is then maintained with the ketogenic diet.

In those patients who were receiving anticonvulsant medication which had proved to be somewhat effective in the control of their seizures, I generally continue with the same dosage of this medication with the ketogenic diet. However, in those patients who were taking anticonvulsant medication which had proved to be completely ineffective, I start decreasing the dosage of this medication at the beginning of the preliminary starvation period and subsequently completely withdraw the medication at the time the diet is started.

During the period of starvation, the child may be up and about and should be encouraged to participate in hospital play activities. For obvious reasons, the patient should not be present when meals are served to the other children.

After the second or third day of starvation, some patients complain of nausea and may even vomit. If this occurs, the patient should be put to rest and encouraged to take cracked ice by mouth. If the nausea persists, he may be given 30 cc. of orange juice and this may be repeated in one hour if necessary. This amount will usually relieve the nausea and although it diminishes the degree of ketosis, it does not materially affect the desired results of starvation.

The patient should be weighed before starvation is instituted and subsequently each day during the entire period of starvation. It is advisable to weigh the patient at about the same time each day. The urine should be examined daily, preferably in mid-afternoon or evening, for the presence of urinary ketosis. The patient should not be started on the ketogenic diet until he has lost at least 10 per cent of his body weight and the urinary tests for ketosis are strongly positive.

CALCULATION OF THE DIET

A ketogenic diet, to be effective, must be rigidly controlled and must be a weighed diet. The child should receive the number of calories per day necessary to maintain body growth. The amount of fat (in grams) should be four times that of the amount (in grams) of carbohydrate and protein combined. This is known as a standard 4:1 ketogenic diet.

I have found the following methods of calculation of the ketogenic diet to be most satisfactory.

(1) The number of calories required per day is calculated by multiplying the child's weight (in kilograms) by the average number of calories per kilogram required daily. For a two to five year old child, this is generally between 60 to 80 calories per kilogram per day. Undernourished children may receive a greater number of calories.

(2) Calculation of the diet is made by using what I term the "dietary unit." Thus a unit of the usually employed 4:1 diet contains four grams of fat (36 calories) and one gram of carbohydrate and protein combined (4 calories). A gram of fat yields nine calories and a gram of protein and carbohydrate yields four calories; therefore, this dietary unit will contain a total of 40 calories. The number of calories the child requires per day (as calculated in 1) is divided by 40 (the number of calories per unit as calculated in 2). This gives the number of dietary units required daily.

Example: A four year old child who weighs 18 kilograms to be put on a diet of the 4:1 ratio: 18 kilos $\times$ 70 calories per kilo = 1,260 calories per day; 1,260 calories per day $\div$ 40 calories per unit = 31.5 units. In a 4:1 diet, each of these units contains 4 grams of fat. Therefore, the number of grams of fat can be calculated by multiplying the number of units (31.5) $\times$ 4 = *126.0 grams of fat required for the daily diet.*

Each dietary unit contains one gram of protein and cabrohydrate combined. It is important, however, that the patient receive sufficient protein to maintain body growth. The amount of protein is set at one gram per kilogram body weight, which has been found quite satisfactory. Therefore, the body weight in kilograms is multiplied by one to obtain the required number of grams of protein (18 $\times$ 1 = *18 grams of protein per day*). The amount of carbohydrate is obtained by subtracting the number of grams of protein in the diet from the total number of dietary units (31.5 units — 18 grams of protein = *13.5 grams of carbohydrate per day*).

The 4:1 diet calculated in the example would then be:

Fat	126 grams
Protein	18 grams
Carbohydrate	13.5 grams

An alternative method may also be used for rapid calculation of 4:1 ketogenic diet. It happens that the number of *grams* of fat required is 1/10 the number of calories needed per day. In the example used above 1,260 calories per day require 1/10 of 1,260 or *126 grams of fat.* Each gram of fat yields nine calories, 126 grams $\times$ 9 calories per gram = 1,134 calories in the form of fat. Subtract this from the total number of calories: 1,260 — 1,134 = 126 calories to be supplied in the form of protein plus carbohydrate. Since both protein and carbohydrate yield four calories per gram, the number of grams of these two combined is calculated by dividing the number of calories by four: 126 ÷ 4 = 31.5. But, as already explained a child needs one gram of protein per day for each kilogram of body weight. Thus the 18 kilogram child of the example needs *18 grams of protein per day*. Subtract this figure from the total grams of protein plus carbohydrate to determine the number of grams of carbohydrate: 31.5 − 18 = *13.5 grams of carbohydrate*.

Calculated diet:

Fat	126 grams
Protein	18 grams
Carbohydrate	13.5 grams

If the 4:1 ketogenic diet proves to be a satisfactory therapeutic regimen, it should be *continued for two years*. After two years the diet should be changed to a 3:1 ketogenic-antiketogenic ratio. The method of calculation is similar to that described for the 4:1 diet except that each dietary unit contains 31 calories instead of 40: (3 grams fat × 9 = 27 plus 1 gram protein-carbohydrate × 4 = 4) = 31. Therefore, the number of grams of fat required is calculated by multiplying the number of dietary units by three. The number of grams of protein is calculated as for the 4:1 diet, that is, one gram of protein per kilogram of body weight. The number of grams of carbohydrate is computed by subtracting the grams of protein from the number of dietary units.

The patient is continued on the 3:1 diet for six months, after which time a 2:1 ratio is substituted. The calculation is as follows: the dietary unit now contains 22 calories: (2 grams fat × 9 calories = 18 plus 1 gram protein-carbohydrate × 4 = 4) = 22. The number of dietary units is multiplied by two to give the number of grams of fat required. On a 2:1 diet it is feasible to give one and one-half grams of protein per kilogram of body weight. This calculated number of grams of protein subtracted from the number of dietary units gives the number of grams of carbohydrate.

After six months on a 2:1 diet, the patient may be given a normal diet as desired. During the period of reduction of the ketogenic-antiketogenic ratio, there will be a progressive diminution in the degree of ketonuria. This may be disregarded and testing of the urine discontinued after ketosis is no longer present. The reason for the gradual reduction in the ketogenic-antiketogenic ratio is to lessen the likelihood of inducing status epilepticus.

PRESCRIBING THE DIET

The total daily amount of fat, protein and carbohydrate is divided into three equal parts to be served at each of the three meals. For example, the total daily amount of fat, protein and carbohydrate contained in a 4:1 ketogenic diet for a four year old child weighing 18 kilograms would be: 126 grams of fat, 18 grams of protein and 13.5 grams of carbohydrate. Therefore, each one of the three meals would contain one-third of these amounts which would be: 42 grams of fat, 6 grams of protein and 4.5 grams of carbohydrate.

It is best to offer the patient only one-third of the total calculated amount of food for the meals given on the first day; on the second day, only one-half of the total calculated amount is offered and on the third day, the child may be given the full diet. When the diet is administered in this fashion it frequently avoids upsetting a previously fasting gastrointestinal tract.

The following general figures are used in calculating the amount of each type of food to be included in a meal.

	Protein	Fat	Carbohydrate
100 Gm. 40% cream	2	40	3
100 Gm. 36% cream	2	36	3
120 Gm. 20% cream	3	20	4
200 Gm. group A vegetables	2	—	7
100 Gm. group B vegetables	2	—	7
100 Gm. 10% fruit	1	—	10
30 Gm. meat, fish, poultry	7	5	—
20 Gm. American cheese	6	7	—
50 Gm. egg	6	6	—
10 Gm. bacon	2	7	—
5 Gm. fat	—	5	—
100 Gm. peanut butter	26	48	22
100 Gm. cottage cheese	20	1	2
28 Gm. cream cheese	2.8	10.6	0.1

Table 13 shows the relative amounts (in grams) of protein, fat and carbohydrate contained in a given weight (in grams) of various foods. Starting first with cream, calculate the number of grams of

TABLE 13

RELATIVE AMOUNTS (IN GRAMS) OF PROTEIN, FAT AND CARBOHYDRATE IN A GIVEN WEIGHT (IN GRAMS) OF VARIOUS FOODS

Meat, Fish, Poultry (Fresh, Frozen, Canned)

Wt. in Gms.	Protein	Fat	Carbohydrate
5	1.2	0.8	0
6	1.4	1.0	0
7	1.6	1.2	0
8	1.9	1.3	0
9	2.1	1.5	0
10	2.3	1.7	0
11	2.6	1.8	0
12	2.8	2.0	0
13	3.0	2.2	0
14	3.3	2.3	0
15	3.5	2.5	0
16	3.7	2.7	0
17	4.0	2.8	0
18	4.2	3.0	0
19	4.4	3.2	0
20	4.7	3.3	0
21	4.9	3.5	0
22	5.1	3.7	0
23	5.4	3.8	0
24	5.6	4.0	0
25	5.8	4.2	0
26	6.1	4.3	0
27	6.3	4.5	0
28	6.5	4.7	0
29	6.8	4.8	0
30	7.0	5.0	0
31	7.2	5.2	0
32	7.5	5.3	0
33	7.7	5.5	0
34	7.9	5.7	0
35	8.2	5.8	0
36	8.4	6.0	0
37	8.6	6.2	0
38	8.9	6.3	0
39	9.1	6.5	0
40	9.3	6.7	0

Cheese* (American, Cheddar, Swiss)

Wt. in Gms.	Protein	Fat	Carbohydrate
5	1.5	1.7	0
6	1.8	2.1	0
7	2.1	2.4	0
8	2.4	2.8	0
9	2.7	3.1	0
10	3.0	3.5	0
11	3.3	3.8	0
12	3.6	4.2	0
13	3.9	4.5	0
14	4.2	4.9	0
15	4.5	5.2	0
16	4.8	5.6	0
17	5.1	5.9	0
18	5.4	6.3	0
19	5.7	6.6	0
20	6.0	7.0	0
21	6.3	7.3	0
22	6.6	7.7	0
23	6.9	8.0	0
24	7.2	8.4	0
25	7.5	8.7	0
26	7.8	9.1	0
27	8.1	9.4	0
28	8.4	9.8	0
29	8.7	10.1	0
30	9.0	10.5	0
31	9.3	10.8	0
32	9.6	11.2	0
33	9.9	11.5	0
34	10.2	11.9	0
35	10.5	12.2	0
36	10.8	12.6	0
37	11.1	12.9	0
38	11.4	13.3	0
39	11.7	13.6	0
40	12.0	14.0	0

Eggs

Wt. in Gms.	Protein	Fat	Carbohydrate
15	1.8	1.8	0
16	1.9	1.9	0
17	2.0	2.0	0
18	2.2	2.2	0
19	2.3	2.3	0
20	2.4	2.4	0
21	2.5	2.5	0
22	2.6	2.6	0
23	2.8	2.8	0
24	2.9	2.9	0
25	3.0	3.0	0
26	3.1	3.1	0
27	3.2	3.2	0
28	3.4	3.4	0
29	3.5	3.5	0
30	3.6	3.6	0
31	3.7	3.7	0
32	3.8	3.8	0
33	4.0	4.0	0
34	4.1	4.1	0
35	4.2	4.2	0
36	4.3	4.3	0
37	4.4	4.4	0
38	4.6	4.6	0
39	4.7	4.7	0
40	4.8	4.8	0
41	4.9	4.9	0
42	5.0	5.0	0
43	5.2	5.2	0
44	5.3	5.3	0
45	5.4	5.4	0
46	5.5	5.5	0
47	5.6	5.6	0
48	5.8	5.8	0
49	5.9	5.9	0
50	6.0	6.0	0

Crisp Bacon

Wt. in Gms.	Protein	Fat	Carbohydrate
5	1.0	3.5	0
6	1.2	4.2	0
7	1.4	4.9	0
8	1.6	5.6	0
9	1.8	6.3	0
10	2.0	7.0	0
11	2.2	7.7	0
12	2.4	8.4	0
13	2.6	9.1	0
14	2.8	9.8	0
15	3.0	10.5	0
16	3.2	11.2	0
17	3.4	11.9	0
18	3.6	12.6	0
19	3.8	13.3	0
20	4.0	14.0	0
21	4.2	14.7	0
22	4.4	15.4	0
23	4.6	16.1	0
24	4.8	16.8	0
25	5.0	17.5	0
26	5.2	18.2	0
27	5.4	18.9	0
28	5.6	19.6	0
29	5.8	20.3	0
30	6.0	21.0	0
31	6.2	21.7	0
32	6.4	22.4	0
33	6.6	23.1	0
34	6.8	23.8	0
35	7.0	24.5	0
36	7.2	25.2	0
37	7.4	25.9	0
38	7.6	26.6	0
39	7.8	27.3	0
40	8.0	28.0	0

TABLE 13 (Continued)

RELATIVE AMOUNTS (IN GRAMS) OF PROTEIN, FAT AND CARBOHYDRATE IN A GIVEN WEIGHT (IN GRAMS) OF VARIOUS FOODS

Group B Vegetables (Note: Use twice as much for Group A Vegetables)				Group A Vegetables								10% Fruits							
Wt. in Gms.	Pro-tein	Fat	Carbo-hydrate	Wt. in Gms.	Pro-tein	Fat	Carbo-hydrate	Wt. in Gms.	Pro-tein	Fat	Carbo-hydrate	Wt. in Gms.	Pro-tein	Fat	Carbo-hydrate	Wt. in Gms.	Pro-tein	Fat	Carbo-hydrate
10	0.2	0	0.7	41	0.8	0	2.9	72	1.4	0	5.0	10	0.1	0	1.0	41	0.4	0	4.1
11	0.2	0	0.8	42	0.8	0	2.9	73	1.5	0	5.1	11	0.1	0	1.1	42	0.4	0	4.2
12	0.2	0	0.8	43	0.9	0	3.0	74	1.5	0	5.2	12	0.1	0	1.2	43	0.4	0	4.3
13	0.3	0	0.9	44	0.9	0	3.1	75	1.5	0	5.2	13	0.1	0	1.3	44	0.4	0	4.4
14	0.3	0	1.0	45	0.9	0	3.1	76	1.5	0	5.3	14	0.1	0	1.4	45	0.5	0	4.5
15	0.3	0	1.0	46	0.9	0	3.2	77	1.5	0	5.4	15	0.2	0	1.5	46	0.5	0	4.6
16	0.3	0	1.1	47	0.9	0	3.3	78	1.6	0	5.5	16	0.2	0	1.6	47	0.5	0	4.7
17	0.3	0	1.2	48	1.0	0	3.3	79	1.6	0	5.5	17	0.2	0	1.7	48	0.5	0	4.8
18	0.4	0	1.3	49	1.0	0	3.4	80	1.6	0	5.6	18	0.2	0	1.8	49	0.5	0	4.9
19	0.4	0	1.3	50	1.0	0	3.4	81	1.6	0	5.7	19	0.2	0	1.9	50	0.5	0	5.0
20	0.4	0	1.4	51	1.0	0	3.5	82	1.7	0	5.7	20	0.2	0	2.0	51	0.5	0	5.1
21	0.4	0	1.5	52	1.0	0	3.6	83	1.7	0	5.8	21	0.2	0	2.1	52	0.5	0	5.2
22	0.4	0	1.5	53	1.0	0	3.6	84	1.7	0	5.9	22	0.2	0	2.2	53	0.5	0	5.3
23	0.5	0	1.6	54	1.1	0	3.7	85	1.7	0	6.0	23	0.2	0	2.3	54	0.5	0	5.4
24	0.5	0	1.7	55	1.1	0	3.8	86	1.8	0	6.1	24	0.2	0	2.4	55	0.6	0	5.5
25	0.5	0	1.7	56	1.1	0	3.9	87	1.8	0	6.1	25	0.3	0	2.5	56	0.6	0	5.6
26	0.5	0	1.8	57	1.1	0	3.9	88	1.8	0	6.2	26	0.3	0	2.6	57	0.6	0	5.7
27	0.5	0	1.9	58	1.2	0	4.0	89	1.8	0	6.3	27	0.3	0	2.7	58	0.6	0	5.8
28	0.6	0	2.0	59	1.2	0	4.1	90	1.8	0	6.4	28	0.3	0	2.8	59	0.6	0	5.9
29	0.6	0	2.0	60	1.2	0	4.2	91	1.9	0	6.4	29	0.3	0	2.9	60	0.6	0	6.0
30	0.6	0	2.1	61	1.2	0	4.3	92	1.9	0	6.5	30	0.3	0	3.0	61	0.6	0	6.1
31	0.6	0	2.2	62	1.3	0	4.3	93	1.9	0	6.6	31	0.3	0	3.1	62	0.6	0	6.2
32	0.6	0	2.3	63	1.3	0	4.4	94	1.9	0	6.6	32	0.3	0	3.2	63	0.6	0	6.3
33	0.7	0	2.3	64	1.3	0	4.5	95	1.9	0	6.7	33	0.3	0	3.3	64	0.6	0	6.4
34	0.7	0	2.4	65	1.3	0	4.5	96	2.0	0	6.8	34	0.3	0	3.4	65	0.7	0	6.5
35	0.7	0	2.5	66	1.3	0	4.6	97	2.0	0	6.9	35	0.4	0	3.5	66	0.7	0	6.6
36	0.7	0	2.6	67	1.4	0	4.7	98	2.0	0	6.9	36	0.4	0	3.6	67	0.7	0	6.7
37	0.7	0	2.6	68	1.4	0	4.8	99	2.0	0	7.0	37	0.4	0	3.7	68	0.7	0	6.8
38	0.8	0	2.7	69	1.4	0	4.8	100	2.0	0	7.0	38	0.4	0	3.8	69	0.7	0	6.9
39	0.8	0	2.7	70	1.4	0	4.9					39	0.4	0	3.9	70	0.7	0	7.0
40	0.8	0	2.8	71	1.4	0	5.0					40	0.4	0	4.0	71	0.7	0	7.1

fat, protein and carbohydrate contained in the weight of an arbitrary amount of cream to be given for one meal. Complete the total carbohydrate for the meal using fruits or vegetables or both. Then adjust the total remaining protein for the meal in terms of foods such as meat, egg or cheese. With both carbohydrate and protein accurate, add fat such as butter, margarine or mayonnaise to achieve the necessary total for the meal. The total amount of protein, fat and carbohydrate in each meal should not vary more than a few tenths of a gram from the exact amount specified; the 4:1 ratio should be maintained at each meal. *If a child should not eat all of the food contained in one meal, the remainder of the food should be disposed of. It should not be given in conjunction with the calculated amount specified for the subsequent meal.*

The child usually remains in the hospital for about four or five days after he has been started on the full ketogenic diet to make certain that he is able to tolerate the diet satisfactorily.

During this period, the parent or guardian should be given complete instructions in regard to the preparation of the diet. In our hospital, each parent is given at least one hour of instruction on each of two days by a competent dietitian. The parent is taught how to prepare the food, is given samples of diets and is taught how to weigh the food. The parents must secure a scale which weighs in grams and has a movable face.

The ketogenic diet is not only custom made for each individual but varies for the same child as his weight increases with normal growth. From time to time such an increase requires a new calculation of the diet by the physician.

After the ketogenic diet has been started, the amount of water allowed should be minimal (the amount necessary to satisfy the patient's thirst). The parents should be instructed not to force fluids in excess of the amount necessary to maintain the daily requirements of the child.

In translating each diet order, the parent or dietitian should use exact proportions so that the ratio of the fat to the combined protein and carbohydrate is constant. As long as this ratio is maintained, the amount of food ingested from meal to meal or day to day can be varied without altering the fixed ketogenic effect of the diet. By simply changing the amount of each item in the meal by the same percentage, the daily appetite of the child can be satisfied in most instances. A 50 per cent increase in each item in the meal or a 25 per cent decrease of each item will enable increased appetite or anorexia to be managed. Such a proportioned diet has the advantage that once it has been accurately planned, whole meals can be interchanged or repeated, since they are all equal in the production of ketosis. The ratio of the planned meal also should be preserved at the time of feeding by limiting additions of any one food until all of the meal has been eaten.

The fixed ratio of the diet requires that its translation into planned meals be rigid. There is room, however, and psychologically there is great necessity for consideration of a child's likes and dislikes regarding the form in which his food will be offered. Before any diet is actually written, the person responsible for the child's feeding should fully discuss this situation with the physician. It is most important that the child's taste for cream and butter be determined, for these two foods are the framework of every meal. Only occasionally can either substance be completely omitted, but it is relatively easy to supply most of the fat in the more palatable form. The remainder of the meal includes small amounts of meat-fish-poultry or egg or cheese plus fruits or vegetables. Menus with bacon, cream cheese, cottage cheese and peanut butter can be planned if the patient wishes.

A point of importance to remember is that the percentage of butter fat varies considerably in cream from various localities. The cream used in the diet must have a butter fat content of 36 per cent to 40 per cent. This type of cream is known as whipping cream.

Since cream and fat are used in relatively large amounts for the limited bulk of the other foods, the main problem becomes how to incorporate these foods into the meal. The use of imagination in the preparation of the diet is of great importance. Cream may be given undiluted or with water. If desired, it may be flavored with a few drops of vanilla or with an infusion of boiled cocoa nibs. It can be used in soups, creamed vegetables, whipped cream toppings and salad dressings, or to make "ice cream," custard or certain Cellu desserts. Fat may be used to cook foods such as eggs and meats, as mayonnaise in either fruit, vegetable, egg or fish salad, to season vegetables and soups and as an oil dressing. Many young children willingly eat butter by itself.

Certain Cellu foods can be introduced into a ketogenic diet with psychologically beneficial effects. Care must be taken to distinguish between those which are relatively food valueless and those which must be calculated into the meal because of the protein and carbohydrate they contain. For the percentage composition of Cellu Products, the interested person should consult the descriptive pamphlet available from that company.

An "ice cream" may be prepared with part of the cream allowance and Cellu Freezette. This ice cream powder is supplied in vanilla and chocolate flavors and has no food value.

Cellu hard gum drops, lollipops, cough drops and jelly may be used sparingly, as may Cellu Cool Sip. The latter beverage is available in assorted flavors. The Cellu gum drops, lollipops and Cool Sip may be eaten between meals if desired, as they have practically no food value. Cellu Cocoa Nibs when boiled with water for several hours makes a pleasant tasting infusion which may be used as such or together with cream and saccharin to make a palatable cocoa.

Cellu Breakfast Crisp, Pudding Powder, D'Zerta (gelatin) Macaroons, and Muffin Flour can contribute in selected cases to the flexibility of the diet, but these products have small amounts of protein or carbohydrate and must be calculated into a menu when served.

The ketogenic diet is rich in the fat soluble vitamins A and D, but is deficient in the water soluble B and C vitamins and in calcium. Therefore, it is necessary to supplement the diet with the daily administration of these deficient vitamins and also additional calcium. Before any supplementary preparation is administered it must be established that the preparation contains no carbohydrate substances.

Patients receiving the ketogenic diet frequently complain of hunger between meals for the first several weeks, even though the caloric intake is adequate. This is largely due to the fact that, because of the high fat content, the bulk of the ketogenic diet is considerably less than that of a normal diet of the same number of calories. The caloric content of the diet should not be increased

ANY OF THE FOLLOWING MAY BE GIVEN IN
ADDITION TO PRESCRIBED MENUS

3 Ripe Olives
1 English Walnut
1 Brazil Nut   *One* each day
2 Butternuts
2 Pecans
3 Filberts
Mushrooms
Spices
Lettuce—small amount
Salt—small amount in cooking only
Pepper
Vanilla Flavoring (15 drops each meal)
Lemon Flavoring (15 drops each meal)
Saccharin—Saxin—Sucaryl

FAT SUBSTITUTIONS

Butter	Mayonnaise
Oleomargarine	Meat Fat
Wesson Oil	Bacon Fat
Mazola	Chicken Fat
Olive Oil	Lard

MEAT SUBSTITUTIONS

Beef	Liver
Lamb	Fish
Veal	Poultry
Pork	Allmeat Frank
Canned Salmon, Tuna (drained)	

FRUITS AND JUICES

Fruits and fruit juices may be either fresh or canned without sugar; in the
latter case the juice must be included in the weight.

Ten per cent fruits (100 grams contains approximately 10 grams
of carbohydrate and 1 gram of protein).

Blackberries	Pear
Cantaloupe	Pineapple
Grapefruit	Plum
Honeydew melon	Raspberries (red)
Orange	Strawberries
Papaya	Tangerine
Canned fruit salad	Watermelon
without cherries	Peach

Fifteen per cent fruits (100 grams contains approximately 15 grams
of carbohydrate and 1 gram of protein).

Apple	Cherries
Apricot	Grapes
Raspberries (black)	

Fresh, canned, or frozen vegetables may be used. The prescribed weight may
be divided among several vegetables of the same class.

GROUP A vegetables (100 grams contains approximately 3.5 grams
of carbohydrate and 1 gram of protein).

Asparagus	Leeks
Beans (young, tender)	Green pepper
Beet greens	Kale
Broccoli	Mustard greens
Brussel Sprouts	Okra
Cabbage	Poke
Cauliflower	Radishes
Celery	Rhubarb
Chicory	Sauerkraut
Collards	Spinach
Cucumbers	Squash (summer)
Dandelion greens	Swiss Chard
Eggplant	Tomatoes or juice
Escarole	Turnip greens
Endive	Watercress

GROUP B vegetables (100 grams contains approximately 7 grams
of carbohydrate and 2 grams of protein).

Beets	Peas
Carrots	Pumpkin
Kohl-rabi	Rutabagas
Onions	Squash (winter)
Oyster plant	Turnips

unless absolutely necessary, such as in the case of a completely
uncooperative patient. I have found that most children will adjust
to the initially prescribed diet after several weeks or so.

Problems of hunger can generally be minimized by permitting
the child to partake of the non-nutritious gum drops and other
products such as Cellu candies.

It is important to understand that the diet will be successful in
maintaining ketosis only if all of the food is consumed. Foods
cannot be saved from one meal to be included in the next or to be
eaten between meals.

Since the efficacy of the ketogenic regimen rests on the maintenance of ketosis, the urine should be tested for the presence of
ketone bodies. The parents should be supplied with materials and
instructions so that this test can be performed at home.

INSTRUCTIONS FOR USE OF
ACETEST® REAGENT TABLETS

Acetest (BRAND) Reagent Tablets make testing for ketonuria* both simple and convenient—no special equipment, no external heating and no undesirable fumes. Results are both reliable and specific; negatives and positives are readily differentiated.

TO MAKE A TEST

1 Place tablet on a clean surface, preferably a piece of paper.

2 Put **one** drop of urine on tablet.

3 Take reading **at 30 seconds.**† Compare to color chart below.

†The drop of urine should be completely absorbed within 30 second period. If not, tablet has been exposed to moisture and may give faulty reading.

INTERPRETATION OF TEST

NEGATIVE: Tablet color will remain unchanged or turn cream-colored from wetting.

POSITIVE: Within 30 seconds, color of tablet will change. Depending on amount of Ketone bodies present, color varies from lavender to deep purple. Results may be recorded as, small, moderate or large amount.

*Although primarily designed for the detection of ketonuria, a similar technic employing serum or plasma has been recorded as suitable for use. References are available to physicians upon request.

Colors shown below are approximate values and are for use with **Acetest** Reagent Tablets only.

SMALL	MODERATE	LARGE

SAMPLE KETOGENIC DIETS FOR 18 KILOGRAM CHILD

Meal Plan

(Content of protein, fat and carbohydrate are in the same ratio at each meal and therefore the meals may be used interchangeably. All foods must be weighed after cooking or as directed on menus)

Meal No. 1	*Meal No. 2*
32 grams Egg	17 grams Meat, Fish or Poultry
15 grams 10% Fruit	43 grams Group B Vegetable
100 grams 36% Cream	50 grams 36% Cream
2 grams Fat	21 grams Fat

Meal No. 3	*Meal No. 4*
12 grams American Cheese	11 grams Meat, Fish or Poultry
44 grams Group A Vegetable	86 grams Group A Vegetable
100 grams 36% Cream	50 grams 36% Cream
2 grams Fat	22 grams Fat
	½ serving D-Zerta

Meal No. 5	*Meal No. 6*
18 grams Egg	10 grams Crisp Bacon
24 grams 10% Fruit	27 grams 10% Fruit
70 grams 36% Cream	30 grams 36% Cream
7 grams Fat	24 grams Fat
11 grams Crisp Bacon	1 Cellu Muffin (1 envelope with 100 grams Egg makes 6)

Meal No. 7

26 grams Egg
22 grams 10% Fruit
50 grams 36% Cream
18 grams Fat
25 grams Cellu Breakfast Crisp

The Acetest Reagent Tablet provides a standardized and reliable colorimetric test for ketosis. A colorimetric chart supplied with each Acetest package has three colors ranging from lavender to deep purple representing small, moderate, or large amount of ketone bodies.

Directions for Performance of Test

1. Place tablet on clean surface, preferably a piece of white paper.
2. Put *one* drop of urine on tablet.
3. Take reading at *30 seconds.* Compare color of tablet to color chart.

Interpretation of Results of Test

Negative: Tablet color is unchanged or turns cream color.

Positive: At 30 seconds, color of tablet varies from lavender to deep purple. Results may be recorded as trace, moderate or strongly positive.

I recommend that the urine be tested for ketosis each day for the first month following the institution of the ketogenic diet. Subsequently, the urine should be examined two or three times a week. Children on a ketogenic diet show the maximum degree of urinary ketosis during the latter part of the day and not during the early morning hours as might be expected. Therefore, the parents should examine the patient's urine in the late afternoon or in the early part of the evening. Although the degree of urinary ketosis may fluctuate slightly, any consistent diminution requires investigation.

The most common cause for loss of ketosis is the ingestion of foods other than those included in the diet. This factor should be investigated thoroughly, particularly in the case of the older child who has occasion to be exposed to prohibited foods while at school or in the company of his playmates. I have also encountered other instances of loss of ketosis which resulted from defective scales and improper preparation of the diet itself.

In those instances where the ketonuria is found to be negative or very slight, the child should be given nothing by mouth except water until the urinary test for ketosis becomes positive. In most cases this can be accomplished by the omission of one or two meals.

The parents should be warned that no medications such as elixirs, syrups, cough medicines, cough drops or laxatives should be given to the child except when instructed to do so by the physician. Articles such as toothpaste and mouth washes should be guarded very carefully. I have had several patients who, in spite of a carefully measured ketogenic diet, failed to maintain ketosis. It was finally established that these children had eaten large amounts of toothpaste daily. To prevent such situations, I recommend the use of a sugarless toothpowder, such as Py-Co-Pay.

Constipation is generally not troublesome in patients receiving the ketogenic diet. Since most of the foods are low in roughage, a bowel movement every two or three days is sufficient in most instances. An enema, mineral oil, unsweetened agar preparations, epsom salt or unsweetened fluid extract of cascara may be prescribed when indicated.

If, during an illness, the patient should refuse to take solid foods, the diet should be temporarily discontinued and the child given light nourishment in the form of a special (4:1 ratio) eggnogg solution. The directions for preparing this solution are:

Dissolve ¼ grain of saccharin in a teaspoon or two of water and add to 60 grams of 36% cream. To this mixture add 25 grams of lightly beaten raw egg and 10 drops of vanilla. A little nutmeg may be sprinkled on top if desired. This mixture may be diluted with water to patient's taste.

COMPLICATIONS OF THE KETOGENIC REGIMEN

During the period of starvation, the patient must be observed closely for untoward signs of acidosis or dehydration. The pulse rate should be counted every four hours after a short period of rest in a recumbent position. If signs or symptoms of cardiac distress appear, the patient should be given an intravenous injection of 5 per cent dextrose solution (not to exceed 20 cc. per kilogram). Children frequently complain of nausea, usually during the second or third day of starvation, at which time the acidosis and ketosis have usually reached their peak. If this occurs, the patient is put to rest and encouraged to suck on cracked ice. If nausea persists, 30 cc. of orange juice may be given and repeated in one hour, if necessary. This amount usually will relieve the nausea, and although it diminishes the degree of ketosis, it does not materially affect the desired results of starvation.

Vomiting, attributable to the ketogenic regimen, may occur during the preliminary starvation period and also at any time while the patient is on the diet. Thorazine is helpful in some instances. If vomiting should become intractable during the starvation period, it may be necessary to interrupt the starvation and resume it again at a later date. However, I have found that this rarely happens. If vomiting occurs when the patient is on the diet and is not relieved by Thorazine, it is usually advisable to discontinue all foods for twenty-four to forty-eight hours and to give the patient nothing but water for this period.

It is noteworthy that in most patients the physical growth is moderately retarded during the time they are on the diet. However, it has been my experience that this is only a temporary disturbance. I have observed many patients who manifested impairment of growth while on the ketogenic regimen. I subsequently reexamined these patients some fifteen to twenty years after they had completed the ketogenic diet treatment and the physical growth of all of them was within limits of normal for their chronologic age.

Kidney stones developed during the course of the ketogenic regimen in about 1 per cent of our patients.

I have frequently been asked the following question by physicians, "Doesn't the ketogenic diet adversely affect the blood vessels?" This question was obviously stimulated by the fact that the ketogenic diet is exceedingly high in fat content. I know of several physicians who were reluctant to prescribe the ketogenic diet regimen to their epileptic patients for fear that the high fat content might injure their vascular systems and subsequently render them susceptible to disorders such as hypertension and coronary disturbances.

I have had the opportunity to see some adults who had been treated during their childhood with the ketogenic diet by Drs. Lawson Wilkins and Edward M. Bridge, former Directors of the Epilepsy Clinic of The Johns Hopkins Hospital. The ages of these patients ranged from forty to fifty years. I have also had contact with many adults to whom I administered the ketogenic diet for epilepsy during their early childhood. My findings did not reveal evidence that the vascular systems of these patients had been adversely affected by the high fat content of the ketogenic diet. These patients did not present evidence of arteriosclerosis; blood pressure readings were normal; and electrocardiographic studies did not reveal abnormalities. Blood cholesterol determinations performed on many of these individuals revealed normal findings.

BIBLIOGRAPHY

Livingston, S.: *The Diagnosis and Treatment of Convulsive Disorders in Children.* Springfield, Ill., Thomas, 1954.

Livingston, S.: Convulsive Disorders in Infants and Children, in *Advances in Pediatrics.* Chicago, The Year Book Publishers, Inc., 1958.

Chapter 10

SURGICAL TREATMENT OF CONVULSIVE DISORDERS

THE primary treatment for an individual suffering with an epileptic disorder is medical, consisting of anticonvulsant therapy, psychotherapy and social and occupational rehabilitation. It is worth emphasizing that medical treatment should be given an adequate trial in all cases of epilepsy and considered unsuccessful only when all appropriate therapeutic agents have been administered alone and in combination without beneficial results. Surgery should be considered only when these measures have failed. Obviously, if the seizures are symptomatic evidence of a progressive cerebral lesion such as tumor, abscess or hematoma, surgery is the method of treatment.

It is of interest to note that surgical procedures for the relief of epilepsy were performed in prehistoric days according to many authorities. An excellent historical review of the surgical treatment of epilepsy is presented by Dr. A. Earl Walker in a relatively recent writing.

When is an epileptic patient a candidate for surgical consideration?

There are four characteristic clinical types of epileptic seizures: major motor (grand mal), petit mal, minor motor (infantile spasms) and psychomotor. A description of these seizures is presented in the section of this book entitled Classification of Epileptic Seizures (Chapter 4). Petit mal and minor motor seizures are rarely, if ever, amenable to surgical therapy.

A patient who presents focal clinical seizures or focal electro-encephalographic abnormalities should always be considered as a potential candidate for surgical treatment. However, I generally do not subject such patients to surgical investigation unless they

163

fail to respond to medical therapy. It is obvious that surgical treatment should be carried out as soon as feasible in those patients in whom there are definite signs or symptoms of a progressive cerebral disorder, such as a brain tumor.

I have treated hundreds of patients who had focal clinical seizures or focal electroencephalographic abnormalities or both with medical therapy and followed them for many years, some for as long as twenty to twenty-five years. Many of these patients were completely controlled of their seizures; others continued to have focal seizures or focal electroencephalographic abnormalities without manifesting specific signs or symptoms indicative of a progressive cerebral lesion. Pneumoencephalographic studies and cerebral arteriography revealed normal findings in these patients.

It is important to call attention to the fact that focal electroencephalographic discharges are frequently found in epileptic patients in whom no other evidence of a cerebral lesion can be demonstrated. It is also not uncommon to find normal electroencephalographic tracings or generalized electroencephalographic abnormalities in patients who have focal clinical epileptic seizures.

I have observed that in many patients, particularly children, electroencephalographic foci migrate from one hemisphere to the other and then disappear completely. Similar findings have been reported by Gibbs and co-workers and by Lundervold and Skatvedt.

I would like to emphasize these findings because it has been my experience that many physicians have the impression that a patient who presents a focal clinical seizure or a focal electroencephalographic abnormality should *immediately* be subjected to surgical investigation. I cite the following instance as an example.

A general practitioner recently phoned me to discuss one of his patients, a fourteen year old boy with major motor epilepsy. He told me that several years ago I performed an electroencephalographic examination on this patient and the findings were normal. He stated that he recently obtained another electroencephalogram at a different laboratory which revealed a spike focus in the left occipital area of the brain. This physician was strongly in favor of referring the patient to a neurosurgeon for surgical investigation and he asked my opinion. This patient had been completely free of clinical seizures since he was started on anticonvulsant medication and presented no other signs or symptoms indicative of a cerebral lesion.

It is true that the physician should maintain a constant suspicion and vigilance for any signs or symptoms which might reveal evidence of a progressive cerebral lesion in all patients with convulsions especially those who present focal clinical seizures or focal electroencephalographic abnormalities. However, I can see no medical reason why the heretofore mentioned patient should be subjected to the inconvenience and expense of consulting a neurosurgeon merely on the basis of an electroencephalographic spike focus. I may add that I have had many similar inquiries concerning epileptic patients.

The general policy in our Epilepsy Clinic is to investigate the feasibility of surgical treatment in all patients who fail to respond to medical therapy, particularly those with grand mal or psychomotor epilepsy who present one or more of the following findings:

(1) Focal characteristics in the clinical manifestation of their seizures;

(2) Localized abnormalities in the electroencephalogram;

(3) Focal neurological abnormalities such as a monoplegia or hemiplegia.

We also consider the possibility of surgical intervention in those patients whose seizures become alarmingly more frequent and more severe, in spite of the fact that they had been treated with only one or two of the available medical therapeutic agents.

How does the neurosurgeon determine whether an epileptic patient is a candidate for surgical treatment?

The neurosurgeon must first attempt to ascertain which part of the brain is most likely the site of the epileptic discharge. He employs various diagnostic techniques such as pneumoencephalography, cerebral arteriography and electroencephalography in this attempt.

Electroencephalographic examinations are initially performed in the routine manner as described in another section of this book entitled Electroencephalography (Chapter 3). If the routine electroencephalogram reveals localized abnormalities and the neurosurgeon considers that the patient may be a candidate for epileptic surgery, more extensive electroencephalographic investigations are carried out by applying the electrodes directly to the brain tissue. In some instances, electrodes in the form of long fine wires are inserted directly into the brain tissue.

Pneumoencephalographic or cerebral arteriographic studies or both are performed to determine the presence of structural defects of the brain which might give a clue as to the causation of the seizures.

Surgical therapy is performed only when the neurosurgeon determines that the site of the cerebral abnormality (electrical or other) is in an accessible area of the brain, the removal of which would be compatible with life and would not cause the patient more of a handicap than the seizures themselves.

The operations most frequently used for the treatment of epilepsy are:

(1) Excision of localized cortical areas exhibiting constant abnormal electric discharge. In such cases, the excision is based on the premise that a single, localized cortical area is responsible for the seizures.

(2) Temporal lobectomy for patients with clinical psychomotor seizures associated with focal, temporal lobe electroencephalographic abnormalities. This operation has been used mainly in adults.

(3) Hemispherectomy, more accurately termed hemicorticectomy, is the newest development in the surgical treatment of certain cases of epilepsy associated with unilateral cerebral atrophy.

Surgery for epilepsy is a highly specialized field and at the present time is practiced by only a very few neurosurgeons in this country. It is also necessary that the operating room be especially equipped for this type of operative procedure. Figure 10 is a photograph of an operating room which is arranged for a craniotomy to ablate an epileptic focus. I make special mention of the fact that surgery for epilepsy is practiced by few neurosurgeons and that the operating room must be specifically equipped for this procedure because I have experienced considerable difficulty

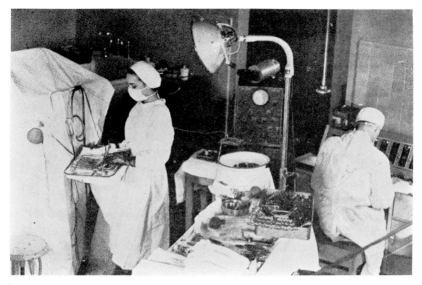

Figure 10. Photograph of operating room arranged for a craniotomy to ablate an epileptic focus. The almost vertical frame holding the drapes allows observers to see the patient's entire body and extremities below the neck. By this means the motor effects of cortical stimulation can be easily determined. The electro-encephalograph at the right and the cathode ray oscilloscope are within the operator's view as he stimulates the cortex. (Dr. A. Earl Walker's operating room at The Johns Hopkins Hospital).

convincing some of my patients that their personal neurosurgeons would not be able to carry out the surgical procedure because: (1) they were not trained for this type of surgery, or (2) they were associated with hospitals in which the operating rooms were not equipped for this type of surgery.

RESULTS OF SURGICAL THERAPY FOR EPILEPSY

During the four year period from 1958 through 1961 my associate, Dr. Lydia Pauli, and I studied, treated and followed approximately 5,000 epileptic patients. About 1,500 of these patients were new to us and the others had been followed by me for a period of years. Approximately 30 per cent of these 5,000 patients were adults and the others were children of varying ages. We considered the practicability of surgical treatment in all patients with severe epilepsy who did not respond to adequate medical therapy. We did not consider those patients whose epilepsy did not cause them a major handicap which was measured by factors such as frequency, severity and time of occurrence of seizures. Also, we did not consider those patients whose general condition was so poor that one did not feel justified to submit them to extensive surgical investigations. This latter group consisted mostly of severely mentally retarded patients, particularly those with minor motor epilepsy.

Sixty-one of these 5,000 patients were referred to Dr. A. Earl Walker, Professor of Neurological Surgery, The Johns Hopkins University School of Medicine, for investigations relative to the possibility of surgical intervention. In spite of intensive medical therapy, these patients continued to have attacks so frequently that they constituted a major handicap. Dr. Pauli compiled the results of Dr. Walker's findings and reported as follows:

(1) Fifty-five of these sixty-one patients were considered by Dr. Walker as unsuitable candidates for surgical therapy.

(2) The other six patients underwent cerebral surgery and the results are as follows: the seizures were completely controlled in two; in two, the seizures were markedly reduced in frequency; and in two, the frequency of seizures remained essentially unchanged.

These six patients were continued on anticonvulsant medication after their operations. I would like to emphasize this fact since the surgical excision of an epileptogenic focus does not terminate the treatment. It is only an intermediate stage, and medical therapy must be continued after the operation.

In 1955, Penfield and Paine reported on 203 patients who had adequate follow-up subsequent to surgical treatment for epilepsy. Treatment was stated to be successful in 45 per cent, the patients either having no attacks or one attack per year. Good control was obtained in an additional 20 per cent; these had up to six seizures a year. In 35 per cent, there was no improvement.

Penfield's findings could give the casual reader a false impression of the practicability of surgery in the control of epilepsy per se. His group consisted of exceedingly selective patients referred from various centers throughout the world (most of these patients presented the ideal criteria for epileptic surgery).

It is true that Penfield's results and also our surgical findings indicate that epileptic surgery is of value in highly selected patients. On the other hand, I believe our total investigation definitely indicates that cerebral surgery is of very little value as a treatment for the overall epileptic population. Our total group of epileptic patients (approximately 5,000 over a 4 year period) represents a good cross-section of the total epileptic population, adults and children of varying ages. The geographical distribution of the patients seen in our Epilepsy Clinic is given in the preface of this book.

I believe that the results of the surgical treatment of epilepsy will improve with the passage of time. For the present, however, conservative treatment should be the first recourse, even in patients with focal clinical seizures and focal electroencephalographic abnormalities. Surgery should be considered only for those patients who have been resistant to intensive medical therapy.

BIBLIOGRAPHY

Gibbs, E. L., Gillen, H. W., and Gibbs, F. A.: Disappearance and Migration of Epileptic Foci in Childhood. *A.M.A. J. Dis. Child.*, *88:*596, 1954.

Lundervold, A. and Skatvedt, M.: Migration of Spike Foci from One Hemisphere to the Other in Children. *J. Pediat.*, *48:*457, 1956.

Penfield, W. and Paine, K.: Results of Surgical Therapy for Focal Epileptic Seizures. *Canad. M.A.J.*, *73:*515, 1955.

Walker, A. E.: Surgical Treatment of Epilepsy, in Livingston, S.: *The Diagnosis and Treatment of Convulsive Disorders in Children.* Springfield, Ill., Thomas, 1954.

Chapter 11

SERVICES AVAILABLE FOR THE EPILEPTIC PATIENT

M Y experiences over the past twenty-six years have made it clear to me that many patients and also many physicians are unaware of many of the services available for the epileptic patient. For example, at a conference in Washington, D. C., in 1961, an administrative official of the Federal Office of Vocational Rehabilitation informed me that a recent survey conducted among physicians by his office revealed that less than 50 per cent of the practicing physicians were cognizant of the fact that help for the epileptic could be obtained from this source at the local level.

The following are some of the important services which are available to the epileptic patient:

(1) Personal physician and physicians who specialize in convulsive disorders;

(2) Special epilepsy clinics;

(3) Vocational rehabilitation centers;

(4) Lay (non-medical) organizations dealing with epilepsy;

(5) Special hospital schools and institutions.

PERSONAL PHYSICIAN AND PHYSICIANS WHO SPECIALIZE IN CONVULSIVE DISORDERS

An individual with a convulsive disorder should first consult his personal physician in regard to "what to do and what not to do." This is the most important service available to any patient, regardless of the nature of his medical disorder.

The attitude that epilepsy is primarily a problem for the neurologist was almost universally present in the past and still exists to a great degree today. I am convinced that this is definitely not true. I believe that most physicians can adequately care for an

170

epileptic patient if they desire to do so. It is true that some general physicians may wish to feel more secure by consulting a neurologist or a physician who specializes in convulsive disorders to establish a diagnosis and to assist in the management of the more complicated cases.

My observations over the past years have convinced me that general physicians and pediatricians are becoming progressively more interested in the disorder of epilepsy. I believe that this is progress in the right direction. Certainly, there is not a sufficient number of neurologists and physicians who specialize in convulsive disorders to care for the vast number of epileptic patients. In view of this it is obvious that the general physician and pediatrician must take the major part in the treatment of the epileptic.

SPECIAL EPILEPSY CLINICS

There are clinics which offer overall medical assistance to the epileptic patient in most of the larger cities in the United States. These clinics are designated by various terms such as Seizure Clinics, Epilepsy Clinics and Anticonvulsive Clinics. In some hospitals the epilepsy clinic functions as a separate unit; in others, the epileptic patient is cared for in the neurology clinic, and in still others, in the psychiatric clinic. Some of these specialized clinics serve only as a diagnostic center. However, in addition to this service, many of them also have facilities for follow-up care.

Crippled Children's Services

Each State has an official Crippled Children's agency which provides a variety of services to handicapped children under twenty-one years of age. The crippled children's programs are supported by Federal, State, and local funds. The Federal share is from grant-in-aid funds administered by the Children's Bureau under the provisions of Title V, part 2 of the Social Security Act and represents for the States as a whole approximately 25 per cent of the total expenditures for crippled children's services.

The administration of crippled children's agencies in the different States and Territories varies—31 crippled children's programs are in State departments of health, 10 in State departments of welfare, 2 in combined State departments of health and welfare, 3 in State departments of education, 4 in State universities and 4 in separate commissions.

A broad program of care encompassing a wide range of services is provided by State crippled children's agencies. They include case-finding, prevention of diseases or disability, diagnosis and re-evaluation, treatment in or outside the child's home by medical specialists as well as related professional personnel, hospitalization, convalescent care including rehabilitation and follow-up care. Appliances, braces, and drugs which are prescribed by the physician are also provided by the State crippled children's agencies.

In States which have developed special programs for children with epilepsy, such as Maryland, q.v., the pattern for giving care usually consists of a central or primary specialized clinic attached to a medical center and several secondary clinics located throughout the State.

In the central or primary clinic(s) expert diagnostic and treatment services are available; also hospitalization, when needed, is an integral part of the program. The most difficult cases may be followed or reevaluated at intervals in this clinic. Consultation service to physicians or secondary clinics is provided. In special programs for children with epilepsy psychological and social appraisal is an integral component of the diagnostic evaluation; referral for educational, prevocational or vocational counselling is part of the follow-up services which are provided.

The secondary or local clinics screen new cases and refer special problems to the central clinic; they regulate medication and provide continuous supervision for children who do not have their own physician.

A total of forty State crippled children's agencies reported services to 7,331 children with epilepsy in 1960, which was 2.1 per cent of the total children served by crippled children's agencies that year. Fifteen States served over one hundred children with a primary diagnosis of epilepsy in their programs (Table 14). Two of these States, it will be seen from this table, served well over one thousand children. Nine States served from under 100 to over twenty-five; sixteen States reported fewer than twenty-five cases.

The information pertaining to the Crippled Children's Services was supplied to me in July, 1962, by Dr. Alice D. Chenoweth,

TABLE 14

States with 100 or More Children with a Primary Diagnosis of Epilepsy in the Crippled Children's Program, 1960

State	*Number of Children with Epilepsy*
Alabama	440
Colorado	255
District of Columbia	242
Georgia	448
Hawaii	115
Illinois	292
Iowa	400
Maryland	841
Massachusetts	248
Mississippi	130
New York	1,438
Puerto Rico	509
South Carolina	116
Virginia	1,136
West Virginia	129

The data contained in this table was prepared by Dr Alice D. Chenoweth.

Chief, Program Services Branch, Division of Health Services, Children's Bureau, Department of Health, Education, and Welfare.

Maryland Epilepsy Program

In July, 1950, with the help of the Children's Bureau of the Department of Health, Education, and Welfare, the Maryland Epilepsy Program was inaugurated primarily to extend the benefits of modern advances in the therapy of epilepsy to patients living in rural areas. This program provides complete diagnostic work-up and arrangements for follow-up care for individuals with epilepsy under twenty-one years of age who are eligible for assistance. It also provides special medication, hospital and related services to these patients. The over-all administrative responsibility for the Crippled Children's Program, of which the Epilepsy Program is a part, is in the Division of Crippled Children of the State Health Department. However, there is a close working relationship between the State Health Department and the two medical schools and their hospitals in Maryland.

In 1957, the Maryland Epilepsy Program was reviewed by Dr. Jean Rose Stifler, Chief, Division for Crippled Children and Heart Disease Control, Maryland State Department of Health. Dr. Stifler stated that the Maryland Epilepsy Program has: "(1) made adequate diagnosis and better control available to all children; (2) developed a feeling of complete acceptance on the part of the schools for these children; (3) given the community a better understanding of the problems involved; (4) helped to eliminate the stigma of this condition; and (5) provided a setting in which doctors and educators can combine their efforts toward the best possible results with children."

I have been actively participating in the Maryland Epilepsy Program since its inception in 1950 and definitely concur with the favorable comments presented in Dr. Stifler's paper. In fact, it is my opinion that the inauguration of the Maryland Epilepsy Program was one of the most significant advances ever made in behalf of the epileptic children in the State of Maryland.

VOCATIONAL REHABILITATION CENTERS

The following resume of the services available to all handicapped individuals, including those with epilepsy, was prepared by W. Bird Terwilliger, Assistant Director, Division of Vocational Rehabilitation, State of Maryland.

> Vocational rehabilitation is a public service provided by all of the states in cooperation with the Federal Government to preserve, develop, or restore the ability of the disabled person to work. All services to the disabled are provided by state agencies. The Federal Government, through the Office of Vocational Rehabilitation, administers grants in aid and provides technical assistance and national leadership for the program. Due to local needs and conditions there are minor differences among the various state programs, but the availability of services and the procedures for providing them are fairly uniform throughout the nation.
>
> Vocational rehabilitation services are available to all citizens of working age (there is no upper age limit, but since 16 is the minimum age for legal employment, children under 16 are seldom considered for service) who present the following conditions:

1. The presence of a physical or mental disability, including epilepsy, with resulting functional limitations or limitations in activities.

2. The existence of a substantial handicap to employment caused by the limitations resulting from such a disability.

3. A reasonable expectation that vocational rehabilitation services may render the disabled person fit to engage in a remunerative occupation.

Counselors employed by the state rehabilitation agencies work on an individual basis with each disabled person who is referred for service. The counselor provides certain services himself and arranges for those which must be purchased outside the agency. One or more of the following services may be necessary to rehabilitate a handicapped person:

1. *Medical Examinations*

Every applicant receives, without charge, a general medical examination, which includes standard laboratory tests and chest and x-ray examinations. Its purpose is to determine the applicant's eligibility for service and his need for further medical, surgical, or special diagnosis. These diagnostic procedures provide the counselor with essential information for counseling the client regarding his limitations, and his capacities, to follow specific training and to do particular jobs. The examinations frequently indicate the need for physical restoration before training or other services are attempted.

2. *Guidance and Counseling*

The counselor considers the previous employment record of the client, his vocational interests and abilities, his educational background, and the availability of training and placement opportunities. There is careful study of his social and economic environment to determine to what extent his family and dependents are involved. Various standardized tests supply helpful information. On the basis of all these criteria, including the medical diagnosis and prognosis, the agency and the applicant develop a complete rehabilitation plan.

3. *Physical Restoration*

If it appears that the physical or mental condition of the disabled person can be materially improved by medical, surgical, psychiatric, or other treatment to such an extent that his vocational possibilities are thereby increased, the agency will secure such treatment through the cooperation of physicians and hospitals. All treatment looks definitely toward employment.

When a hearing aid, artificial leg or arm, glasses, or other artificial appliance is needed to improve the vocational ability of the disabled person, such prosthesis is secured from a reliable manufacturer. In this part of the program, medical advice is followed implicitly. Careful supervision is given during the fitting of each appliance and for a reasonable time afterward.

Use of rehabilitation funds for these purposes depends upon the economic need of the client.

4. *Vocational Training*

A client who needs to acquire certain manual or academic skills to fit him for the chosen job objective is given a course of training in a public or private school or "on the job." Only approved schools or training agencies are used for rehabilitation trainees. Through the entire process, from time of planning the course of instruction to the completion of the job requirements, a rehabilitation counselor provides helpful advice and supervision. All tuition costs may be paid from public funds. Payment for training supplies and equipment, however, is dependent upon the economic need of the client.

5. *Maintenance and Transportation*

When it is impossible for a disabled person to pursue a training or physical restoration program because of his lack of funds for room and board or transportation, and if these necessary funds are not available from other sources, the agency may provide the financial assistance necessary to carry out the chosen objective. Such assistance is based on the "dollar standard" prevalent in the community where rehabilitation service is given, and through constant supervision, is strictly limited to the period absolutely necessary for the attainment of the objective.

6. *Placement*

The agency is not a placement agency, but it assumes the responsibility of finding satisfactory employment, if possible, for every disabled person accepted for service. The agency maintains contact with all public, private, and individual sources that might offer job opportunities to its clients and follows up continuously on their performance in employment in order to make necessary adjustments, to provide further medical care that may be needed, and to furnish desirable supplementary training.

7. *Follow-up on the Job*

Each client who is placed in employment is followed on the job by the counselor until he is assured that the employment is satisfactory in every way.

Vocational rehabilitation agencies also serve employers in assisting them in making job studies to determine the suitability of jobs for persons with various disabling conditions.

Disabled persons are referred to vocational rehabilitation agencies from every conceivable source. Some of the more common sources of referral are physicians, hospitals, public and private health and welfare agencies, and schools.

If the vocational rehabilitation agency is not listed in the local telephone book, information regarding it can usually be obtained from the local office of the county or state health department.

LAY (NON-MEDICAL) ORGANIZATIONS DEALING WITH EPILEPSY

There are four voluntary *national* lay organizations currently in operation in the United States:

> The Federal Association For Epilepsy
> 1729 F Street, N.W.,
> Washington 6, D.C.

> The National Epilepsy League
> 203 N. Wabash Ave.
> Chicago 1, Illinois

> United Epilepsy Association
> 111 West 57th Street
> New York 19, New York

> The American Epilepsy Federation
> 77 Reservoir Road
> Quincy, Massachusetts

These organizations serve many useful and important purposes and can offer valuable help both to the epileptic patient and his physician. Some of the many services and programs offered by these organizations are enumerated as follows:

1. Referral Services

These organizations maintain complete, up-to-date files of community services, seizure clinics and other resources throughout the country which are equipped to help the epileptic patient. Patients who request assistance through correspondence are directed to available local help in familial, social, recreational, psychological, educational and medical problems.

2. Counseling and Personal Information

The national organizations annually answer thousands and thousands of letters from epileptic patients, their families and their physicians. Requested information pertaining to marriage laws, insurance, employment and other non-medical problems of vital concern to the epileptic is promptly forwarded.

3. Research

These organizations stimulate, sponsor, promote, conduct and contribute to research projects investigating the medical and social aspects of the epileptic disorder.

4. Consultation Services

The national organizations provide without fee consultative services to professions, individuals and agencies, ranging from relatively simple inquiries to complex, time-consuming projects.

5. Professional Education

The national organizations provide appropriate professional materials and information to physicians, clinics and specialized agencies such as public health departments, special education departments, State Crippled Children's Services and state employment services.

6. Public Education

Because of the vast amount of misinformation about epilepsy existing among both professional workers and the general public, the national organizations conduct broad and intensive programs of professional and public information. All mass media are utilized in the constant battle against the misunderstanding and fear that surround the epileptic disorder. Each of the national lay organizations prepares, publishes and distributes leaflets, pamphlets and brochures dealing with various facets of epilepsy. In addition to their own respective literature, these organizations distribute appropriate reprints appearing in journals, magazines and government publications. Factual reference material has been supplied to every daily newspaper and to every science writer in the nation. The organizations are constantly acquiring new films relative to epilepsy which are available for group viewing (See Appendix No. 1). Requests for information pertaining to epilepsy are stimulated by the national lay organizations in the belief that through repeated exposure to the facts regarding epilepsy, the public will eventually accept the disorder as any other medical illness.

7. Educational and Job Opportunity Development

Through research, legislative reform and the dissemination of factual information, the national organizations constantly strive to create an atmosphere of acceptance for epileptics among prospective employers and educational administrators.

8. Legislation

These organizations attempt to attain revocation or modification of unwarranted legislation which discriminates against epileptics. They sponsor and promote new enlightened legislation which reflects current medical knowledge of the epileptic disorder.

These organizations also publish newspapers which may be obtained by any individual upon request. The purposes of these newspapers are to keep the epileptic patient abreast of the current advances in epilepsy and advising them of the multitude of organizational activities.

The national voluntary epilepsy organizations have affiliate chapters which operate at a local level in many communities throughout the United States. The epileptic patient can determine if there is a local affiliate in his community by contacting his physician or the local health department or by contacting the national organization itself.

It has been my experience that the epileptic patient gains much personal help and also can contribute much to the promulgation of a better understanding of the epileptic disorder by associating himself with one of the lay epilepsy organizations. In addition to the many benefits which the epileptic patient receives from the services and programs previously enumerated, he will also benefit greatly from the intangible support derived from the knowledge that large national organizations are concerned with his type of disorder and the many associated problems.

SPECIAL HOSPITAL SCHOOLS AND INSTITUTIONS

There are many resident hospital schools and institutions in the United States which offer comprehensive programs for the medical, emotional and social management of epileptic patients, both children and adults.

The names of these schools and institutions may be obtained by contacting one of the national lay epilepsy organizations or its local chapter, or by consulting the *Directory for Exceptional Children*, which presents a state-by-state listing of the names and programs of the various schools. This book is available at most medical libraries.

Individuals interested in a particular resident hospital school or institution should first obtain information and a descriptive brochure or catalog from the respective school or institution. If it appears that the school or institution might be appropriate for the patient and if the patient or his family are capable of fulfilling the financial requirements, the school or institution should be visited for a more comprehensive evaluation. The patient's physician and the physician associated with the school or institution can then determine if it meets the requirements of the patient in question. Some of the hospital schools and institutions conduct special resident camps for epileptic children.

Unfortunately, the cost of many of the hospital schools is far above the financial means of many individuals. Therefore, in certain instances, the only recourse is admission to one of the state sponsored institutions. Many of the state operated institutions which house epileptic patients offer well-defined programs.

The general impressions of the public that state institutions are for "crazy people" only, are of inferior quality, do not provide proper medical care and treat all patients on an "impersonal basis," are definitely not true. This fact should be explained and emphasized to the candidate for admission and to his parents.

BIBLIOGRAPHY

Directory for Exceptional Children, 3rd edition. Porter Sargent, Publisher, 11 Beacon Street, Boston 8, Mass., 1958.

Services for Children with Epilepsy. The American Public Health Association, Inc., 1790 Broadway, New York 19, N. Y., 1958.

Stifler, J. R.: A Review of the Maryland Epilepsy Program. *Am. J. Public Health, 47:*587, 1957.

Wheeler, M. P.: *Study of Services Available to Children with Epilepsy*. Cleveland Health Council, June 1959. 14 p.

Chapter 12

INTELLIGENCE OF THE EPILEPTIC

Y EARS ago it was almost a universal opinion of the general public and also of many physicians that all, or at least most, epileptics were or eventually would become mentally retarded or "insane." The many misunderstandings relative to the intelligence of the epileptic which were so prevalent in the past are presented in the writings of Kanner and Temkin.

These misconceptions regarding the intelligence of the epileptic are totally unwarranted and stem primarily from the time when there were no effective remedies for seizures. Epilepsy was then regarded as a hopelessly incurable condition. For this reason, some intellectually normal patients with epilepsy were placed in institutions which housed mental defectives, idiots and other patients with serious mental illnesses. Because of the confinement of epileptics in mental institutions, the belief that all epileptics were mentally deficient became widespread.

Another factor responsible for the promulgation of such misconceptions was the paucity of reliable, comprehensive and scientific determinations of the intellectual performance levels of epileptic patients. Several decades ago the only available information relative to the intelligence of patients with seizures was that obtained in the evaluation of institutionalized patients. Most of these individuals were severely brain damaged patients with seizures and obviously, intellectual studies made on such groups revealed exceedingly low levels of intelligence. The very poor intellectual performances of these institutionalized patients led many individuals to assume that all epileptics were of low intellectual capacity. However, this group of epileptic patients constituted but a very small fraction of the total epileptic population, and the interpretation of its intellectual performance as representative of the general overall epileptic population was definitely fallacious. Such an interpretation is analogous to that of the woman who witnessed an epileptic seizure in a child whose mental status was that of an idiot and immediately assumed that all persons with seizures were mentally retarded.

One might as well believe in a relationship between genius and epilepsy as between mental retardation and epilepsy. Among the great men of history who are reported to have had epileptic seizures are: The Apostle Paul, Buddha, Socrates, Alexander the Great, Julius Caesar, Mohammed, Blaise Pascal, Peter the Great, Handel, Gustave Flaubert, Paganini, George Gordon (Lord) Byron, Feodor Dostoyevski, Edward Lear, Algernon Charles Swinburne, Sir William Pitt, Napoleon Bonaparte, Alfred the Great, Louis XIII of France, Swedenborg, and Vincent van Gogh. The reader may wish to refer to the book by Bryant which gives brief sketches of great men who possessed both genius and epilepsy. Actually, one can say there is no consistent relationship between epilepsy and mental retardation or genius. An epileptic may possess other infirmities or he may be richly endowed.

Even today many people including some physicians have expressed the attitude that the vast majority of epileptics are "intellectually deficient." This definitely is not true of the overall epileptic population. I have not observed a significant relationship between epilepsy and mental deficiency except in those children who have minor motor epilepsy. This type of epilepsy constitutes a very small percentage of the total epileptic population; less than five per cent of our patients suffered with minor motor epilepsy. A description of minor motor epilepsy is presented in another section of this book entitled Classification of Epileptic Seizures (Chapter 4).

The incidence of mental retardation in patients with minor motor epilepsy is exceedingly high. I have followed many patients with this form of epilepsy over a period of years and have observed that only an occasional patient presented normal intelligence. Most of them revealed evidence of mental retardation when the seizures first appeared; in others, mental retardation did not become apparent until the child became older. The degree of retardation varied from moderate to severe; the vast majority, however, showed evidence of rather severe mental retardation.

It is important that the parents of children with minor motor epilepsy be cognizant of the most likely final outcome, so that they can prepare to make arrangements for the care of their children. In many instances, institutionalization is the most appropriate recourse.

On the other hand, I have not observed a high incidence of mental retardation in our patients who suffered with other forms of epilepsy. I have treated thousands of epileptic patients for many years and can definitely state that the vast majority, including those who continued to have seizures, maintained normal intellectual capacities.

My findings in regard to the intelligence of the epileptic are supported by the results of a detailed study carried out by Lennox. In his study of twins, Lennox found that "the member with repeated seizures is as well off with respect to his I.Q. as his twin who has not had that handicap," and concluded that "seizures in and of themselves do not weaken the intelligence."

These findings should be emphasized to the parents of normally intelligent children who develop epilepsy, since many of them fear that their children will eventually become mentally retarded.

I have seen many epileptics who gave a gross impression of low intelligence which was initially assumed by their physicians to be due to organic brain damage. However, after investigating these patients thoroughly with neurological examinations and psychological tests, it was concluded that they did not present demonstrable evidence of organic brain damage and were not basically mentally retarded. In some instances, the poor intellectual performances were related to the fact that the patients were emotionally disturbed because of their illness and in others, it was due to excessive antiepileptic medication.

Many of those patients who were able to "readjust their emotions," either of their own accord or with appropriate psychiatric assistance, subsequently performed at a normal intellectual level. The various emotional difficulties encountered in epileptics are discussed in another section of this book entitled Behavior and Personality of the Epileptic (Chapter 13). Many of the other patients also performed at a normal intellectual level when their antiepileptic medication was regulated to the proper dosage.

BIBLIOGRAPHY

Bryant, J. E : *Genius and Epilepsy*. Old Depot Press, Concord, Mass., 1953.

Kanner, L.: Folklore and Cultural History of Epilepsy. *Medical Life, 37:*167-214, 1930.

Lennox, W. G.: *Epilepsy and Related Disorders*. Vol. II. Little, Brown and Co., Boston, 1960.

Temkin, O.: *The Falling Sickness—A History of Epilepsy*. The Johns Hopkins Press, Baltimore, 1945.

Chapter 13

BEHAVIOR AND PERSONALITY OF
THE EPILEPTIC

MUCH has been written in the past about the existence of an "epileptic personality." Almost every type of behavioral and personality aberration has been assigned to the epileptic as a manifestation of his "epileptic personality," such as criminal tendencies, sexual perversions, paranoid traits, suicidal tendencies, perseveration and numerous other psychotic disorders. The reader may refer to the writings of Clark, Kanner, and Temkin for descriptions of behavior and personality deviations which have been classified as expressions of epileptic personalities.

Even today many laymen and also some physicians express the attitude that most epileptics have or will subsequently develop "psychopathic personalities." Dr. Walter C. Alvarez, for example, in his widely published syndicated column which appeared in the *Boston Daily Globe*, stated that many epileptics are intelligent, and others, because of their tendency to violence, or psychosis, or criminality, or their constant seizures and inability to earn a living, have to be confined to an institution.

I do not believe that many, if any, medical authorities in the field of epilepsy would concur completely with Dr. Alvarez's statement. I can definitely state that I have not been impressed with the occurrence of psychosis or criminality in my group of patients. My observations are in agreement with the findings of Alström who investigated the relationship between criminality and epilepsy and reported as follows: "In a modern text-book of neurology published in 1946 we read that the impulsive equivalents in epileptics 'have many crimes to their account' such as 'arson, unmotivated homicide, theft and exhibitionism.' This gloomy view of the criminality of epileptics by no means conforms with the conditions that have been found to obtain in the present investigation . . . .. The correspondence with the figures for the general population is good: at any rate there can be no decisive difference between this group and the general population in regard to criminality. . . . The so-called impulsive equivalents in psychically unchanged epileptics are greatly exaggerated in respect to their dangerousness for the general public. It is therefore remarkable that precisely epileptics should have been made the scapegoats around whose necks these frightful descriptions of criminality should have been hung in the text-books. The explanation for this is probably extremely complicated. An important, if not the only, role is doubtless played by the old superstitious attitude to the epileptic seizure as such."

There are, in my opinion, no reports in the current literature which prove that there is a higher rate of criminal action among epileptics than among other individuals.

An article which appeared in the Saturday Evening Post was presented in a manner that certainly could convey a false impression of the outcome of the overall epileptic population to the average reader. A half-page photograph at the beginning of this article shows a physician and four epileptic patients behind bars. The statement below the picture indicates that the physician is examining four of the epileptics ordered by the courts to be locked up with the criminally insane in Wisconsin's Central State Hospital. It is quite possible that the casual reader could get a completely false impression of the relationship of epilepsy and criminal insanity because of this outstanding and dramatic photograph.

I recently received a letter, parts of which are subsequently quoted, from the executive director of a large charitable organization in which he questioned the attitude of their medical director concerning the emotional stability of epileptics.

"Our Medical Committee in considering adoptive applicants were concerned about their physical condition and were ruling out certain applicants on the basis of current or previous illness . . . There was some discussion of epilepsy and it was the opinion of the chairman of our Medical Committee that any person who had had epilepsy in childhood, even though there might be no seizures present as an adult, should be ruled out. His thinking was that even though the

child was 'supposedly cured,' there was certain emotional damage
. . . . There were two of our Board members who have epileptic
children and apparently have had considerable experience in dealing
with their children's problems. They also had obtained a great deal
of information about the illness and took marked exception to the
recommendations of our chairman of the Medical Committee."

I believe that one could reasonably question whether an individual with active seizures, regardless of how infrequently they
recur, should be allowed to adopt a child. However, I can see no
reason why a patient who has been completely free of seizures for
many years should not be evaluated on the same basis as anyone
else, that is, on his physical, mental, emotional and financial
ability to care for a child properly. The statement by the medical
director of the adoption organization: ". . . even though the child
was 'supposedly cured,' there was certain emotional damage," is
definitely not true in my experience. I have been in contact with
hundreds of my patients who have been seizure free for many
years and have not observed that their "emotional status" was
significantly different from that of any other group of people.
I do not believe that there is a specific syndrome such as the
"epileptic personality" which is mentioned so often in the older
medical literature.

It is true that some epileptic patients present a behavior or
personality which is at variance with that considered normal.
However, I do not believe these aberrations in behavior or personality are due directly to the epilepsy, except those which are
manifestations of the seizures themselves such as psychomotor
epileptic seizures or those which occur immediately following a
grand mal convulsion. In those epileptic patients where there is
definite evidence of brain damage, I believe the emotional difficulties are more likely related to the brain damage than to the
epileptic seizures.

The emotional disturbances encountered in many epileptics are,
by and large, essentially the same as those observed in many
patients who suffer with other disturbances which have a tendency
to be chronic such as heart disease and asthma, and consist primarily of anxiety and/or depressive states, feelings of insecurity
and inferiority, and anti-social tendencies. From a recent study,

Anderson and co-workers concluded that "the epileptic person-ality" as a distinguishing characteristic of the epileptic did not exist in their study group. They stated that the epileptic patient, as well as the patient with other chronic illnesses, does seem to develop what might be termed "the chronic disease personality."

I believe the emotional and personality deviations observed in many epileptics are due mostly to factors such as: (a) fears and anxieties associated with the anticipation of having a seizure; (b) the many unwarranted restrictions and social stigmas directed toward the overall epileptic population; (c) the mismanagement of the patient at home or in the community, and; (d) idiosyncracy, overdosage or adverse reactions of antiepileptic drugs.

FEARS AND ANXIETIES ASSOCIATED WITH THE ANTICIPATION OF HAVING A SEIZURE

The most common of the behavioral difficulties observed in epileptics are those related to anxiety and/or depressive states which stem in most instances from the following: fear of being out of contact for a period of time, of injury or of death as a result of a seizure; or fear of having their disorder exposed to the general public. Therefore, epilepsy, as it manifests itself to the personality development of the individual, is a psycho-social disturbance rather than a physiological one, because of the insecurity resulting from the anticipation of experiencing a seizure and its accom-panying social implications.

Life, for many epileptics, consists of an almost endless number of obstacles which, even if evaded or surmounted, may inflict varying degrees of emotional damage. The epileptic patient may experience a variety of emotional difficulties relative to his fear of a recurrence of seizures.

Many epileptics live in a constant state of anxiety due to the fear of sustaining an injury during a seizure. Some epileptics have even expressed a fear of dying during, or as a result of, a seizure. The physician can alleviate these fears in many instances by informing the patient and his family that epilepsy is not generally associated with a high incidence of injuries and deaths. The reader may refer to the section of this book entitled Prognosis of

Epilepsy (Chapter 17) for a more detailed discussion of injuries and deaths associated with epileptic seizures.

The epileptic is ever fearful of being suddenly thrust into a state of unconsciousness. This fear of loss of contact with reality is one of the most disturbing problems with which the epileptic "must learn to live." The suddenness and unpredictability of most seizures certainly tend to make many epileptics tense and apprehensive. It is exceedingly distressing for the epileptic to realize that one minute he may be engaged in the performance of some activity and the next minute he may be unconscious. This loss of consciousness, regardless of its duration, constitutes a source of never-ending embarrassment and apprehension for many epileptic patients.

Epileptic patients frequently exhibit continual anxiety related to the recurrence of seizures because of the pronounced effect which epileptic seizures, especially grand mal convulsions, exert on the family or persons witnessing an attack. There is no other physical handicap, the manifestation of which is so dramatic and fear-provoking as a grand mal convulsion. The effect which such seizures produce on observers may be reflected in their attitude toward the patient. In many instances, epileptics recovering from major seizures are subjected to ridicule, mockery and insults by misinformed observers. These adverse attitudes, of course, greatly magnify the epileptic's already intense embarrassment and regret.

Repeated seizures with concomitant loss of contact with the environment cause some epileptic patients to become frustrated and disheartened. The physician and the family should exert every effort to prevent the epileptic patient from becoming discouraged because of his epileptic disorder. Some epileptics have expressed a fear of being "put away in an institution" because of their recurrent seizures. The physician and the family frequently can dispel such fears and anxieties by displaying affection and love for the afflicted individual and making him feel "wanted."

Cognizant of the adverse social implications associated with an epileptic disorder, many adult epileptics adopt a policy of strict secrecy regarding their condition. I have known some individuals who have resorted to extreme measures to conceal their epileptic disorder because of the fear of exposure and its resultant social rejection and isolation. Such individuals live in a state of perpetual fear and tension engendered by their maintenance of secrecy relative to their epilepsy. Individuals who are obsessed with keeping their epileptic disorder secret may suffer, sooner or later, emotional damage because of the realization of the inevitability of the exposure of their condition. Fearful of having a seizure in public, some such patients restrict their activities to the confines of their homes, and consequently develop marked anti-social tendencies. In some instances, public exposure has resulted in a beneficial effect upon the epileptic who had previously adhered to secrecy regarding his epileptic disorder. Tensions and anxieties related to the fear of disclosure of his condition disappeared following a seizure in public and more constructive attitudes were then afforded an opportunity to become manifest.

Because the overall epileptic population is too often regarded as unemployable, the individual with a history of epilepsy may be reluctant to disclose the nature of his condition to a prospective employer. Epileptics who conceal their disorder from their employers frequently exhibit marked attitudes of insecurity, bitterness and frustration which stem from the realization that exposure of their condition may be tantamount to dismissal. It is not difficult to understand why some epileptics who have been repeatedly denied employment or who have been discharged four or five times because of their epileptic disorder manifest behavioral or personality problems.

BEHAVIORAL DISTURBANCES RELATED TO THE SOCIAL STIGMAS ASSOCIATED WITH EPILEPSY

It is quite obvious that any individual, epileptic or non-epileptic, who is continuously exposed to obstacles created by social and economic rejection and who is denied privileges which are considered basic human rights, such as marriage, education and employment, is certainly likely to develop emotional difficulties. Even those epileptics who have been free of seizures for many years encounter social and economic obstacles of great magnitude.

It is of prime importance to understand that most of the emotional disturbances observed in many epileptic patients are not manifestations of the disorder itself, but are results of a hostile society which has discriminated against the epileptic since the dawn of recorded history. Some of the social and economic problems encountered by the epileptic patient are discussed in detail in the sections of this book entitled General Management of the Epileptic Patient (Chapter 7) and Socio-Economic Aspects of Epilepsy (Chapter 15).

MISMANAGEMENT OF THE PATIENT

Epilepsy makes its initial appearance in the vast majority of instances during childhood; at least 90 per cent of all epileptic patients experience their first seizure during this period. Therefore, I believe it is reasonable to assume that the emotional problems encountered in many epileptic patients probably began at home.

Children are, of course, greatly influenced by the attitudes and reactions of their parents. It is generally recognized that the early life experiences with parents and the ensuing relationships are of great importance, since they determine to a large extent the child's later social and emotional patterns and capabilities.

The parents of an epileptic child should be convinced that their efforts must be directed toward raising a "normal child" within the limits of the disability. This obviously requires an atmosphere of natural, relaxed affection in which the child can develop "normal" emotional traits which, in later years, can aid him in coping with the adverse attitudes of a misinformed society.

Since emotional security is a human need common to all individuals, and particularly to the person with epilepsy, the parents and family must exert every effort to provide an atmosphere in which the epileptic feels "wanted." Patients, particularly children, may react to poor management by developing withdrawn, dependent and submissive personality patterns or by developing an aggressive, demanding and hostile attitude to their environment. Relieving the tension which surrounds the patient may actually lessen the number of seizures, improve his ability to learn and decrease his hyperactivity and restlessness.

The home environment is often dependent upon the effect which the seizures have on the parents and the other members of the family. Families who live in constant fear of a recurrence of seizures create an atmosphere of continual tension and anxiety which, obviously, has an undesirable effect upon the patient. Because epilepsy is still considered by many to be a "shameful and disgraceful disease," the epileptic patient, in many instances, is resented by his parents and rejected by his brothers and sisters. Such adverse intra-family attitudes can but magnify the epileptic's feelings of being unwanted and "different."

In many instances, the attitudes of the parents are influenced by their personal feelings in regard to their child's epileptic disorder. Feelings of embarrassment and shame and the fear of social rejection cause some parents to resort to a policy of secrecy with respect to their child's epileptic condition. Such parents may restrict their child's social and physical activities to the extent that the child is denied the necessary normal social contacts. Epileptic children, particularly teen-agers, whose activities and social contacts have been rigidly curtailed tend to manifest marked attitudes of belligerence and inferiority; many of these teen-aged epileptics develop pronounced anti-social tendencies.

It is well known that the tendency of parents to over-protect a child is greatly increased by the existence of any physical or mental handicap. Aware of the many adverse attitudes concerning epilepsy and because of the possibility of injury associated with a seizure, many parents exert an even greater effort to protect their epileptic child from emotional and physical trauma. Over-protection by the parents may manifest itself in constant, strict surveillance, in preventing the child from engaging in any activity on his own, in supplying his requirements in excess of his actual physical and mental requisites, or in protecting him from any type of disappointment.

Too frequently an epileptic child in a family is treated as "something special" and allowed to do as he pleases, pampered and over-protected by his parents. Unreasonable demands are granted because of a mixed emotion that the epileptic child is a pitiful, unfortunate person who should be given the greatest possible happiness, and that an emotional upset might precipitate a seizure. Most parents have the impression that if the seizures are aggravated by circumstances which "excite" the child, he should live in as quiet and sheltered a manner as possible. Within limits, there may be justification for such an attitude, but in the majority of cases such failure of authority to institute reasonable limits carries the more serious risk of establishing a lifelong neurosis based on lack of security and the concomitant feelings of antagonism, resentment and inferiority. It is important to impress upon the parents or guardian of an individual with epilepsy that great endeavors should be made to prevent the occurrence of emotional problems which are so prone to develop in epileptic patients, since these emotional problems frequently are more difficult to control than the seizures of epilepsy themselves.

In many cases parents of a child who has had only an occasional epileptic seizure consider him ill in the same respect as if he were afflicted with active tuberculosis or acute rheumatic fever. Such a child is encouraged and, in many instances, forced to rest and take daily naps. Such attitudes should be discouraged. The parents should be instructed to allow their children to play and conduct themselves, if possible, in the same manner as their normal associates. Contrary to the general belief, physical activity favorably affects an epileptic disorder in most instances. It is generally known that epileptic patients experience fewer seizures when they are participating in normal physical activities, such as football, baseball or other games. It has also been demonstrated that abnormalities in the electroencephalograms of epileptic patients frequently become more numerous during the resting state.

I have seen many epileptic patients who had been instructed by their previous physicians not to swim, ride a bicycle, play baseball, or participate in any of the activities usual for their age groups. Even though a patient may have an occasional convulsion, there is no valid reason for such an edict. There is always a certain hazard in life for everyone and in some instances this may be greater for the epileptic. However, the disadvantage of the increased hazard, if it is a reasonable one, is offset by the advantage of a normal life.

I explain to the parents that there is a small, calculated risk when they allow their child to participate freely in all normal childhood activities. However, they must weigh this against the greater risk of instilling attitudes of inferiority and of being "different" which would handicap the child more severely and more surely than the convulsions. My recommendations in regard to the physical activities for the epileptic are discussed in detail in another section of this book entitled General Management of the Epileptic Patient (Chapter 7).

It is of utmost importance for both the physician and the layman to understand and differentiate between the emotional problems which occur in many epileptic patients because of mismanagement at home or by society, and (a) those behavioral disturbances produced by antiepileptic drugs, and (b) those behavioral-like performances which are actually manifestations of the epileptic disorder, such as psychomotor seizures. A description of psychomotor epilepsy is presented in another section of this book entitled Classification of Epileptic Seizures (Chapter 4).

It is important to understand that some patients will present abnormal behavior for a varied period of time following a grand mal epileptic seizure. In some instances the abnormal behavior may last for a short period of time, five or ten minutes or so, or it may last for hours or even for days. It is imperative for the parents to realize that the patient is not responsible for his bizarre activities during this period. Reprimanding the patient and/or attempting corrective measures are of no avail, since these behavioral aberrations represent a definite phase of the seizure itself.

I have observed many patients, particularly children, whose behavioral patterns were essentially normal when they first consulted me; they were having periodic seizures at this time. Soon after the seizures were controlled with antiepileptic medication, they presented abnormal behavioral patterns. When the medication was either reduced or withdrawn and the patient began having seizures again, the behavioral pattern returned to that of a normal child. This phenomenon has also been observed by other physicians. It is the concensus of opinion that the behavioral difficulties occurring under such circumstances are not functional in origin or related to the antiepileptic medication, but actually are manifestations of cerebral dysfunction similar to that which is the basis of the frank epileptic seizures themselves. In many instances behavioral difficulties presented by such children when they are rendered completely free of seizures are much more of a problem than the seizures themselves. In such cases it is probably better for all concerned to allow the individual to have an occasional seizure and normal behavior between these seizures than to be made completely free of seizures with concomitant uncontrollable behavior.

IDIOSYNCRASY, OVERDOSAGE OR ADVERSE REACTIONS OF ANTIEPILEPTIC DRUGS

Emotional and personality aberrations observed in some epileptic patients are undoubtedly related to their antiepileptic medications. In order to affect an adequate control of seizures, some patients require dosages of medication which keep them constantly drowsy and dull; this may cause them to be somewhat irritable. I would like to emphasize the fact that the proper dosage of medication for each patient is that amount which controls his seizures but does not produce untoward reactions which interfere with his general well-being. Most patients would be better off leading a normal life between occasional seizures than being seizure-free in a perpetual state of drug-induced drowsiness or confusion.

Phenobarbital causes many patients, particularly children, to become exceedingly restless, belligerent and hyperactive. Dilantin occasionally produces behavioral changes; I have seen a few patients who became markedly euphoric while receiving this drug and several others who presented psychotic symptoms. Phenurone is notorious for causing behavioral and personality aberrations.

It is important that the physician investigate the possibility of the antiepileptic medication being the causative factor in those patients who present behavioral or personality deviations subsequent to the administration of the drug. The reader may refer to the section of this book entitled Medical Treatment for Epilepsy (Chapter 8) for detailed descriptions of adverse reactions of antiepileptic medications.

Some patients, particularly teen-agers, become markedly disturbed because they must take medication daily over a period of years. Some of my patients have told me that the fact that they must take medication "annoys them considerably"; others have stated that taking medication makes them feel "different from their associates"; and still others have expressed anxieties because they feel they must conceal the fact that they are taking anti-epileptic medications.

I have observed that within recent years emotional difficulties associated with epilepsy are becoming less frequent and less severe because of early diagnosis and treatment, better management at home, and a somewhat better understanding of the disorder of epilepsy by the general public. The development of an educational program which would dispel the many misunderstandings and stigmas associated with epilepsy is essential to the emotional welfare of the epileptic. In fact, I believe it would be reasonable to assume that most persons with epilepsy could live completely normal lives were it not for the psychological and social side reactions to their disorder.

In conclusion, I would like to state emphatically that I do not believe an "epileptic personality" as such exists. If there were such a syndrome as an "epileptic personality," one would then be able to identify an epileptic in a group of people. However, I am definitely convinced that this cannot be done. Many of my epileptic patients are currently engaged in all spheres of endeavor—as physicians, lawyers, clergymen, educators, etc.—and function both professionally and socially without their associates' knowing of their epileptic disorder, unless they should happen to have a seizure in their presence.

It is true that many epileptics present emotional problems. However, these are, by and large, no different in character from the emotional difficulties observed in patients with other disorders which have a tendency to be chronic, such as heart disease and asthma. This so-called "chronic disease personality" may be slightly more marked in the epileptic because he has a two-fold handicap: (1) he must cope with the potential hazards of an epileptic seizure, per se, and (2) he must cope with the many obstacles and restrictions imposed upon him by society.

THE HYPERKINETIC SYNDROME

Children with epilepsy frequently exhibit a stereotyped pattern of behavior, consisting essentially of marked restlessness, increased irritability, belligerence and short attention span. This disturbance is not limited to epileptic children; it is also observed in mentally retarded children and in children who are otherwise normal. It is also occasionally caused or aggravated by drugs, particularly phenobarbital.

Hyperactive behavior is frequently an important consideration in the treatment of the epileptic child. In many cases, it is more of a problem to the parents than the seizures themselves. Epileptic seizures usually occur relatively infrequently, whereas the hyperkinetic syndrome manifests itself almost continuously.

It has been my experience that the hyperkinetic syndrome is frequently difficult to control with the available therapeutic agents. There are many so-called tranquilizing drugs currently being employed for the treatment of this disorder. I have given many of them an adequate trial, but did not observe significant benefit. However, I have encountered a few good results with the use of the amphetamines. One of my associates, Dr. Dennis Whitehouse, has observed some beneficial results with the use of Ritalin.

The most beneficial therapeutic regimen for the hyperkinetic syndrome which I have encountered is the ketogenic diet. However, I have never prescribed this form of therapy for a patient with the hyperkinetic syndrome unless there was an associated seizure disorder. The reader may refer to the section of this book entitled Dietary Treatment for Epilepsy (Chapter 9) for a more detailed discussion relative to the ketogenic diet as a tranquilizing agent.

In many instances the hyperkinetic syndrome is aggravated by improper parental management or other adverse environmental conditions. Therefore, treatment should also be directed towards establishing as satisfactory a parent-child relationship as possible. The parents should be told that the child cannot "control" his restlessness. They should also be informed that harsh disciplinary measures are of no value and frequently make the condition worse. I frequently tell the parents that they must "learn to live with the disorder," and that "there is a good possibility that it will disappear as the child grows older." I have seen hundreds of epileptic children with the hyperkinetic syndrome and have observed that in the vast majority of these patients the marked restlessness disappeared when they reached puberty.

As stated previously, the hyperkinetic syndrome is frequently observed in epileptic children. However, it has been my experience that this disorder is relatively rare in the epileptic adult.

An excellent resumé of how the physician can help the hyperactive child is presented by Dr. W. Hugh Missildine in the Ross Laboratories publication, *Feelings and Their Medical Significance*, vol. 3, no. 4, April 1961 (Dr. Stella Chess, Guest Editor).

Dr. Missildine states, "Hyperactivity in a child needs careful investigation into its possible causes. It may be physiologic, symptomatic of something awry within the brain substance, indicative of noxious attitudes in the parent-child relationship, or a combination of these. The physician can:

1. Take a careful history for possible insults to the child's brain before, during or after birth. He can ask about illness or bleeding during the mother's pregnancy, prematurity, jaundice, difficulty in breathing or feeding after birth. He can ask whether there has been head injury or high fever with convulsions, meningitis or encephalitis.

2. He can investigate the parent-child relationship, looking for possible abnormal parental attitudes—oversubmission, overcoercion, punitiveness, neglect, distrust or rejection—to which the child may be reacting with increased restlessness.

3. He can give drugs which have a calming effect, especially on those children whose hyperactivity derives from an organic or physiologic basis.

4. He can make sure that the parents accept the child as hyperactive and provide opportunity for the child's motor discharge.

5. He can be sure the parents limit the child firmly, isolating him whenever necessary, when the child's excessive activity interferes with the rights of others.

6. He can see to it that the parents have an active recreational life away from the child, so that they can accept the child's hyper-

activity with the balanced respect and firmness that insures the child's optimal development.

7. There are some hyperactive children whose problem is so complex or the attitudes of whose parents are so intense that these measures will not suffice, and the assistance of a psychiatrist must be sought."

BIBLIOGRAPHY

Alström, C. H.: *A Study of Epilepsy in Its Clinical, Social and Genetic Aspects.* Copenhagen, Munksgaard, 1950.

Alvarez, W. C.: *The Boston Daily Globe,* page 11, column 6, Monday morning, June 8, 1953.

Anderson, W. W., Guerrant, J., Weinstein, M., and Fisher, A.: The Epileptic Personality—Does It Exist?. *Neurology, 12:*301, 1962.

Clark, L. P.: *Clinical Studies in Epilepsy.* Utica, State Hospitals Press, 1917.

Delay, J., Pichot, P., Lemperiere, T., and Perse, J. (translated by Rita and A. L. Benton): *The Rorschach and the Epileptic Personality.* New York, Logos Press, 1958. 265 pp.

Forster, F. M.: Personality Problems Associated with Seizures. *General Practitioner, 14:*5:90-96, Nov. 1956.

Kanner, L.: Folklore and Cultural History of Epilepsy. *Medical Life, 37:*167-214, 1930.

Lennox, W. G.: Epilepsy and Related Disorders. Vol. II. Boston, Little, Brown and Co., 1960.

Liberson, W. T.: Emotional and Psychological Factors in Epilepsy: Physiological Background. *Am. J. Psychiat., 112:*2:91-106, Aug. 1955.

Loveland, N., Smith, B., and Forster, F. M.: Mental and Emotional Changes in Epileptic Patients on Continuous Anticonvulsant Medication: A Preliminary Report. *Neurology, 7:*12:856-865, Dec. 1957.

Spencer, S. M.: No Wonder Epileptics Are Bitter. *The Saturday Evening Post,* page 26, March 28, 1953.

Temkin, O.: *The Falling Sickness—A History of Epilepsy.* Baltimore, The Johns Hopkins Press, 1945.

Chapter 14

SHOULD EPILEPSY BE PUBLICIZED?

WHAT SHOULD THE PHYSICIAN TELL THE PATIENT AND THE PARENTS?

IT HAS been my experience that the vast majority of parents and even some of the older children will think about epilepsy when they consult a physician in regard to a seizure disorder. This is true even in the case of the individual who has had only one seizure. In many instances they do not ask the physician about the possibility of this diagnosis at the beginning of the initial interview. I believe that this is due mainly to the fact that they are fearful of the word epilepsy. My experience has been that most of them will eventually, during the course of the interview, or at a subsequent visit, ask the physician "Do I have epilepsy?" or "Does my child have epilepsy?"

I do not believe that it is wise in most instances for the physician to withhold the term "epilepsy" from the parents and some of the older patients, and cite the following case as an example. The mother of one of my patients stated that she took her child, who had suffered with several convulsions, to a physician. After a thorough examination, the physician told the mother that he was unable to demonstrate a cause for her child's convulsions. The mother then asked the doctor, "Does my child have epilepsy?" The physician in turn answered, "Mother, I do not know what the term epilepsy means. In fact, the term epilepsy does not exist in my dictionary. So far as I am concerned, your child suffers with convulsions of undetermined cause." The mother left this doctor's office quite confused. She became even more confused when her neighbor, who knew that the child had suffered with convulsions, asked whether she thought the child had epilepsy.

The mother remembered from the interview that her doctor had said that the word epilepsy did not exist in his dictionary. When she was able to find the word in Webster's dictionary as well as in several textbooks from the library, she became more upset. She then called her doctor and told him he had confused her, that she did not have any confidence in his diagnosis, and also that she did not think his dictionary was a very good one because the term epilepsy was in Webster's dictionary and in books by many famous doctors.

I do not believe that one can "hide" the word epilepsy from parents and older patients. The term is used in medical textbooks, is seen by the public in newspapers and magazines, and is heard on radio and television broadcasts. I believe that it is best to face this problem honestly. [I explain first that the term epilepsy is derived from the Greek word "epilepsia" which, when translated into English, means "seizure."] I also tell them that the term epilepsy is assigned to those patients in whom a definite cause cannot be established for their convulsions. I explain to them that epilepsy is a disease which should differ in no way in its social implications from other diseases such as diabetes, heart disease and rheumatic fever. I also explain to them that the many stigmas which are currently attached to the disorder of epilepsy are totally unwarranted and stem from many misconceptions which have been carried down throughout the ages.

The emotional difficulties which arise in some of the parents and older patients or both are undoubtedly related to the public's attitude toward epilepsy. Because of this, I recommend that the diagnosis of epilepsy should not be generally publicized.

I believe that it is unwise to tell the younger child and even some of the teen-agers about the diagnosis of epilepsy, unless they specifically ask the physician. It may be that the term "epilepsy" can be explained more clearly to these individuals when they get older.

If the child should happen to ask the physician specifically about the word epilepsy, then the physician should explain the term to the child in words appropriate for the individual child's intelligence. I have found that the terms "dizzy spells" and "fainting spells" are suitable for the younger child. The exact nature of the disorder of epilepsy can be better and more clearly explained to these young children when they get older. I have encountered one instance where a very young child was told by his physician that he had epilepsy. He told his playmates that he had epilepsy and they subsequently told their parents. The parents of the playmates did not understand the nature of the disorder of epilepsy and forbade their children to play with the epileptic child. They also told their children that epileptics were "crazy" and "insane" and, therefore, they should not play with epileptics.

It is important that the term epilepsy not be concealed from the child when he gets older. I have found that, generally, the time that the child can best accept and understand the term epilepsy is when he reaches his early teens. It is important that the child be told about the diagnosis of epilepsy when he reaches this age, or he may become emotionally upset if informed of the fact that he has or did have epilepsy by someone other than his physician or parents. I know of several instances where individuals were informed by outside sources about the diagnosis of epilepsy; because of this, they "held it against" their parents or guardians and "never forgave" them for concealing this information.

It is best that an epileptic be told about the nature of his disorder and also of possible restrictions sometime before he reaches the usual age for certain activities, such as automobile driving and service in the Armed Forces. For example, I begin discussing the question of automobile driving with a child who is still having seizures when he reaches fourteen or fifteen years of age. I periodically tell him that in all probability he will not be allowed to operate a motor vehicle when he reaches the age of sixteen. Also, in the case of military service, I begin explaining at least two or three years before the usual age of acceptance in the armed services that the peacetime regulations forbid acceptance of individuals with a history of epilepsy. I have found that preparing an individual for these restrictions gradually is much less of an emotional insult than that which occurs when the individual is abruptly informed of the restrictions at the age when these activities are usually performed.

WHAT SHOULD THE PARENTS TELL THEIR CHILD?

The first reaction of many parents to a diagnosis of epilepsy in their child is one of "horror" and frequently of disbelief. Also, many parents have an intense feeling of guilt which stems from a belief that they brought a child into the world "with this horrible disease." This is a moment requiring tact and sympathetic understanding. The general belief that epilepsy is a shameful disease is often foremost in the minds of the parents and the physician should clearly emphasize several points to them. Firstly, the parents should be told that there is no definite proof that epilepsy is unquestionably an inherited disease; secondly, that there is no reason why epilepsy should carry a stigma; and thirdly, that they should look upon epilepsy as a disease differing in no way in its social implications from other diseases such as rheumatic fever, tuberculosis and diabetes.

The parents must be made to realize that nothing they have done or have not done has contributed to the development of epilepsy in their child. This is very important. I have observed that parents frequently believe that the condition has resulted from some error of omission or commission on their part. In many instances the development of epilepsy in a child is considered by parents as "punishment for their sins." Such guilt feelings are seldom expressed openly, but, nevertheless, they affect the parents' attitude towards the child. I have found that such feelings may seriously impede a wholesome relationship between parents and the epileptic child.

In many instances parents are reluctant to discuss the word epilepsy with their child and frequently ask the following question, "What and how much should I tell my child about his illness?" The parents will invariably say, "I certainly do not want to tell him that he has epilepsy. I do not even want to mention the word epilepsy to him."

From the standpoint of the patient the implications of his handicap should not be minimized. Instructions given in each case must be individualized, depending upon the patient's likelihood of understanding the situation.

I usually advise the parents to tell the young child that he has some sort of disorder such as "fainting spells" or "dizzy spells." Occasionally, I suggest the use of the term convulsions. As the child grows older he should be acquainted with the responsibilities imposed by his condition. Generally, by the time the patient reaches fourteen or fifteen years of age, he can be given a thorough account of his disorder.

Young children are sometimes thoughtless and "cruel." The following is an example. A young boy learned that one of his classmates had epilepsy. During recess on the playground, in the presence of the epileptic child, he shouted, "Don't play with Johnny because he has epilepsy. Johnny has epilepsy and that's very bad." He later stated to the school principal that his parents told him that all epileptics are "dumb and crazy."

When a child has been subjected to and disturbed by such ridicule, the parents should explain to him as simply as possible the meaning of the word epilepsy. They may tell him that the word epilepsy is a "foreign word" or a "Greek word," which, in English, means "fainting or convulsions." The parents may also tell the child that some people do not understand the meaning of the word epilepsy and think that it has a "bad meaning" but that it does not. The childhood saying, "Sticks and stones can break your bones, but names can never hurt you" has also been helpful in some instances.

If a child has already been accepted by other children, the commotion associated with his disorder soon dies away. However, if he is a newcomer to a group, unpopular or in any other way an "outsider," the attitudes of playmates can become an almost insuperable obstacle to an epileptic child.

When restrictions, such as forbidding participation in activities usual for their age, are imposed on young children, they very quickly get the impression that they are *completely* different from other children. This attitude can be prevented in many instances by encouraging the epileptic child to participate in certain activities in which he can excel. For example, in those instances where the epilepsy is so severe that the child cannot compete physically with this playmates, parents should encourage, but not force, hobbies such as photography, music or model building. The patient's ego and pride can frequently be enhanced in this manner. The epileptic child should be praised for his accomplishments; the emphasis should never be on "you can't do this," but rather on "you can do this."

WHAT SHOULD THE PARENTS AND THE PATIENT
TELL THEIR RELATIVES AND FRIENDS?

Despite the most skilful handling of an epileptic patient on the part of the physician and parents, many problems may arise from the attitude of an ill-informed population. Since Biblical days, epilepsy has carried with it the idea of uncleanliness, ungodliness and even of insanity. Today some parents still warn their children to stay away from a schoolmate who has epilepsy. Even when such advice is prompted only by the desire to spare the young child the unpleasant sight of a seizure, it creates problems for the patient. For the present, the epileptic child and his parents will have to accept this community attitude.

The adverse attitudes of the public are generally much more of a problem in small towns than in larger cities, because of the closer contact of individuals within a small community. Some families have found it necessary to leave communities in which they had enjoyed good jobs and good reputations for many years, because they could not cope with the ridicule and many insults to which they were subjected because of their epileptic child.

Keenly aware of the adverse attitudes of the public in regard to the epileptic disorder, many parents have asked me, "My relatives and close friends are so interested in my child, I am sure they will ask about his condition. What should I tell them?" It is obvious that the physician cannot give the parents a direct answer to this question since a specific response would depend upon the make-up and understanding of the individuals in question. Therefore, each such situation must be evaluated and answered on an individual basis. The parents could limit their discussion by merely telling their friends and relatives that their child suffers with fainting spells or convulsions, omitting the term epilepsy entirely. Obviously a more sensible approach would be for the parents, in appropriate instances, to reveal the nature of the disorder and attempt to "teach" their friends and relatives what they learned from the physician about epilepsy. They should emphasize that epilepsy is not a hopelessly incurable and shameful disease. This latter approach must be considered the more meaningful since, in addition to answering the questions of friends and relatives, it constitutes one method of helping to correct the many misconceptions and fallacious ideas which now exist in regard to the disorder of epilepsy.

It is probably best that very close associates be told of the diagnosis of epilepsy and the condition explained to them in detail, so as to preclude their becoming unduly alarmed in case the child should have a seizure in their presence. This, of course, would be better not only for themselves, but also for the epileptic patient.

WHAT SHOULD THE PARENTS AND THE PATIENT TELL THE TEACHER AND THE SCHOOL AUTHORITIES?

A frequent question asked by parents is, "Shall I tell the teacher or the school authorities that my child suffers with epilepsy?"

I have been informed by some parents that other physicians have advised them not to mention the word epilepsy to the school teacher or school authorities, but merely to tell them that the child suffers with convulsions or seizures. I believe that this is futile since today most of the school authorities and teachers are familiar with epilepsy as a disorder characterized by "seizures" or "convulsions," although some of them do not realize the exact nature of the disease.

As with all types of treatments and also all types of general advice, each case must be individualized. Generally, however, I believe that in the case of a young child who suffers with infrequent seizures and who has never had a spell at school, it is best not to mention the disorder in any manner to the school teacher or school authortiies. This is particularly true in those instances where the seizures have only occurred at night during sleep. It is quite possible that such children would never have an attack at school.

While this course may seem "morally wrong," I justify it by considering the adverse effects such knowledge might produce. Since many teachers and other members of the school faculty do not themselves completely understand the condition of epilepsy, they may treat the child in a manner which sets him apart from other children. I have found in some instances that even when a teacher apparently understood the condition, she over-protected the child and looked upon him as someone different from the other children. Every time the child did something which appeared to be "out of order," the teacher attributed it to the epilepsy. Many of the teachers were in a constant "state of tension" for fear that the child might have a seizure in class. Obviously, this is not good for the child.

However, if a patient suffers with frequent seizures or manifests side reactions from drug therapy, such as drowsiness, it is best that the teacher and the school authorities be told about the condition in detail. It has been my experience that much is gained when the parents have a personal interview with the school teacher and also consult him periodically at times such as Parent-Teachers Association meetings in regard to the child's progress and general activity in class.

Older patients, in the higher schools, should have the condition fully explained to them. When the patient has a good understanding of the disorder, then it is advisable to inform the school authorities of the condition. For the good of the child the school authorities should know the actual situation, and with the consent of the parents this appraisal should be submitted by the physician. He should state honestly that the child is an epileptic and also what frequency of convulsions might be expected. It may take some persuasion to convince a principal or teacher that no material upset in school routine will result if the child should have an occasional seizure.

WHAT SHOULD A TEACHER TELL THE CLASSMATES ABOUT AN EPILEPTIC PATIENT?

It is quite obvious that the teacher should not tell the classmates about the presence of an epileptic in the classroom unless he should have a seizure in their presence. I have found that the following explanation has been very satisfactory in those instances where a child has an epileptic seizure in school.

The teacher should first explain to the other students (in the absence of the patient) that the afflicted individual has a "disturbance" and that the seizure which the child experienced is a manifestation of his illness.

The teacher should definitely tell the other students that the illness is not contagious. This may appear to be ridiculous, but I have on numerous occasions been told by some intelligent individuals that they were afraid to allow their children to play with an epileptic for fear that their own children would "catch" the disease.

The teacher should also have a private interview with the patient to determine whether he is disturbed in any manner by the actions or attitudes of any of his classmates, whether they have refused to play with him, called him "bad names," etc. If no troublesome situations are apparent, the teacher should not continue with further discussions. However, in instances where the patient shows evidence of having been disturbed, the teacher should have a conference with the other students. In appropriate instances, he should define in simple terms the meaning of the word epilepsy; that is, of course, if the word has been mentioned. He should tell them to associate with the patient in the same manner as anyone else and explain that people with seizures are not "crazy," "different" or "peculiar," as has been expressed by many misinformed people in the past. It is obvious that the teacher should not call attention to these adverse designations unless they have been expressed by the classmates.

The success which any teacher has in coping with and handling situations involving epileptic pupils is governed largely by his attitude and understanding of the disorder of epilepsy. The teacher sets the pattern in the classroom, because the other children will reflect the attitudes and feelings of the teacher in most instances. Whether the other students consider a convulsive episode as a horrible major catastrophe or as a relatively insignificant incident, is usually based upon the actions, understanding and attitude of the teacher.

I have been told by the school authorities that, in some instances, teachers absolutely refused to have an epileptic child in the classroom. Some teachers stated that the appearance of the seizures per se frightened them considerably, and others expressed the fear that the child might hurt himself or even die as a result of a seizure. Some teachers said that their past experiences with a seizure was that it disturbed some of the other pupils to the extent that they were unable to perform satisfactorily for the remainder of the school day.

Obviously, these attitudes, in many instances, stem from misconception and ignorance of the disorder of epilepsy. The physician can frequently clarify the problem by a personal interview with the teacher. If this is not feasible, he should relay his advice to the teacher via a school nurse or school counselor.

The teacher should be informed that the chance of severe injury resulting from a seizure is minimal and that the chance of death is essentially nil. He should be told that, except for the word epilepsy, the "upsetting" effect of a seizure on the other pupils, if the situation is handled properly, should not be very different from that of a fainting spell, short temper outburst or even a vomiting spell.

Specific instructions concerning the management of a patient at the time of a seizure are presented in the section of this book entitled General Management of the Epileptic Patient (Chapter 7).

Chapter 15

SOCIO-ECONOMIC ASPECTS OF EPILEPSY

EMPLOYMENT FOR THE EPILEPTIC

IT HAS been my experience that in many instances an epileptic's capacity for work is definitely confused with his acceptability for work. I am in complete agreement with the following statements which appeared on pages 58 and 59 of the April 8, 1961 issue of the *Journal of the American Medical Association*: "Individuals with a neurological disorder constitute a vast and potentially valuable reservoir of manpower. In considering these individuals for employment, their *capacity* for work should not be confused with their *acceptability* for work. Acceptability is affected not only by capacity for work, but by factors inherent in the job under consideration and by the attitude of prospective employers and fellow workers."

It is unquestionably true that the unacceptability of the epileptic for employment stems in most instances from misconceptions of the disorder of epilepsy on the part of prospective employers and fellow workers. In many instances this is true even for patients who have been free of symptoms for many years. Case Histories 10 and 11 demonstrate instances of patients who were disqualified from employment solely because of a past history of epilepsy. In fact, of all of the common medical disorders, epilepsy is the only one where the name of the disorder frequently causes the patient more handicaps than the disturbance itself. Therefore, the epileptic patient faced with the problems of an occupation must be made to understand that, at least for the present, he is likely to encounter difficulties which at times may be quite severe.

There is no doubt in my mind that most epileptics are employable provided that their seizures are adequately controlled and their placements are selective ones. Hibbard screened 250 ambulatory epileptics looking for employment placement and found that 80 per cent were employable under normal conditions. Of the

211

remaining 20 per cent, about half required vocational rehabilitation for employment, and half were not employable because of associated defects.

I believe that the classification of persons with neurological disorders in regard to employment which appeared in the same issue of the *Journal of the American Medical Association* is very appropriate for the epileptic patient. This classification is as follows:

"CLASS N-1*—An individual with a neurological disorder, which is of slight severity or which is constantly under such control that, without aggravating this disorder, he can perform the work normally expected of any employee.

EXAMPLE: A person with controlled epileptic seizures.

CLASS N-2—An individual with a neurological disorder, in the control of which there may be transient symptoms and/or who has residual defects. These persons may range from those who have only occasional symptoms, which if satisfactorily anticipated by proper placement would allow performance of work normally expected of any employee, to those who have frequent symptoms. The severity of the symptoms in the latter may require careful supervision and specific placement.

EXAMPLES: An individual with occasional epileptic seizures, with or without an additional impairment such as hemiplegia, or an individual with moderately severe myasthenia gravis.

CLASS N-3—An individual with a neurological disorder of such severity and constancy as to incapacitate him for gainful employment, except possibly under limitations, e.g., in sheltered workshops or home-bound employment.

EXAMPLE: An individual with traumatic paraplegia.

SUB-CLASS "X" (Under N-1, N-2, or N-3). An individual with a neurological disorder, the nature of which is such as to warrant his classification in any one of the first three classes, but which is of such changing nature as to require or justify special arrangements for his employment and more frequent reevaluation.

EXAMPLES: An individual with recent onset of a hemiplegia who may be moving to complete return of function, or those in the

---

*The "N" is used in this neurological classification to distinguish this system from other systems used by industry to classify workers.

early stages of amyotrophic lateral sclerosis where progression of the condition may be expected."

In the case of the epileptic, the problem of employment arises in two distinct groups of patients. The first group consists of those individuals who have never worked before; and the second, of those who develop epileptic seizures after having been established in vocations not suitable for individuals with seizures.

The first group usually consists of younger individuals. In those instances where an individual has been free of seizures for a prolonged period of time (at least four years), he should be encouraged to prepare for the future in the same manner as if he never had epilepsy. However, he should be made to understand that for the present even the controlled epileptic encounters some difficulties relative to employment and that there are certain specific types of employment from which he is automatically excluded because of a past history of epilepsy, such as the Military Services.

In the case of the individual who continues to have seizures in spite of medical therapy, it is best to assume that this situation will, in all probability, continue. Therefore, such patients should be prepared at an appropriate early age for certain possible restrictions as far as future employment is concerned. They should be told that, in all probability, they will not be suitable for certain vocations because of their disorder, and that they may not be acceptable in other instances because of the many unwarranted misconceptions concerning the disorder of epilepsy. Of course, the controlled epileptic also encounters these same problems on many occasions.

It is the responsibility of the parents, the physician, the school teacher and the school counselor to see that advice in regard to employment is forthcoming. It has been my experience that generally the most appropriate time to direct the patient's attention towards his future vocation is during the first or second year of high school. I have found that many patients are helped considerably when they are informed of the possibility of restrictions several years or so before they reach the contemplated age of employment. When patients are so advised, they have sufficient time to reorient their "way of thinking." As examples, I cite two of my patients, both high school students: one had his "heart set" on becoming an airplane pilot, and the other, a surgeon. After several years of repeated discussions, these students were made to realize that, in all probability, they would not be able to go into these fields.

The second group (those who had been previously employed) frequently presents a much greater problem. Many of them are "forced" to change their employment because of the attitude of the employer or the inherently dangerous characteristics of the occupation. This may necessitate extensive rehabilitation and can cause the individual considerable financial and emotional difficulty. Some of my patients were helped with psychiatric guidance during this period of rehabilitation. Sometimes these patients can be given a little encouragement if the physician mentions the names of outstanding individuals who were "forced" to change their employment because of disorders other than epilepsy. An excellent example is that of Roy Campanella, the outstanding major league baseball player, who became paralyzed in both legs as a result of an automobile accident.

Some of the occupations which I consider as suitable and not suitable for patients with infrequent seizures are listed in Tables 15 and 16, respectively.

There is no doubt that the epileptic has considerable difficulty obtaining employment. As an example, the degree of success achieved by Veterans Administration personnel in vocational rehabilitation and placement of epileptic veterans probably is lower than that for any other major disability group. The controlled epileptic experiences less difficulty in securing employment than the patient who is still having seizures.

It has been my experience that at the present time the epileptic patient is more likely to secure employment in small organizations (out of sympathy or friendship in many instances) and most likely to obtain his financial livelihood from a vocation, profession or business of his own.

I have discussed the problem of the employment of the epileptic with executives of many of the major industries and learned that most of these individuals were not in favor of employing epileptics because they considered them as "sick individuals with a disorder

TABLE 15

TYPES OF OCCUPATIONS WHICH ARE SUITABLE* FOR PATIENTS WITH
INFREQUENT EPILEPTIC SEIZURES

Farmer	Cabinetmaker
Gardner	Draftsman
Salesman	Jeweler
(not requiring auto driving)	Plumber
Clerk	Forester
Mechanic	Florist
(manually controlled equipment)	Dog breeder
Laborer	Photographer
Electrician	Physician
(repairing or bench work)	(one who does not deal directly
Technician	with patients)
Librarian	Lawyer
Psychologist	(one who does not participate in
Stenographer	court activities)
Veterinarian	Tailor
Accountant	(manually controlled equipment)
Pharmacist	†School teacher

*Many of my patients are currently engaged in the various occupations designated as suitable and are performing well.

†For adult education. Discussed in a subsequent section of this chapter entitled Education for the Epileptic (Training for the Future).

TABLE 16

TYPES OF OCCUPATIONS WHICH ARE NOT SUITABLE FOR
PATIENTS WITH INFREQUENT EPILEPTIC SEIZURES

Surgeon	**Armed Services
*Those which necessitate operation	**Roman Catholic Priest
of a motor vehicle	Those which necessitate altitude or
Those which involve automatically	ladder work
controlled machinery or equipment	Solitary watchman or look-out
Policeman	Swimming instructor or lifeguard
Fireman	Nursery maid
	Baby sitter

*Exceptions—An individual whose employment necessitates the operation of an automobile should be allowed to drive if his seizures have always occurred in association with sleep. Also, a farmer should be permitted to operate a tractor or motor vehicle on his own property, if he cares to do so.

**Epileptics are *not acceptable.* Discussed in a subsequent sections of this chapter entitled Attitude of the Armed Services Toward Epilepsy and Education for the Epileptic (Training for the Future).

of the type which would make them very prone to accidents and excessive absenteeism; they would be relatively non-productive and might be too disturbing to the other employees." Many of these executives stated that "insurance problems" make the employment of epileptics prohibitive and assumed the following attitude: "Why should I employ an epileptic when I can very easily get a 'normal' person? If I employ epileptics my workmen's compensation insurance premium will be increased."

These assumptions and attitudes are untrue and unwarranted and unquestionably stem from misconceptions concerning both workmen's compensation insurance and employability of epileptics. I would like to call attention to the fact that there is no provision in workmen's compensation insurance policies or rates that penalizes an employer for hiring epileptics. The reader may refer to the section of this chapter entitled Insurance for the Epileptic for a detailed discussion of workmen's compensation insurance.

There is no reason why an individual who is physically, mentally and emotionally capable of working and who has been free of seizures for a prolonged period of time should be disqualified from employment solely because he has epilepsy. Also, many of my patients with infrequent seizures are currently employed in various vocations and professions. They have performed their working duties in the same manner as a similar group of normal people. I have not been impressed with an accident rate any higher than would be expected in any other group of individuals. In fact, I believe there is good reason to predict a lesser accident rate among competent epileptics than among normal individuals. The sensible epileptic realizes his handicap and is therefore exceedingly cautious in performing his working activities, whereas the average worker frequently assumes a more nonchalant attitude and performs automatic movements without "thinking." An excellent example is presented in the section of this book entitled Prognosis of Epilepsy (Chapter 17).

Unfortunately, the idea that the epileptic is a less proficient worker and more prone to accidents has prevailed for many years. However, I would like to emphasize the fact that this is merely an assumption of ill-informed people. It is true that these traits may apply to a given isolated epileptic, but such is also the case with individuals suffering with other disorders. The assumption that these characteristics are applicable to the overall epileptic population has never been documented either by my own experience with epileptics in industry or by other individuals. The following studies bear out these views.

(1) Investigation by the U.S. Department of Labor compared the work performance of epileptics with the performance of matched non-epileptics. The Department concluded that there was no significant difference between the two groups.

(2) Dr. John G. Lione reported that the sickness and accident experience of epileptics in industry is as good if not better than that of the total employee population. Dr. Lione's study consisted of 9,600 employees in an oil refinery; fifty-eight of these employees had epileptic convulsions or loss of consciousness during a period of six years (1954 to 1959), a prevalence rate of six per 1,000. Sickness absenteeism was average or less than average in forty-seven of these fifty-eight workers; the criteria for excessive absenteeism were more than fifteen days total sickness per year or more than four absences per year. Off-the-job disabling accidents were experienced by eight of the fifty-eight employees, and only one had an industrial accident. The one industrial accident was not related to a convulsive seizure.

(3) A recent survey of Veterans Administration hospitals, regional offices and centers showed 122 known epileptic employees. The work performance of this group of epileptics generally was found to be satisfactory; many were considered above average. Some have been promoted to better positions, a few of them supervisory. Their attendance records showed no abnormal pattern. Most significantly, the epileptics have been well accepted by their fellow employees.

(4) In a report by Dr. Fabing which appeared in *Harper's Magazine*, it is stated, "Studies by the U.S. Department of Labor and the Association of Casualty and Surety Companies show that epileptics have no significantly larger number of injuries on the job than other workers, and that they compare favorably in absenteeism and work output."

It is highly significant that the nation's largest employer, the Federal Government, has approved the employment of epileptics in the Federal Service if their attacks are adequately controlled and if their placement is selective. The following is an excerpt from a pamphlet issued by the United States Civil Service Commission, Washington, D.C., August, 1958, C.S.C. Form 614, entitled *Employment of Epileptics in the Federal Service.*

"GUIDELINES FOR EMPLOYMENT IN THE FEDERAL SERVICE"

"Selective placement is extremely important in these cases.

"A history of epilepsy, in itself, will not preclude an individual from working for the government. When an applicant for Federal employment discloses a history of epilepsy, the case is investigated by the Medical Officers of the Commission to determine if the condition is adequately controlled and if the duties of the position can be performed by an epileptic without hazard to himself or others.

"The Commission considers that a person's condition is adequately controlled if: (a) he is under a physician's continuing supervision; (b) he is taking medication designed to prevent seizures, and (c) the seizures are effectively controlled by medication.

"When evidence of adequate control is submitted, the Commission will accept the individual's application for consideration for positions which do not require him to work at heights or around dangerous power-driven machinery, operate motor vehicles, or work in any other environmental situation that would cause the individual to be a hazardto himself or others in the event he did experience a lapse of consciousness.

In addition to these restrictions on placement, it is felt that, wherever possible, employment should be in a small group or area where the occurrence of a seizure would not be disruptive to many employees. These epileptics should be under surveillance of the available health units to insure continuing selective placement and to provide any necessary care.

"Placement is not confined to sedentary or light duty positions since there is no evidence that arduous duties promote seizures. It is felt attacks tend to be fewer when the muscles or mind are employed.

"If a person with a history of convulsive disorder can furnish satisfactory medical proof that he has been free of seizures for a period of at least five years, without the use of medication, he may be authorized to drive motor vehicles.

"With respect to epilepsy, as with all physical defects or deviations from normal, the Commission holds that these conditions alone should not keep a person from being employed in the Federal service if he is able to perform his duties effectively and without hazard to himself or others."

The epileptic should also be encouraged by the fact that many of the city and state governments are now employing epileptics. The State of Maryland, for example, employs epileptics on essentially the same basis as outlined by the Federal Government.

In regard to the employment of epileptics by the State of Maryland, Dr. Nathan E. Needle, Medical Director, Department of Personnel, State of Maryland, has stated:

"An attempt has been made to rehabilitate many epileptics and place them into the various departments of the State service. I have attempted to put them into useful positions so that they can establish an independent socio-economic position in life.

"The selected placement of these people is very important. They should be placed in positions that are not hazardous to themselves or others. We do not expose them to hazardous machinery, open elevator shafts, or in positions requiring them to work above ground level.

"Before acceptance, these people must have been under proper medical supervision and therapy. At least two years must have elapsed since their last attack of grand mal. Continued therapy with their private physician is stressed."

Although the employment situation with respect to the epileptic is not nearly as poor as it was some years ago, there is still much room for improvement. The major obstacle to the employment of the epileptic is the attitude of the employer. Many employers still cling tenaciously to the impression that an epileptic, even one who has been seizure-free for many years, is not a competent individual. Evidence must be presented to the employer and also to the insurance companies documenting the good employment records and low absenteeism of epileptic workers. Emphasis must be placed upon the fact that there is little or no difference in the respective accident rates of epileptic and non-epileptic workers.

My experience, based on the employment records of hundreds of my patients, indicates that the efficiency and work record of both the controlled epileptic and the epileptic with an occasional seizure, is equal to that of any other worker if he is assigned to a suitable employment. My observations indicate that the accident rate in epileptics is no higher than that observed in the general working population.

The experience of a unique industrial plant in California, Epi-Hab, supports my observations that many epileptics are competent workers. Epi-Hab is an organization which provides the epileptic with employment, on-the-job training, technical instruction by credentialed instructors and ultimate placement in private business and industry. Epi-Hab stands for epilepsy rehabilitation and is a non-profit corporation chartered under state non-profit laws.

The following information concerning Epi-Hab was supplied to me by Dr. Frank Risch, Director, Epi-Hab U.S.A., Inc., and Epileptic Rehabilitation Service, V. A. Center, W. Los Angeles, California.

Epi-Hab L.A., Inc., began operation in 1956 and is the outgrowth of a Veterans Administration experimental workshop which was designed to determine the beneficial effects of steady gainful employment on the control of seizures and to further promote the economic rehabilitation of the epileptic. At the time of this writing there were Epi-Habs located in Los Angeles, California, Phoenix, Arizona and Long Island, New York, and co-operating Epilepsy Rehabilitation Workshops in the Veterans Administration hospitals at Los Angeles, California and Northport, Long Island, New York. Epi-Hab has received financial and gratuitous professional support from the Office of Vocational Rehabilitation, Washington, D.C., from private contributions, and from a variety of community organizations.

Early doubts and fears relative to the epileptic's working with basic shop tools led to the encasement of such implements in plastic shields and padding. Today, however, such extraneous and costly shieldings have been eliminated. The work benches, the concrete floor, the brick walls, the tools and the motor-driven machines are all conventional, as are the standard safety guards. In appearance, the Epi-Hab shop looks just about the same as any other small machine shop.

The safety performance record of Epi-Hab L.A. has been good enough to earn a 20 per cent discount on its Workmen's Compensation Insurance premiums and a Safety Plaque from the Pacific Employers Insurance Company for two consecutive years for outstanding safety performance. During the four year period between 1956 and 1960, over 1000 generalized seizures have occurred with but 425 man-hours lost due to seizures; this represents approximately one hour for every 1000 man hours worked. Slightly over 100 industrial accidents have occurred at the Epi-Habs, 25 per cent of which have been associated with seizures.

As of June, 1960, over 1000 applicants have been referred to the Epi-Habs and in excess of 400 have been employed. These employees earned over $1,000,000 and paid over $100,000 in taxes. A survey of the employees' earnings before employment at Epi-Hab and their period of earnings at Epi-Hab, showed a ten-fold increase during Epi-Hab employment.

Approximately ninety-five Epi-Hab employees have been placed in private industry. This represents 25 per cent of the Epi-Hab labor force placed with other companies, the ultimate objective of the Epi-Hab program.

Athletics are stressed at Epi-Hab. Over the years, baseball and bowling teams comprised of Epi-Hab employees have been company policy and have appeared in community leagues.

Improvement in skill and knowledge is another objective of the Epi-Hab organization. In this regard, the Los Angeles Board of Education was asked to sponsor courses in electronic theory for the Epi-Hab employees and to grant certification for completion of the courses.

Epi-Hab performs the following services for industry: wire harness assembly, electronic equipment assembly and sub-assembly; wire prepping, curring and marking; mechanical sub-assembly; machine operation; drilling c'sinking, c'boring, deburring, tapping, nut plate assembly, etc.; overseas and commercial packaging; salvage; and other work requiring labor operations. The Epi-Habs have sub-contracted over 475,000 man-hours of work from a variety of industrial establishments including aircraft, electronic, metal, woodworking, toy, plastic and hardware.

Epi-Hab has become an integral part of the community and participates with other firms in contributing to human welfare by supporting the Community Chest. In fact, Epi-Hab has been the recipient of three consecutive bronze plaque awards for its leadership in contributions, a record unexcelled by the thousands of companies located in Los Angeles.

Case History Number 10

This is the case of a twenty-five year old male graduate civil engineer. About five years before I saw this patient he fell from a horse and for several months thereafter had a short "fainting spell" once or twice a month. His physician diagnosed his disorder as epilepsy and prescribed anticonvulsant medication. He was also classified 4F by the Armed Services at this time. He took the medication for two months and then stopped it on his own accord. For the subsequent five years he did not have the slightest indication of a spell and enjoyed perfect health. He was contemplating marriage and children, but was stymied in this respect because he was unable to secure employment. He said that he had been refused one job after another because of his 4F classification. He told me of one instance which disturbed him considerably. He made application for the position of civil engineer in a large company and was given an appointment for his medical interview. He was seated in the reception room and when it was his turn to see the medical director, the nurse called into the doctor's office and said, "Doctor, the epileptic is here to see you." He was immediately disqualified because of a company regulation prohibiting the employment of epileptics.

Case History Number 11

This is the case of a twenty-six year old male who had infrequent seizures up until he was thirteen years of age. At eighteen years of age he was drafted into the army and shortly thereafter was sent overseas where he participated in combat action for a period of four years. During this interval he did not have a seizure.

Upon discharge from the Armed Services, he obtained a job as an electrician at one of the larger establishments. He had been completely seizure free for about ten years. After he had been working for several months and doing well, his foreman came to him one day and said, "Mister, I am sorry, but because of certain circumstances which we did not know about before, we will have to let you go." He went to the employment bureau where he was told that he was discharged because his employer learned that he was an epileptic.

BIBLIOGRAPHY

Angers, W. P.: Job Counseling of the Epileptic. *J. Psychol.*, *49:*123-132, Jan. 1960.

Fabing, H. D.: Epilepsy and the Law. *Harper's Magazine*, September, 1960, pages 56-59.

Fabing, H. D.: Legal Discrimination Affecting Employment of the Epileptic. *Rehab. Record*, *1:*5:19-22, Sept.-Oct. 1960.

Federation Employment and Guidance Service. Survey of Employers' Practices and Policies in the Hiring of Physically Impaired Workers. New York, The Service, May 1959, 133 p.

Gooddy, W.: Rehabilitation of the Epileptic. *Rehabilitation*, *7:*10-16, Jan. 1953.

Gray, B. H.: The Employment of Epileptics. *Am. A. Indust. Nurses J.*, *4:*3:35-37, Mar. 1956.

Guide to Classification and Employment of Persons with Neurological Disorders. Council on Occupational Health. *J.A.M.A.*, *176:*58, April 8, 1961.

Hammond, H. S.: The Epileptic Cases. The Performance of Physically Impaired Workers in Manufacturing Industries. Bull. No. 927, U. S. Dept. of Labor, Bureau of Labor Statistics, 1948.

Hibbard, B. F.: *Are Epileptics Employable?* National Association to Control Epilepsy, New York, 1945.

Lione, J. G.: Convulsive Disorders in a Working Population. *J. Occupational Med.*, *3:*369-373, August 1961.

Lorbeer, L. T., and Barron, C. I.: Employment of Persons with Epilepsy and Heart Disease. *Calif. Med.*, *88:*2:160-165, Feb. 1958.

Montgomerie, J. F.: Employers and the Epileptic. *Rehabilitation*, *31:*5:7-9, 11-12, Oct.-Dec. 1959.

Olshansky, S. S.: A Plea for the Employment of Epileptics. *Occupations*, *29:*1:51-52, Oct. 1950.

Risch, F.: New Horizons in Rehabilitation of the Epileptic. *J. A. Phys. & Ment. Rehab.*, *14:*5:129-131, 141, Sept.-Oct. 1960.

Schecter, D. S.: Helping Epileptics Into Jobs. *J. Rehab.*, *18:*5:13-14, 29-30, Sept.-Oct. 1952.

Shafter, A. J., and Wright, G. N.: Planning Vocational Objectives with Epileptics. *J. Rehab.*, *27:*2:11-12, Mar.-Apr. 1961.

Tatlow, W. F. T.: Employment of Epileptic Patients. *Occupational Therapy*, *16:*1:8-26, Jan. 1953.

Udel, M. M.: *The Work Performance of Epileptics in Industry*. New York, Columbia University, 1959. 16 p.

U. S. Civil Service Commission: *Employment of Epileptics in the Federal Service*. (CSC Form 614) Washington, D. C.: Govt. Print. Off., Aug. 1958. 5 p.

U. S. Office of Vocational Rehabilitation. Facts in Brief: Persons with Epilepsy Rehabilitated in Fiscal Year 1957. (Rehabilitation service series no. 450, supplement 6.) Govt. Print. Off., July, 1958.

U. S. Dept. of Veterans Benefits. Occupations of Epileptic Veterans of World War II and the Korean Conflict. (V.A. pamphlet 22-6.) Washington, D. C., Govt. Print. Off., Jan. 1960. 62 p.

PREGNANCY AND EPILEPSY

There is some diversity of opinion in regard to the effect of pregnancy on the course of pre-existing epilepsy. For example, Fairfield in her book published in 1954 stated: "The writer had for eighteen years to make arrangements for the care of epileptic women before, during and after confinement and was surprised to find that the fits appeared to be unaltered or diminished with very rare exceptions." On the other hand, in 1961, Huhmar and Jarvinen reported a study of ninety-six women with epilepsy during pregnancy or the puerperium and concluded that pregnancy constitutes a risk for most patients with serious epilepsy.

I have had occasion to observe approximately 300 patients during the course of their pregnancies. Some of these patients had had several pregnancies while under my care for the treatment of their epileptic disorders. Each of the 300 patients took antiepileptic medication regularly throughout the duration of their pregnancy. The frequency of seizures during pregnancy remained essentially unchanged in the vast majority of these patients. In a few instances, the seizure state was worsened, that is, the seizures occurred more frequently and/or became more severe; in a few cases, the incidence of seizures was reduced. The specific details of these observations will be reported at a later date.

It has been my experience that epileptic seizures per se do not cause abortions or adversely affect the unborn child. There are only rare instances where epilepsy of itself provides definite reason for therapeutic abortion. I can cite the case of a young female who suffered with relatively infrequent seizures. During the latter stages of her first two pregnancies, she had severe attacks of status epilepticus which almost terminated in death. The question of a therapeutic abortion arose when she became pregnant for the third time. I definitely consider that epilepsy constitutes an indication for a therapeutic abortion in such an instance and recommended that it be performed during the early stages of this third pregnancy. The problem of sterilization of the epileptic is discussed in the latter part of this chapter.

It is important to bear in mind that convulsions occurring during the course of a pregnancy in an epileptic patient may not necessarily be a recurrence of the epileptic disorder, but may be a manifestation of a toxemia of pregnancy.

Antiepileptic medication should be prescribed during the entire pregnancy. In most instances I maintain the patient on the same dosage of medication which she had been taking prior to her pregnancy. In some instances, however, I recommend that the dosage of the patient's medication be increased during pregnancy, particularly in those patients who have experienced an increase in frequency and/or severity of seizures in association with previous pregnancies.

I have frequently been asked the following question: "Does the anticonvulsant medication have any deleterious effect on the offspring?" I obtained information concerning the immediate and subsequent clinical course of hundreds of offspring of epileptic mothers, many of whom had been taking relatively large doses of anticonvulsant medication including barbiturates. None of these babies appeared to have been adversely affected by absorption of the mother's antiepileptic drugs.

The decision in regard to whether any individual epileptic patient should become pregnant is obviously a personal problem which is best settled by the patient and her physician. In our clinic we do not advise against pregnancy unless the patient's epileptic disorder is such that it would materially interfere with the normal care and management of the offspring. The reader may refer to the section of this chapter entitled Marriage and Epilepsy for further discussion of this subject.

BIBLIOGRAPHY

Fairfield, L.: *Epilepsy, Grand Mal, Petit Mal Convulsions.* London, Gerald Duckworth & Co., Ltd., 1954.

Huhmar, E., and Jarvinen, P. A.: Relation of Epileptic Symptoms to Pregnancy, Delivery and Puerperium, *Ann. chir. et gynaec. Fenniae, 50:*49-64, 1961.

Suter, C., and Klingman, W. O.: Seizure States and Pregnancy. *Neurology, 7:*105, 1957.

MARRIAGE AND EPILEPSY

The three questions which are foremost in the minds of many epileptics when they approach or reach the marrying age are: "Should I marry?", "Can I marry?" and "Should I have children?"

Marriage is one of the accepted goals of adult life and those who feel that they may be deprived of their right or opportunity in this sphere cannot help but be adversely affected, each in his own way. Reasonably normal social contacts and experiences with other people form a basis on which marriage becomes a reality. However, many epileptics, because of over-protection by their families or because of personal fears of having a seizure in public, do not socialize and, therefore, do not get or benefit from normal social contacts. By the very nature of the illness and the feelings which it arouses, epilepsy is often mainly responsible for producing the personal and social isolation which renders marriage unlikely. I know of many young females with mild epileptic disorders who grew up with unfounded fears and conflicts regarding marriage and consequently became almost completely anti-social; because of this, they had little or no opportunity to meet a prospective marriage partner.

Should An Epileptic Marry?

There is certainly no medical reason for the epileptic not to marry. Obviously, this does not apply to the small percentage of epileptics who are severely retarded either mentally or physically or both, or to the epileptic whose seizure disorder is of such severity that it would cause undue hardship on his mate.

I have seen many patients who believed that they should not marry for one or more of the following reasons: (1) they felt that marriage was not "good for their epilepsy;" (2) they did not want to inflict the burden of their illness on their mates; and (3) they feared that their children might develop epilepsy.

My findings definitely indicate that marriage per se does not adversely affect an epileptic disorder. Hundreds of my epileptic patients have married and are leading happy and productive lives. I can definitely state that the emotional satisfaction derived from married life has helped to stabilize many of my patients.

It is the moral responsibility of an epileptic who is contemplating marriage to inform his mate as to the exact nature and extent of his epileptic disorder. This could, in many instances, prevent future misunderstandings and marital difficulties relative to the epileptic disorder and should also lessen the fear and anxiety of inflicting the burden of the illness on their mate. Obviously the non-afflicted individual must realize that marrying an epileptic may possibly cause some socio-economic hardships. I have found that young epileptic males in particular are somewhat reluctant to consider marriage for fear that they may have difficulty in obtaining employment which would enable them to support a wife.

The physician and other qualified persons (social workers, clergymen) can perform a very important service by inviting both partners to a consultation during which questions relative to marriage and epilepsy can be discussed. Of paramount and obvious importance is the necessity that the prospective marital partner be fully aware of the medical and social aspects of the epileptic disorder.

It is my general policy to routinely discuss these questions with younger individuals as they approach the marrying age. I have found that this gradual indoctrination has helped to avoid or at least minimize the problems and difficulties associated with the general misconception that an epileptic should not marry. I endeavor to preclude the development of anti-social tendencies by strongly encouraging my epileptic patients to participate as completely as possible in the social functions appropriate for their age group.

Can An Epileptic Marry?

In July, 1962, I investigated the laws of the fifty states and found that there is some type of restrictive legislation with respect to marriage and epilepsy in the following seven states: Delaware, Michigan, Nebraska, North Carolina, Utah, Virginia and West Virginia.

In addition I would like to call attention to the fact that some of these states also designated the following as a *crime*: (1) for an epileptic to marry; (2) for the solemnizing official to perform the marriage knowing one of the parties is epileptic; (3) for an epileptic to make a false statement regarding his epileptic condition in the application for a marriage license; and (4) for the licensing official to issue a marriage license when it is known that one of the parties is epileptic.

It is difficult for me to accept the fact that in these modern times there are still seven states which have restrictive legislation relative to the marriage of an epileptic. I can understand why such laws were formulated in ancient times, since epilepsy was then considered to be an unquestionably inheritable disorder. Today, however, I would classify these restrictive legislative measures as definitely archaic and unwarranted.

It is my definite belief that these measures are ineffective and may be considered "absurd," since they are not rigidly enforced in most of these states, and also, many individuals with epilepsy marry in these states without revealing the fact that they have epilepsy to the legal officials. In addition, the known epileptic who wishes to marry can move to a section of the United States which has no such prohibitive marital regulations.

On the other hand, the existence of these statutes does "harm" to the overall epileptic population by perpetrating the many existent stigmas associated with epilepsy. These restrictive laws do not reflect the current enlightened medical opinion and there is certainly no medical basis for their continuance. This restrictive legislation can cause a great deal of unnecessary emotional damage to the epileptic who is denied the marriage right. It is known that the epileptic is faced with many unwarranted socio-economic problems, such as employment and acceptance as a "first class citizen," and denial of the privilege of marrying obviously adds to his difficulties.

I am of the opinion that the legislators of the heretofore mentioned seven states just "have not gotten around" to removing these discriminatory legislative measures from the statutes of their respective states. However, I feel quite certain that in the not too distant future epileptics will be permitted to marry in all sections of the United States.

I have frequently been asked whether the concealment of epilepsy constitutes ground for divorce or annulment of a marriage. The legal interpretation of this problem is presented in *American Jurisprudence*, Vol. 35, 1941, page 255, as follows:

"Statutes may, and frequently do, prohibit marriages of epileptics, or of epileptics under a certain age, but the marriage of an epileptic is not void where the statute merely forbids it under penalty of imprisonment.

The view has been taken that false representations at the time of marriage as to the cessation of epilepsy constitute no ground for annulment of the marriage, at least, fraudulent concealment of epilepsy is no ground for annulling a consumated marriage. But where marriage by an epileptic is penalized by statute, an annulment or divorce may be granted for concealment of the disease as for fraud, the reasoning being that there was a concealment of an incapacity to marry, which constituted a fraud on the law and on the other party. However, under a statute declaring that no marriage shall be contracted between persons either of whom is epileptic, a marriage is not voidable at the suit of the husband on the sole ground that the wife was an epileptic at the time of the marriage, in the absence of any showing of fraud or concealment, where it does not appear that the wife ever knew that her trouble was epilepsy."

Should An Epileptic Have Children?

In our present state of knowledge, this question is difficult to answer, because no positive information is available. In fact, from the results obtained in a recent survey conducted in our clinic, we could not prove or disprove hereditary transmission of epilepsy.

In dealing with the problem of inheritability with couples contemplating marriage, it is better to present the facts and leave to them the decision concerning the advisability of having children. This is a personal problem; some individuals would prefer a calculated risk rather than be denied the satisfaction of parenthood. The possibility of having an abnormal child is not restricted to epileptics. There is a calculated risk that the offspring of any couple may be abnormal in any one of many respects. I do not believe that the chances of an epileptic's having an epileptic offspring are very much greater than that which exists in the normal population. The hereditary aspects of epilepsy are discussed in another section of this book entitled Heredity and Epilepsy (Chapter 16).

I base my decision in regard to marriage and children primarily on the frequency of the patient's seizures and his or her physical and mental ability to raise a family. Obviously, an individual who has frequent epileptic seizures would most likely be unable to care adequately for a family.

EDUCATION FOR THE EPILEPTIC

Even in these modern times many epileptic individuals are prohibited from attending public schools and colleges merely on the basis of a diagnosis of epilepsy. In 1958, Wallace made a survey of the 106 cities in the United States with a population of 100,000 or more concerning the educational provisions for children with epilepsy. He states that "twenty-two (22.4%) of the ninety-eight responding urban school services reported that they had no provision for children with epilepsy," and also that 33.7 per cent or "thirty-three school systems delay admission of children with epilepsy beyond the usual age or school admission of 'normal children'."

The rejection of a qualified epileptic from school is not only unfair, but it is not the attitude to assume with respect to any medical disability. The intellectual and physical capabilities of each person should be measured and the decision in regard to school attendance should be governed accordingly.

I have found that too often children with epilepsy are automatically considered to be "material" for a "special class" and no attempt is made to evaluate them on an individual basis. It is true that some epileptics should not and cannot attend regular public school classes with normal children. Some do not have the intelligence necessary for normal school work; others have seizures so frequently that they cannot perform normal scholastic activities, in addition to the fact that the occurrence of the seizures themselves would disrupt the activities of both the teacher and the other pupils.

It has been my experience, however, that most epileptic patients can be placed in a regular class with normal children. Lennox investigated the type of schooling received by children with epilepsy in the Massachusetts public schools. An analysis of his findings reveals some encouraging facts. In 1942, 21 per cent of the epileptic school population were attending regular classes, whereas in 1958, 76 per cent of the epileptic school population were attending regular classes. In 1942, 63 per cent of the epileptic children received home instruction, whereas in 1958, only 6 per cent of the epileptic children received home instruction. It is of interest to note that Wallace also reported that "most school children with epilepsy are in regular classes."

I believe that every effort should be made for children with epilepsy to attend regular schools and that home instruction and special schools should be utilized only when absolutely necessary. The names of some of the special schools and institutions may be obtained by contacting one of the national lay epilepsy organizations or its local chapter, or by consulting the *Directory for Exceptional Children*, which presents a state-by-state listing of the names and programs of the various schools.

Certainly, it is obvious that attendance in regular schools will help insure the development of the epileptic child to the fullest of his capacity. Competent educators agree that there is no question as to the desirability for education of the epileptic child with normal children in regular classrooms. An epileptic child whose seizures are under control and who has no co-existing mental defect or illness needs no special school facilities. Also, most children who have only an occasional seizure can be taught effectively in a regular classroom with normal children. An occasional seizure in the classroom need not, and does not, interfere with the conduct of the class if the teacher and the other students are instructed how to cope with such a situation. Placing an intelligent and emotionally stable epileptic child in a school environment other than normal can do irreparable damage to his emotional stability.

An epileptic child, like any other child, needs and is also entitled to an education. Most of my school age patients who have normal intelligence attend public schools and colleges and do well scholastically. Obviously, the patient with frequent seizures (daily, weekly) could not, in most instances, be educated in a public school because of the frequent interruptions caused by the seizures. However, it is important to note that this does not necessarily apply to patients whose seizures occur only in association with sleep. These individuals should be permitted to attend public schools. Educable patients with frequent seizures which occur during the daytime can obtain their education from home teachers or at so-called private hospital schools. The mentally retarded child with or without seizures will have to attend a special school or a custodial institution of some type.

I know of an instance where a qualified epileptic child was refused admission to the only public school in his community. He was told by the school authorities that the refusal of admission was due primarily to the fact that the teacher absolutely refused to have an epileptic in her class. My initial discussion with this teacher revealed that she was exceedingly poorly informed in regard to the disorder of epilepsy. However, after several consultations during which the nature of the condition was explained, she agreed to accept epileptic students in her classes. The reader may refer to the specific section of this book entitled What Should a Teacher Tell the Classmates about an Epileptic Patient? in Chapter 14 (Should Epilepsy be Publicized?) for some suggestions in regard to the management of an epileptic in the classroom.

I would like to call attention to the fact that in some instances the school personnel is not responsible for the exclusion of normally intelligent epileptic students from the public schools. I have encountered some instances where the parents refused to send their epileptic child to regular schools and made provisions for him to receive his education at home from a special private tutor. The parents did this, so I was told, to preclude any possible social repercussions either to themselves or to their child which might result from exposure of their child's epileptic condition. I know of several other instances where socially prominent parents sent their epileptic children to out-of-town resident schools for this same reason.

I have met several school teachers who had made a practice of giving special privileges to the epileptic children in their classes. They were exceedingly over-protective and lenient and never employed the normal scholastic disciplinary measures in the case of an epileptic pupil. When I asked why they assumed such an attitude, these teachers stated that they had the impression that emotional stress and strain can cause seizures in some patients. I do not believe that normal scholastic disciplinary measures create significant psychological distress in most epileptic patients. Handling a child in an unfair or discriminatory manner can cause more emotional harm than a fair punishment. Therefore, I generally recommend that the epileptic child receive the "same normal discipline" as other children. I have observed that this procedure has not increased the frequency of epileptic seizures in any of my patients.

Many years ago, we did experience instances where intellectually normal epileptics were prohibited from attending regular public schools in Maryland. However, at the present time this problem is non-existent and patients with epilepsy are admitted to the regular public school classes; in fact, hundreds of my patients are attending public schools in the State of Maryland at the present time. There are occasions, however, when it is necessary to remove an epileptic from the regular public school system, such as in the case of the individual who has seizures so frequently that he cannot function in a normal school environment. In such instances, the patient's physician is contacted and a decision as to "what is best for the child" is determined by the physician and the school authorities. These patients, if educable, generally receive their education from home teachers supplied by the public school system. The child is returned to the regular school environment as soon as his seizures are brought under control. In those instances where there is an associated mental retardation, the child may have to be placed in a school for mentally retarded children—not because of his epilepsy, but because of his mental capacity. Many of my patients have had occasional seizures in class and, by and large, the situation was handled appropriately by the school teacher and the classmates.

In the past many of my patients, including those who had been free of seizures for years, were refused admission to some colleges and universities merely on the basis of a diagnosis of epilepsy. In many instances, the general policy of a university was automatic rejection of individuals with a history of epilepsy. This rejection was undoubtedly due to misunderstanding of the disorder of epilepsy. It was my opinion that some administrative officials of various universities had the impression, which was so widespread in the past, that the epileptic did not have the mental capacity to achieve a higher education.

I have observed, however, that within recent years many colleges have adopted a more lenient, and also a more realistic, attitude in regard to the admission of epileptic students. This enlightened policy is probably based on a better understanding of the epileptic disorder by the administrators of colleges and universities.

Many of my patients are currently attending colleges in all sections of the United States, in spite of the fact that some of them still experience periodic seizures. Also, many of my epileptic patients have already successfully completed their college careers and are performing very well in all vocations and professions.

It has been my experience that, generally, the larger colleges are less reluctant to admit epileptic pupils than the smaller ones. I have also observed that state universities and colleges usually admit epileptic students more readily than private universities. Since there are great variations in the individual admitting practices of colleges and universities, the interested person should contact the school in question to ascertain its specific policy in regard to the admittance of epileptics.

In his book published in 1960, Lennox relates similar experiences in regard to higher education for the epileptic.

Training for the Future

One of the most important factors in planning the educational program of an individual who suffers with epilepsy, and one which in my experience has been very much neglected, is that he acquire the training and education which are needed for a suitable remunerative occupation. This is of particular importance in the case of males. An individual's scholastic endeavors should be directed toward a vocation or profession, the performance of which will not be adversely affected by the occurrence of seizures.

It is obvious that the occurrence of seizures will exclude the epileptic from certain types of employment. Therefore, an individual who has had seizures for many years, regardless of how infrequently they recur, should not undertake an educational program whose ultimate goal, for example, is surgery. Such an individual's educational training should be directed towards a type of employment which would be essentially unaffected by his disease.

It is the responsibility of the parents, the school counselors and the physician to see that advice in these matters is forthcoming. Discussions concerning the patient's future vocation should be started at an early age, so that he can adjust his scholastic training accordingly. I have found that, generally, the most appropriate time to initiate such discussions is during the first or second year of high school.

The types of employment which I consider suitable and unsuitable for the epileptic are listed in Tables 15 and 16 which are presented in the section of this chapter entitled Employment for the Epileptic.

It will be noted in Table 15 that there are many professions and vocations listed as being suitable for the epileptic with infrequent seizures. However, it is obvious that in each instance the choice of any specific occupation must be made on a selective basis, depending upon the frequency, character and duration of the individual's seizures. For example, it will be noted that school teaching is recommended for adult education only. It is obvious that the calculated risk of causing a panicky situation and disrupting classroom activities would be quite great if a teacher were to have a seizure in the presence of very young children, such as those in the elementary grades and even those in the first year of high school. However, I do not believe that such would be the case in classrooms consisting of adults. In fact, several of my patients are currently teaching in the upper grades of high school and at college and have had seizures periodically without causing any undue inconvenience or alarm. I advise my adult educators that they should inform the members of their classes of their disorder at the beginning of the school term and also that they should briefly discuss the disorder of epilepsy.

It will be noted in Table 16 that epileptics are listed as being unsuitable for the Armed Services and also for the Roman Catholic priesthood. Actually, it would be more appropriate to say that epileptics are not acceptable for such vocations. My comments in regard to the suitability of epileptics for the Armed Services are presented in the section of this chapter entitled Attitude of the Armed Services Toward Epilepsy.

The following information relative to the epileptic and the Roman Catholic priesthood was supplied to me by Reverend James H. Brennan, S.S., J.C.D., St. Mary's Seminary, Baltimore, Maryland.

"Those who are, or who have been epileptics," are forbidden to receive orders, or to exercise orders that have been already received. (Canon 984, # 3; *Codex Juris Canonici*).

However, permission to receive orders is sometimes granted by competent ecclesiastical authority especially in the case of epilepsy contracted in childhood but which has ceased and, in the judgement of medical authorities, a total cure has been effected. But if the epilepsy is contracted after adolescence permission to receive orders is seldom granted. (Cappello, *De Sacramentis*, Vol. II, pars. III, ## 482-489.)

If epilepsy is contracted after ordination, the ordained priest's superior may permit him to exercise his orders after satisfying himself that the priest is free of the disease. (Canon 984, # 3; *Codex Juris Canonici*.)

BIBLIOGRAPHY

Abraham, W.: Educational Problems of College Age Persons with Seizures. *Exceptional Children*, 22:4:147-151, 174, Jan. 1956.

Beck, H. S.: A Comparison of Convulsive Organic, Nonconvulsive Organic, and Nonorganic Public School Children. *Am. J. Mental Deficiency*, 63:5:866-875, Mar. 1959.

Illinois Epilepsy League: *The Child with Epilepsy in Your School*. Chicago, The League 1956. 20 pp.

Lampe, J. M.: Education and Epilepsy. *J. School Health*, 29:6:220-223, June 1959.

Lennox, W. G.: *Epilepsy and Related Disorders*. Vol. II. Boston, Little, Brown and Co., 1960.

Directory for Exceptional Children, 3rd Edition. Porter Sargent, Publisher, 11 Beacon St., Boston, Mass.. 1958.

Wallace, H. M.: School Servces for Children with Epilepsy in Urban Areas. *J. Chron. Dis.*, 12:654, 1960.

INSURANCE FOR THE EPILEPTIC

Life Insurance

I have discussed the problem of life insurance for the epileptic with executives of many insurance companies in the United States and I also talked to the Chairmen of the Mortality Committees of the Society of Actuaries and of the Medical Directors Association concerning the problems of insurance for epileptic patients. These Committees are charged with the responsibility of compiling the available mortality statistics on different classes of risks insured at standard or extra premium rates who have medical histories or impairments of possible mortality significance.

I was told that the field of extra premium life insurance has gradually broadened in scope over a period of the last thirty to fifty years. Substandard (extra premium) insurance, so I was told, was issued on a very limited basis by one company prior to the turn of the century when selected individuals were insured with experimental extra premiums to cover an expected extra risk because of certain medical histories or physical defects. The comparative success of this early experimental practice encouraged gradual growth until today it is a fact that most companies will accept a broad range of special risks at some increase over the premium charged for standard policyholders. It extends to a great many medical impairments or disease entities as well as to physical impairments and defects.

I was informed by the Chairmen of the heretofore mentioned Committees that available statistics to date relative to the mortality of epileptics are not substantial in volume, but show some impairment of longevity of epileptics compared with individuals without such a history. Many of the large insurance companies utilize these statistics in evaluating the insurability of epileptics. I examined this data and agree with Lennox who stated in his book published in 1960 that ". . . the reader is puzzled by the scarcity of the cases and the slim criteria on which mortality ratios are based." It is my opinion that these statistics are not only insignificant because of the exceedingly small number of cases, but also that many of the conclusions derived from this small study group would not be accepted by experts in the field of epilepsy. In addition, these statistics definitely do not reflect modern treatment and control methods available to epileptics today.

I am certain that insurance companies are cognizant of the fact that they are unknowingly insuring many epileptic patients. I have encountered many individuals with epilepsy who obtained life insurance without acknowledging the fact that they have or have had epileptic seizures. These patients had their insurance applications filled out by physicians who were not aware that these individuals had epilepsy. Since the statistical data utilized by the insurance industry does not include the mortality experiences of the large number of insured individuals who have not revealed their epileptic condition, it is obvious that this statistical data definitely does not give a true picture of the mortality ratios of the insured epileptic population. Actually, I believe that the statistical data currently being utilized by many insurance companies in the evaluation of the mortality of the epileptic is worthless, misleading and definitely should be discarded. The reader may refer to this data which is included in the "Impairment Study" conducted by the Society of Actuaries for the years 1935-1949 and published in 1954 by Peter F. Mallon, Long Island City, New York.

My experience has been that, by and large, the mortality rate of the overall epileptic population is not significantly higher than that of the non-epileptic population. The reader may refer to the section of this book entitled Prognosis of Epilepsy (Chapter 17) for a discussion in regard to the mortality of the epileptic.

I believe that the insurance industry at large is many years behind in their understanding of the outcome of the overall epileptic population and because of this, many epileptics are denied the privilege of life insurance or penalized by higher premium rates. I believe that much could be gained, both by the patient and the insurance company, if the insurance industry would follow the policy adopted by many Motor Vehicle Departments relative to the issuing of driving licenses to epileptics. Under these programs, epileptics are screened by physicians who are experienced in the diagnosis and prognosis of epilepsy.

It is my belief that it will not be too long before all, or at least most, of the major insurance companies will become more interested in the disorder of epilepsy. I agree with Lennox who states, "Insurance companies have contributed substantially to the lowering of morbidity and mortality, especially in 'big name' diseases. They have taken little interest in epilepsy." The improvement in the status of these "big name" diseases has been accomplished through various media such as pamphlets and booklets made available to the general public. I believe that the same beneficial effects would result if the insurance companies would utilize similar programs for the disorder of epilepsy.

I am definitely convinced that with the accumulating mortality statistical evidence from insurance being issued currently and to be issued in the future, proof of the improved mortality outlook for epileptic patients will undoubtedly become available. This, together with the opinion of specialists on the convincingly more favorable outlook for the treatment of epilepsy, will result in more and more favorable terms for life insurance for epileptics as time goes on. This somewhat improved attitude toward liberality for life insurance for epileptics is exemplified by the fact that some companies are already issuing this type of insurance to epileptics at premiums varying from standard to moderately sub-standard extra premium charges, depending upon the particular factors in an individual case. The following are the current attitudes of some of the insurance companies in regard to the insurability of the epileptic.

Dr. F. R. Stearns, Vice President and Medical Director, the Security Benefit Life Insurance Company, Topeka, Kansas, stated:

"As to the insurability for life insurance of epileptics, the approach of various companies differs. Most companies do not accept epileptics under age of fifteen. The mortality ratings, although not well founded statistically, are made dependent on the time lapsed since last epileptic seizure, the type of seizures, the frequency of seizures, and the response to treatment. Post-traumatic and Jacksonian epilepsy is appraised differently from idiopathic epilepsy; type of injury, neurological deficit, success of operation, and control of seizures determines the mortality rating. Most companies consider petit mal seizures less life shortening than grand mal seizures apparently because of the lesser accident risk. Very little attention has been paid to the appraisal of psychomotor seizures and focal epilepsy because statistics are hardly available and because these cases very rarely come to the attention of Medical Departments of life insurance companies.

"In the approach of the Medical Department of our own Company, we accept children with idiopathic epilepsy after the age of five years. We are of the opinion that idiopathic epilepsy has no higher mortality in children when response to treatment is satisfactory, and we only postpone or decline children in whom seizures are not controllable, where serious behavior problems are present, or where epilepsy is complicated by other physical impairments. Taking into account the mortality rate of epilepsy in comparison to the mortality rate of the entire population, we find that the mortality rate of epileptics is only slightly higher than the mortality rate of the population at large. However, those patients who generally apply for life insurance are not the best controlled cases; and although no statistics are available for the various degrees of control in epilepsy as to mortality rate, we have to assume that the mortality in these cases is somewhat higher than the mortality in the total epileptic population. However, we have adjusted our excess mortality rating to the fact that the mortality statistics of epileptics are quite favorable and that, therefore, our own excess mortality ratings in epilepsy are lower than that of most other companies. We rate patients with grand mal seizures slightly higher than those with petit mal and psychomotor seizures only because of the fact there is greater danger of accident or injury. As to Jacksonian seizures, we do not rate them differently from grand mal or petit mal seizures depending on the type of attack, whether with or without loss of consciousness; when successfully operated on and well controlled, we accept these cases with lower mortality ratings and, several years after successful management, even without any extra rating. As to convulsive disorders after brain tumor, the brain tumor and not the convulsive disorder is the determining factor in the mortality consideration. Epileptic equivalents generally are considered in the same way as petit mal or psychomotor epilepsy.

"Our approach to the life insurance of patients with convulsive disorders has not essentially changed in the last twelve years. Although our experience has remained limited both in number of insured persons and in years of exposure, we have had only one death attributable to epilepsy (status epilepticus) among several hundred of insured persons with convulsive disorders."

Dr. W. H. Scoins, Vice President and Chief Medical Director, The Lincoln National Life Insurance Company, Fort Wayne, Indiana, stated:

"Let it be said first that our company has been offering insurance to individuals with a history of epilepsy for many years. As would be expected our underwriting practices have changed gradually, being influenced by the advances in diagnostic and treatment facilities, a generally better understanding of all the convulsive disorders, to some extent by mortality studies on insured lives and also a company philosophy which strives to insure as many as possible at as fair a price as possible. You will understand, of course, that for us in insurance, classification of these cases is often difficult. Our policyholders, patients of private practitioners, come to us from all social and economic classes and present a variety of diagnostic and treatment backgrounds. All too frequently we are unable to develop as complete a history as can be developed in a specialty practice such as yours. In other words, the heterogeneity characteristic of epilepsy as a risk group for insurance will itself have an adverse influence on the mortality of the insured epileptic population. In all probability, were we able to develop a more homogeneous risk group of true idiopathic epileptics, as would be obtained in your clinic, our mortality experience might be better. Finally it should be noted that the majority of so-called epileptics applying for insurance are over the pediatric age range.

"With respect to life insurance coverage our underwriting attitude concerning epilepsy has not changed materially since about 1950. Many, if not all, individuals with a history of epilepsy are considered insurable. For those with a history of grand mal seizures we feel it necessary to refuse the more hazardous situations such as children under sixteen, those whose first attack has occurred within a year of application, those with more than six attacks per year or with a history of status epilepticus within the preceding five years, those with demonstrable mental or personality changes, those with circulatory impairments and those in occupations subject to unusual accident hazard.

"In accepting individuals with grand mal seizures the essential point is the duration of time during which seizures have been controlled or prevented. Relatively high ratings are required when seizures have occurred within the recent past, but as more and more time elapses without seizures, lower ratings can be used. When treatment has prevented seizures for more than ten years, only minimum ratings are required.

"Similarly, in those cases with a history of petit mal seizures the length of time the individual has been free of seizures is the most important underwriting factor. Those with recent seizures require moderate ratings. Those free of seizures for more than five years can be issued insurance with quite low ratings and, in some cases, on a standard premium basis.

"Individuals with Jacksonian seizures not treated by operation are handled in accordance with the individual circumstances but usually on about the same basis as those with a history of grand mal seizures. Following successful surgery they may be treated in about the same fashion as those with petit mal seizures."

Dr. L. Gordon LaPointe, Vice President and Medical Director, The Manhattan Life Insurance Company, New York, New York, stated:

"A summary review of our underwriting practice in relation to victims of epilepsy reveals the following:

"(1) We will consider epileptics at any time, in relation to the onset of the disease, after a definitive diagnosis as to type has been established.

"(2) We require a routine examination and an attending physician's statement outlining the nature of the treatment and the response thereto.

"(3) In the case of children under ten, since we do not write children under ten on a rated contract, according to Company rules they can usually be insured on the Family Member Plan.

"(4) The amount of rating or extra charge is dependent upon the number of attacks, their frequency and the occupation of the individual and his response to treatment.

"(5) In general, severe grand mal epileptics would probably be rated at age twenty, anywhere from $5.00 to $15.00 a thousand; at age thirty, about $10.00 to $20.00; at age forty, $15.00 to $25.00.

"(6) As a rule, petit mal or Jacksonian epilepsy would rarely be rated at any age more than $3.00 or $4.00 per thousand.

"(7) Usually, we will exclude Waiver of Premium and Double Indemnity.

"(8) Lastly, the Company's usual rules as to amount of insurance, according to the rating, always apply—although, I imagine we would go as high as $50,000 in most instances."

Health, Accident and Hospitalization Insurance

Very few of the insurance executives with whom I consulted would commit themselves to a specific attitude concerning health and accident insurance for the epileptic. However, I concluded that in all probability the epileptic would encounter considerable difficulty in obtaining this type of insurance.

The epileptic usually does not have too much difficulty obtaining some type of hospitalization insurance. It is my understanding that the Blue Cross Plan is the most widely utilized form of insurance for this purpose. Many hospitalization policies are also available from private insurance companies.

The following is an expression from Dr. W. H. Scoins, Chief Medical Director, The Lincoln National Life Insurance Company, Fort Wayne, Indiana:" For accident and sickness coverage, we have not been attempting to handle any grand mal histories. Petit mal and Jacksonian cases are handled on essentially the same basis as for life insurance although the ratings are substantially higher and the period of time free of seizures required for consideration at lower rating levels is considerably longer than is felt necessary for life insurance."

Dr. Clement G. Martin, Medical Director, Continental Casualty Company, Chicago, Illinois, stated: "In 1954 Continental Casualty Company first began to write 'rated' or 'sub-standard' A and H and hospitalization insurance. As Continental is proud of being first in many fields, this was again a First.

"At that time we began to write coverage for epileptics. Following a three year adjustment period we will give them a life-time accident and one year sickness indemnity, with a six months maximum benefit for 'disorders of the central nervous system.' We also offer a basic hospital plan up to 90 days for those under age 60 and a 30 day plan for those over 60 to age 79. In each policy there is a 21 day elimination period for 'any disorder of the central nervous system.'

"We also offer a catastrophe policy with a $400 deductible and a $5000 maximum hospitalization benefit. This also has specific provisions in it for 'any disorders of the central nervous system.' Should they be hospitalized because of this, only the board and room charges are acceptable, however, it is the same as any other catastrophe medical plan for illnesses which do not involve the central nervous system.

"As you know, there are many clubs and associations of epileptics. We have insured numbers of these with these types of policies.

"We have a 'Sub-Standard' mechanism for making insurance available to non-standard risks and we are able to insure epileptics with histories of coronaries, diabetes and malignancies."

Workmen's Compensation Insurance

There are two major aspects of workmen's compensation insurance which I would like to clarify. Firstly, I would like to call the epileptic's attention to the fact that while employed, he is entitled to insurance benefits for injuries sustained during working hours in the same manner as any other individual. Secondly, I have discussed the problem of employment of epileptics with executives of many business organizations and found that there existed considerable confusion and misunderstanding concerning workmen's compensation insurance premiums. Many of these employers had the impression that their workmen's compensation insurance premiums would be elevated if they were to hire epileptics. This assumption is definitely untrue.

The problem of workmen's compensation insurance and employment of the physically handicapped is explained very clearly in a pamphlet published by the Association of Casualty and Surety Companies in cooperation with The President's Committee on Employment of the Physically Handicapped. This pamphlet is entitled, *The Physically Impaired Can be Insured Without Penalty*, and states as follows:

"Let this be understood—there is no provision in workmen's compensation insurance policies or rates that penalizes an employer for hiring handicapped workers.

"There appears to be much misinformation on this point. For many employers have been known to say they could not or would not hire disabled applicants because they had been advised that their insurance costs would be increased as a result. Nothing could be farther from the truth. Employers who have such ideas have simply been hoodwinked by scuttle-butt rumours that are easily circulated because of their sensationalism. It is much more difficult to gain acceptance of the cold, stark truth—because its honesty affords no opportunity for gossip.

"Therefore, to erase any misunderstanding, these are the facts. Workmen's compensation insurance rates are determined by two factors. These are the relative hazards in a company's work and it's accident experience. The formulae for determining the premium rates make no consideration of the kind of personnel hired. Whether a company is staffed with workers having two legs apiece or one or none—influences the rates not at all. The insurance contract, therefore, says nothing implied or direct about the physical condition of the workers an insured may hire.

"It is true that a poor accident experience—that is, a relatively high number or cost of claims over a period of time—will cause an increase in an employer's compensation insurance rates. It is equally true that *if* a disabled worker would be more apt to have accidents and consequently suffer greater disability, as some people once believed, then an employer's insurance might eventually go up. BUT, and this should not be forgotten, research studies conducted by governmental agencies, the Accident Prevention Department of the Association of Casualty and Surety Companies and the New York University Center for Safety Education which it endows, have shown that when placed at the proper jobs the handicapped have an accident experience that is as good as their ablebodied fellow workers—and is often superior. So then, this possibility for an increase in an employer's compensation insurance costs is nullified. In order to assist each industry to achieve proper placement of the handicapped and so to be of service to both employers and the physically impaired, the casualty insurance companies have prepared a booklet, *The Physically Impaired—A Guidebook to Their Employment*, which is free to anyone who requests it from his stock insurance broker.

"In addition, these studies have shown that the properly placed disabled are more reliable workers with an equal or better production record.

"All this sums up to an important conclusion. As long as misinformation and untruths concerning the employability of the handicapped are permitted to be circulated, the chance for these workers to prove they can produce successfully will be denied them. But now you know that the frequently voiced objections to their employment—that is, insurance companies forbid it or insurance costs will rise—are unfair, false and illogical.

"The casualty insurance industry refuses to be accused of blocking the employment of the handicapped not only because such an accusation is unjustified, but also because it is even more harmful to the physically impaired than to the insurance companies."

I believe that the epileptic should be given consideration for employment in the same manner as any other physically impaired individual. It has been my experience that when the epileptic is employed on a selective basis, the accident rate is not greater, and may even be less, than that of the non-epileptic worker. The reader may refer to the section of this book entitled Injuries and Longevity (Prognosis of Epilepsy, Chapter 17) and to the section of this chapter entitled Employment for the Epileptic for details relative to injuries and accidents associated with epilepsy.

Social Security

The information concerning Social Security and epilepsy was supplied to me by:

Mr. Edward L. Binder, Chief, Evaluation Policy Section, Division of Disability Operations, Bureau of Old-Age and Survivors Insurance, Social Security Administration; and,

Dr. Joseph Lerner, Chief Consultant in Psychiatry and Neurology, Division of Disability Operations, Bureau of Old-Age and Survivors Insurance, Social Security Administration.

The old-age, survivors and disability insurance program is a work-related social insurance program under which more than nine out of ten workers and self-employed people in the United States are covered. Contributions are paid into trust funds by employers, covered workers and self-employed persons. Benefits are payable out of these funds to retired and disabled workers and their families and to families of insured workers upon their death. Benefits are related to earnings in covered work.

The old-age, survivors and disability insurance provisions of the Social Security Act include three types of disability protection:

(1) The disability freeze;

(2) Disability insurance benefits; and

(3) Childhood disability benefits.

Depending upon the individual case, insured workers who have become disabled because of an epileptic disorder, their families and disabled epileptic children of insured workers may be entitled to disability benefits of the Social Security Act.

The Disability Freeze

The disability freeze is a provision of the Social Security Act which insures the worker against loss of insured status or reduction in the amount of retirement or survivors benefits resulting from total disability which can be expected to be of long-continued and indefinite duration.

To be eligible for the disability freeze a disabled worker must have worked under social security for at least five years out of the ten years immediately before the beginning date of the disability, and he must be "fully insured."

The disability must have lasted at least six months before the earnings record may be frozen. The worker must be disabled on the date he files for the disability freeze.

For purposes of entitlement to the establishment of a period of disability, "disability" means:

(1) Inability to engage in any substantial gainful activity because of any medically determinable physical or mental impairment which can be expected to result in death or to be of long-continued and indefinite duration.

(2) Blindness as defined in the law.

Disability Insurance Benefits

Disability insurance monthly benefits are provided for workers irrespective of age who meet the following definition of disability: inability to engage in any substantial gainful activity because of any medically determinable physical or mental impairment which can be expected to result in death or to be of long-continued and indefinite duration.

Disability insurance benefits can begin no earlier than the seventh month of a worker's disability, that is, after he has been disabled for a waiting period of six full months. A disabled worker may be paid retroactive benefits for as many as twelve full months before the month of his application—but for no further back than the first month in which he met the requirements of the law.

The amount of a worker's disability insurance benefit is calculated as if the worker were of retirement age at the beginning of the waiting period.

The work requirements are the same as for the disability freeze.

Benefits to Families of Disabled Workers

Beginning with the month of September, 1958, cash benefits are payable to the following members of the families of disabled workers who are receiving disability insurance benefits:

(1) Children under age eighteen, and disabled children eighteen years of age or over whose disability began before their eighteenth birthday.

(2) The wife aged sixty-two or over, or the wife under age sixty-two, if she has in her care a child who is entitled to benefits.

(3) The dependent husband aged sixty-five or over.

Childhood Disability Benefits

Under a disability provision of the 1956 amendments to the Social Security Act, cash benefits were made payable to dependent disabled children aged eighteen or over, of retired or deceased insured workers.

Those individuals who can fulfill the following requirements are entitled to receive Childhood Disability Benefits:

(a) The "child" must be the son or daughter of a worker who either: (1) is entitled to retirement or disability insurance benefits, or (2) died after 1939 after working long enough under Social Security to become insured for the payment of survivors benefits.

(b) The child must meet the following definition of disability: inability to engage in any substantial gainful activity because of any medically determinable physical or mental impairment which can be expected to result in death or to be of long-continued and indefinite duration.

(c) The child's disability must have begun before he reached age eighteen.

(d) In addition, the son or daughter must be at least eighteen years of age, unmarried, and "dependent" upon the worker-parent on whose account he is claiming the benefit.

Filing Applications for Disability Insurance Benefits

Applications for disability insurance benefits should be made at a district office of the Bureau of Old-Age and Survivors Insurance. There are almost 600 such offices throughout the United States and Puerto Rico. They are listed in the telephone book under United States Government, Department of Health, Education, and Welfare, Social Security Administration.

The staff of these district offices will assist any person wishing to file his application and will advise him about obtaining the necessary proofs.

Evidence of Disability

The burden of establishing the existence and duration of disability is on the applicant. Opinions regarding prognosis or functional capacity expressed by the applicant's medical sources are not conclusive. If submitted, they should be supported by an adequate summary of the medical history, course, findings and reasons for the opinion.

An applicant must furnish evidence based upon examinations made by a qualified medical examiner to establish the nature and severity of his impairment from the time he claims it prevented him from engaging in substantial gainful work. The Department of Health, Education, and Welfare may, under certain circumstances, purchase medical evidence to reconcile discrepancies in the proof, obtain more detailed findings, etc. However, this may be done only after the applicant has furnished sufficient evidence to establish the reasonable likelihood of disability.

The medical evidence submitted by the applicant should contain an adequate summary of the history, diagnosis, physical and clinical findings, treatment and response. The clinical facts must be adequate to confirm for the reviewing physician the diagnosis, and to describe the severity of the condition, the response to therapy, and the applicant's residual physical or mental capacity. Where appropriate, the applicant's physician is expected to supply results of tests that he has made to establish the diagnosis or describe the applicant's capacity to function. Where an applicant has been examined in connection with an application for benefits under another disability program or has been hospitalized or institutionalized, the report of such findings or treatment is acceptable in support of the applicant's claim. In many cases the Department will be able to assist an applicant to obtain copies or summaries of medical records.

The applicant should also submit evidence as to his education and training, work experience and daily activities both prior to and after the alleged date of onset of disability, efforts to engage in gainful employment or self-employment and any other pertinent evidence showing the effect of his impairment or impairments on his ability to engage in any substantial gainful activity during the time he alleges he was under a disability.

Determinations of Disability

Determinations of disability are made by State agencies, usually the State vocational rehabilitation agencies, under agreements between the States and the Secretary of Health, Education, and Welfare.

The Department of Health, Education, and Welfare makes disability determinations for persons living in States which have not entered into an agreement with the Secretary, for individuals residing outside the United States and for a few other applicants whose cases are specifically excluded from the Federal-State agreements.

After the claimant has filed his application and supporting evidence in a Social Security district office, the case is transferred to a cooperating State agency. Such further field investigations and medical examinations as may be necessary are carried forward at the initiative of the State agency evaluation team, composed of a physician and a vocational specialist, and that team is responsible for making the disability determination.

The determinations of State agencies are examined by the Bureau of Old-Age and Survivors Insurance to assure consistency of understanding of the disability requirements and conformity with national policies. The Bureau may not reverse a State finding that no disability exists, but it may reverse an allowance of disability. In an appealed case, the hearing examiner and the Appeals Council of the Social Security Administration may reverse a State agency determination of no disability.

When a determination of disability has been made by a State agency, the case file is sent to the central office of the Bureau of Old-Age and Survivors Insurance. The Bureau of Old-Age and Survivors Insurance examines the file and adjudicates such non-disability aspects of the claim as age, insured status, and dependency. Benefits are certified for payment by a payment center. Most disability benefit claims are certified from the payment center in Baltimore, Maryland.

Medical Factors in Determining Effect of Impairments

In order to establish that a medically determinable physical or mental impairment is present there should be evidence that medically discernible anatomical, physiological, biochemical or psychological aberrations exist. An alleged impairment is medically determinable only if it can be verified by the use of clinical and laboratory diagnostic techniques.

The medical evidence should be complete enough to support an independent diagnostic, therapeutic and prognostic conclusion by the State agency or the Social Security Administration, and form a clear picture of the individual's functional limitations. The impairment should be described etiologically, pathologically, physiologically, psychologically and therapeutically.

In determining the severity and expected duration of an impairment, consideration is given to:

(1) Whether the disease is of a type affecting one, or more than one body system;

(2) The extent to which the disease interferes with the ability of all body systems to contribute their share to the individual's capacity for walking, sitting, standing, bending, remembering, seeing, speaking, hearing, manipulating and maintaining interpersonal relationships; and

(3) The etiology of the disease (that is, whether neoplastic, infectious or degenerative).

Sections 404.1511 to 404.1519, Subpart P, Part 404, Chapter III, Code of Federal Regulations relate to specific body systems and the medical evidence generally required and the factors considered in determining the effect of impairments which are most frequently encountered. The medical requirements and the factors considered in determining the effect of an epileptic disorder are described in Section 404.1519 entitled "Impairments involving the nervous system."

"Sec. 404.1519 Impairments involving the nervous system.

"(a) General. Disorders of the nervous system include both organic (resulting from disease or injury) and functional (in which disease or injury to the brain or other parts of the nervous system cannot be demonstrated). These disorders may result in impairment of the individual's ability to perform motor functions, such as walking, manipulating; the ability to communicate, such as in speech disturbances; intellectual functions, such as reasoning, memory; the ability to make social adjustments; or emotional stability, such as depression. As in cases involving other body systems, there is a wide range in the impairments resulting from varying degrees of severity of these conditions.

"(b) Neurological disorders. Among these disorders are cerebrovascular accident, epilepsy, poliomyelitis, Parkinson's Disease, multiple sclerosis, cerebral palsy and head injuries:

"(1) Cerebrovascular accident. ....

"(2) Epilepsy. In cases of epilepsy a complete history, description of seizures and physical examination are needed. The etiology should be defined where possible. Reports of electroencephalographic tracings and medical observation during convulsive seizures, ill effects or injuries resulting from seizures are important evidence. The type of medication, dosage, and duration of and response to accepted therapy should be recorded. Consideration is given to the frequency and type of seizures.

"(3) Anterior poliomyelitis. ....

"(4) Other conditions. ...."

Other Factors in Evaluating Disability

The following are additional factors that may influence the extent of handicap imposed by an impairment and which may be considered in the evaluation of a disability: age, education training and experience.

Automobile Insurance

The general policies and laws dealing with automobile driving and epilepsy vary somewhat from state to state and are discussed in another section of this chapter entitled Automobile Driving and Epilepsy.

Those individuals who secure a license from the Commissioner of Motor Vehicles in their respective communities to operate an automobile should not have difficulty obtaining automobile insurance which provides them with the same coverage as other individuals.

It is quite possible that if an epileptic should have an automobile accident which was considered to be due to a seizure, he may experience difficulty having his automobile insurance renewed in spite of the fact that he may be given permission to drive again at a later date by the Commissioner of Motor Vehicles.

Automobile insurance for epileptics with a driver's license is sometimes issued through an "Assigned Risk Pool," a plan by which the state arbitrarily requires a designated insurance carrier to sell the policy. Insurance obtained through this arrangement ordinarily has a higher rate.

BIBLIOGRAPHY

Arieff, A. J.: Epilepsy and Life Insurance. *Neurology*, 7:259-264, 1957.

Boland, J. E.: *Clinical Medicine vs. Insurance Medicine*. Country Life Insurance Company, June, 1955.

Lennox, W. G.: *Epilepsy and Related Disorders*, Vol. II. Boston, Little, Brown and Co., 1960.

Lew, E. A.: Insurance Mortality. Investigation of Physical Impairments. *Am. J. Pub. Health*, 44:641, 1954.

Yochem, D. E.: *Insuring Special Class Risks*. Indianapolis, Indiana, Research & Review Service, Inc., 1953.

Young, G. G.: Underwriting Consideration of Epilepsy and Convulsive Seizures. *Proc. Am. Life Convention, Medical Section, 42nd Ann. Meet.*, p. 190, 1954.

ATTITUDE OF THE ARMED SERVICES
TOWARD EPILEPSY

At the time of this writing the Medical Fitness Standards of the three Armed Services (Army, Navy and Air Force) designated the following as one of the causes for PEACETIME rejection for appointment, enlistment and induction (Army Regulations 40-501, Medical Service—Standards of Medical Fitness, Dec., 1960; Army Regulations 40-501, Medical Service—Standards of Medical Fitness, April, 1961).

"*Paroxysmal convulsive disorders*, disturbances of consciousness, all forms of psychomotor or temporal lobe epilepsy thereof except for seizures associated with toxic states or fever during childhood up to the age of twelve."

The Medical Fitness Standards set forth by the Army for partial and total mobilization exclude individuals suffering with:

"Convulsive disorders except when infrequent convulsions while under standard drugs which are relatively non-toxic and which do not require frequent clinical and laboratory followings."

Partial mobilization means mobilization resulting from action by Congress or the President, under any law to effect a limited expansion of the active Armed Forces from the Reserve components and other manpower resources of the Nation.

Total mobilization means mobilization resulting from action by Congress or the President, under any law, to effect a maximum expansion of the active Armed Forces from the Reserve components and other manpower resources of the Nation.

The Retention Medical Fitness Standards of the Army designate as medically unfit for future military service individuals who have:

"*Convulsive disorders.* (except those caused by and exclusively incident to the use of alcohol): When seizures are not adequately controlled (complete freedom from seizure of any type) by standard drugs which are relatively non-toxic and which do not require frequent clinical and laboratory checks. However, individuals on active duty who have infrequent seizures while under medication may be recommended for continuance on active duty if they are deemed to be of special value to the service."

My Comment on the Medical Fitness Standards of the Armed Services

The epileptic must understand that he is not necessarily being singled out and denied the privilege of serving in the Armed Services solely because of the many unwarranted social stigmas which currently exist in regard to epilepsy. Individuals with other disorders which have a tendency to be chronic, such as asthma, are also disqualified for military service, regardless of whether the disorder is still active or whether there is merely a past history of asthma.

It is true that organizations of the importance and magnitude of the Armed Services must have Medical Fitness Standards which are considered to be as free of risk as possible. However, it is my impression that the medical attitude of the Armed Services toward epilepsy is entirely too rigid. I agree that many individuals with seizures should be classified as medically unfit for military duty. However, I believe that an individual who has been free of epileptic seizures without medication for a prolonged period of time should be evaluated on essentially the same basis as any other individual.

It is well known that the epileptic encounters difficulties in practically every phase of life and because of this, it is no wonder that many of them develop feelings of insecurity, inferiority and "unwantedness." Refusal of admission to the Armed Services certainly tends to enhance these feelings in many patients, particularly in the teen-age boy who would like to believe that he is "just as good" as his non-epileptic colleague.

I believe that an individual who has been free of epileptic seizures without antiepileptic medication for a prolonged period of time and is otherwise, physically, mentally and emotionally fit, should be given the privilege of serving in the Armed Services. I do not suggest that these individuals pilot an airplane or even be assigned to activities, the performance of which could lead to serious consequences if a seizure should occur. I believe it is the general policy of the Armed Services to assign all individuals to duties which are considered to be most appropriate for their physical, mental and emotional make-up. I feel that the controlled epileptic should be considered individually in this same manner and his fitness for induction or enlistment into the Armed Services be judged accordingly.

If controlled epileptics were to be selected in this manner, I do not believe that the calculated risk of serious consequence outweighs the harm that automatic rejection can do emotionally to the individual in question, and even more so, to the overall epileptic population. Certainly, I do not recommend that the Armed Services be employed as a rehabilitation center or therapeutic tool to help alleviate the many unwarranted stigmas which are currently associated with epilepsy. I make the above recommendations in view of the fact that it has been my experience that an individual who has been free of epileptic spells without medication for a prolonged period and is otherwise normal, can perform as well as non-epileptic individuals.

AUTOMOBILE DRIVING AND EPILEPSY

It is quite obvious that an individual with seizures should not drive an automobile for the protection of the lives and property of others and also for his own protection. The patient must be told that he will have to conduct his activities without having this privilege.

Most adult patients will accept this restriction without much difficulty. In some instances they may be "forced" to change their employment, at least temporarily, until the seizures are controlled. The reader may refer to the section of this chapter entitled Employment for the Epileptic for information concerning the types of jobs which are suitable and not suitable for individuals with seizures.

A very important problem related to automobile driving is that which is presented by the teen-ager. Many teen-agers who are not permitted to drive an automobile develop emotional disorders such as belligerent and antagonistic behavior and marked feelings of inferiority and "being different." It has been my experience that teen-age psychological disturbances frequently can be prevented or at least minimized if the physician informs the patient about this restriction several years or so before he reaches the lawful driving age for his community. The child should be told that, in all probability, he will not be permitted to operate a motor vehicle. He should also be reminded periodically of this fact during his return visits to the physician. I have learned that, in most instances, when a child is gradually indoctrinated with this restriction starting at an early age, he does not become nearly as psychologically disturbed as when he is abruptly told that he will not be permitted to drive an automobile after he has already reached the lawful driving age.

The rules and regulations pertaining to epilepsy and automobile driving vary somewhat from state to state. Most states will allow an epileptic to operate a motor vehicle after he has been free of seizures for a period of time. However, Fabing, in 1960, reported that there are some states where epileptics are designated as a group which shall be denied the driving privilege categorically and by law.

In 1958, the United States Civil Service Commission published a pamphlet in which it is stated, "If a person with a history of convulsive disorder can furnish satisfactory medical proof that he has been free of seizures for a period of at least five years, without the use of medication, he may be authorized to drive motor vehicles" (U. S. Civil Service Commission: *Employment of Epileptics in the Federal Service*, CSC Form 614, Washington, D. C., August, 1958).

The general policy in the State of Maryland is as follows. After a patient has been free of seizures for at least three years, he is given his license to operate a motor vehicle. It is renewable for six month periods on recommendation of his attending physician and approval of the Medical Advisory Board of the Department of Motor Vehicles, provided the patient continues under treatment and has no seizures. In appropriate instances, however, the Medical Advisory Board may make exceptions to this three year blanket ruling of freedom from seizures, such as in the case of individuals whose employment necessitates the operation of an automobile and in those instances where the patient's seizures have always occurred only in association with sleep. In such instances, the Medical Advisory Board may recommend that the patient be issued a license to drive after he has been free of seizures for a period of time shorter than three years. The decision rests entirely upon the discretion of the Medical Advisory Board.

I also believe that a farmer with seizures should be permitted to operate a tractor or motor vehicle on his own property if he cares to do so. The physician should explain to the farmer the calculated risk of injury to himself or his property. The patient should then make the decision himself.

Mr. Robert B. Garrett, Secretary of the Medical Advisory Board, advised me, at the time of this writing, that the following are the procedures involved in securing and maintaining an automobile driver's license in the State of Maryland. The patient should first consult his personal physician and obtain a letter stating the length of time he has been free of seizures and, if he is taking antiepileptic medication, the names and dosages of the drugs. The patient should then submit this letter together with an application to the Department of Motor Vehicles. The patient is given an appointment to appear before the Medical Advisory Board. If the application is approved and the patient passes his driving test, he is granted a license on a six months basis. He is instructed to return and reappear before the Medical Advisory Board in six months. At this time it is necessary that he submit a letter from his physician concerning the status of his epileptic disorder. If the patient has had no seizures and has followed the medical advice of his physician, his license is renewed for another six month period.

These six month appearances are continued at the discretion of the Medical Advisory Board. In many instances, the patient is subsequently relieved of these six month return visits and is instructed to complete and return a form (Form A) at yearly intervals to the Medical Advisory Board.

This plan of issuing automobile driving licenses has been in effect in the State of Maryland for approximately twelve years and has proved to be exceedingly effective. Many of my patients are currently driving automobiles and, to my knowledge, the incidence of accidents in this group is no greater than that which would be expected in a similar number of individuals who do not have epilepsy. In 1961, Mr. Garrett told me that "to my knowledge the incidence of accidents in those patients with epi-

TO THE MEDICAL ADVISORY BOARD
Department of Motor Vehicles
Guilford Avenue and 21st Street
Baltimore 18, Maryland

Gentlemen:

In connection with my status as an operator of motor vehicles in Maryland, I hereby affirm that I have not suffered any form of seizure, blackout, loss of consciousness, or other interruption of consciousness since ....

I also certify that I have kept in touch with my physician at regular intervals as suggested by my physician or as required by Medical Advisory Board instructions, and that I am taking regularly, as prescribed, the medication in dosage as described below:

....
....

....
Signature of Applicant

(Notary)

Personally appeared before me, the undersigned, a Notary Public (Justice of the Peace) of the State of ....residing in said State, this .... day of .... 19............, the above named .... who made oath in due form of law that the above statements are true.

Witness my Hand and Official Seal ....

....
Signature of Notary Public or Justice

Form A. This letter is supplied to the patient by the Secretary of the Medical Advisory Board and is to be returned to this Board at yearly intervals.

lepsy who secured their drivers' licenses in the manner heretofore stated has not been any greater than that in a similar group of non-epileptic individuals."

It is my opinion that the issuance of restricted licenses to controlled epileptics in the manner heretofore described could even result in an accident rate lower than that presented by the general population. I make this statement for the following reasons. Most automobile accidents are caused by carelessness or violation of the codes of automobile driving, such as driving while under the influence of alcohol, violating the speed limits and rushing to "make a light" before it turns red. It has been my experience that the epileptic who is issued a license in the manner described previously realizes that he is on probation and for this reason he is exceedingly cautious in his driving activities. On the other hand, many of the so-called normal individuals frequently assume a more nonchalant attitude in their driving activities.

In 1960, Fabing reported that a somewhat similar policy for granting automobile driving licenses had been established in Wisconsin and that during the first five years this law had been in effect, no one to whom a license was granted by the Wisconsin Board had been involved in a motor vehicle accident because of a seizure. He also stated that these drivers can now obtain a full-coverage liability insurance at premiums which are uprated only five per cent for administrative costs. Fabing called attention to the fact that the number of persons admitting a history of seizures rose substantially after the enactment of this law.

BIBLIOGRAPHY

Fabing, H. D.: Epilepsy and the Law. *Harper's Magazine*, September, 1960, pages 56-59.

Fabing, H. D., and Schwade, E.: Discussions Concerning Driver's License, in *Total Rehabilitation of Epileptics*. U. S. Department of Health, Education, and Welfare, Office of Vocational Rehabilitation, Washington, D. C., January, 1962, pages 17-19, 21-23.

STERILIZATION AND EPILEPSY

Sterilization of an individual with epilepsy with the prime purpose of preventing the birth of an epileptic offspring was practiced extensively in the past. At that time epilepsy was considered by most people, including many physicians, to be an unquestionably inheritable disorder. On the contrary, present-day scientific thinking is of the opinion that the genetic factor in epilepsy is insignificant.

Fabing, in 1962, stated: "In 1956 there were seventeen States that called for the sterilization of epileptics. In none of the statutes was 'epilepsy' defined. In fourteen of them the law was restricted to those epileptics confined to institutions. At the present time most epileptics live in open society outside the walls of institutions, so the laws touched few patients. Furthermore, most States had closed their eyes to the existence of the law, allowing it to sleep quietly between the covers of the code. Present scientific thinking is of the opinion that the genetic factor in epilepsy is so slight that no useful purpose can be served by using the legally wielded knife against the patient's reproductive apparatus. These laws proved to be both unused and useless. They served only one purpose: to perpetuate the stigma against the epileptic. We advocated their repeal. As yet nothing has been accomplished."

I am in complete agreement with Fabing's statements in regard to the laws contained in the statutes of some States relative to the sterilization of the epileptic. There are, however, some instances when sterilization should be recommended, such as is the case with other medical disorders. Two such examples are as follows:

(1) an individual who already has children and who subsequently developed frequent and severe epileptic seizures which had not responded to any of the available antiepileptic therapeutic regimens.

I would recommend sterilization in such instances not because of the fear that the patient would produce an epileptic offspring, but because I believe that there would be a great possibility that she would be unable to adequately care for additional children.

(2) an individual whose epileptic disorder during previous pregnancies became so severe that it almost caused death. I would recommend sterilization in such instances to prevent the possible death of the patient during a subsequent pregnancy, particularly in those instances where the individual already had children.

BIBLIOGRAPHY

Fabing, H. D.: Discussions Concerning Sterilization of the Epileptic, *in Total Rehabilitation of Epileptics*. U. S. Department of Health, Education, and Welfare, Office of Vocational Rehabilitation, Washington, D. C., January, 1962, pages 16-17.

Chapter 16

HEREDITY AND EPILEPSY

FOR thousands of years, epilepsy had been considered by most people, including many physicians, to be an inheritable disorder. Throughout the ages, physicians have speculated on the hereditary aspects of epilepsy. Hippocrates in his treatise *On The Sacred Disease* written around 400 B.C. said "its origins are hereditary" and placed the origin of the seizures in the brain. Jules Preuss stated that among the ancient Hebrews marriage to a woman from an epileptic family was prohibited on the grounds that the disease was hereditary. Kanner, in his *Folklore and Cultural History of Epilepsy*, mentioned that among the ancient Scots epileptic males were castrated, females were isolated, and if an epileptic woman conceived, both mother and child were killed, "that his infected blude culd spread na firther." Kanner also tells of the practice prescribed in early times of orchidectomy as a cure for epilepsy and mentions a Jean Taxil, who in 1603 wrote, "Some have advised eunuchism to cure such malady (epilepsy), though I believe not intending to cure thereby, but to prevent its transmission to offspring."

Even today many individuals, including some physicians, regard epilepsy as an inheritable disorder. For example, Dr. Walter C. Alvarez presented a discussion entitled "Significance of Convulsions" in his syndicated column which appeared in the *Baltimore Sun*, Tuesday, July 17, 1962. It is my impression that Dr. Alvarez believes that epilepsy is an unquestionably inheritable disorder and that the hereditary factor is one of the most important considerations in determing the outcome of an individual who suffers with convulsions. I certainly disagree completely with Dr. Alvarez's evaluation of the importance of heredity in epilepsy and I feel quite sure that most authorities would also take exception to Dr.

Alvarez's dogmatic statements regarding the hereditary transmission of epilepsy.

There are some significant studies which have been presented in the medical literature concerning heredity and epilepsy. The following are summaries of the findings of some of the investigators who are considered to be experts in the fields of epilepsy and/or genetics: Lennox, Metrakos and Metrakos, Harvald and Alström. There is also a summary of the investigation carried out in our clinic.

LENNOX

Lennox has conducted extensive investigations into the hereditary aspects of the epileptic disorder. The results of his comprehensive studies of the incidence of electroencephalographic abnormalities in the relatives of epileptics, the incidence of epilepsy in the relatives of epileptics and concordance with regard to epilepsy in monozygotic twins, have been interpreted by some physicians as evidence favoring inheritance as a predominant etiological factor in epilepsy. Lennox is generally regarded as the leading proponent of the concept that hereditary factors assume a major role in the pathogenesis of epilepsy.

To determine the frequency of epilepsy in the relatives of epileptics, Lennox, in 1951, divided his 4,231 patients into two groups: those with evidence of brain damage that predated the first seizure, and those without such cerebral damage. The former group accounted for 23 per cent of the total and the latter group comprised 77 per cent of the total. He investigated the 20,000 relatives and found that 643 or 3.2 per cent revealed a history of seizures. The incidence of epilepsy among the near relatives of the patients without brain damage was 3.6 per cent; the incidence for the group of cerebrally damaged patients was 1.8 per cent.

Employing one per cent as the approximate incidence of epilepsy in the general population, Lennox calculated the incidence of epilepsy among all the relatives to be 3.2 times the normal. The ratio was 3.6 to 1 for relatives of the group with metabolic epilepsy and 1.8 to 1 for relatives of those patients with "some acquired condition." Lennox concluded that "the genetic factor in the organic" (acquired) "group was one-half the genetic factor in the nonorganic" (metabolic).

Lennox investigated the relationship of the age of the patient at the time of the initial seizure to the incidence of epilepsy in the relatives. In the nonorganic series, Lennox reported that the incidence of epilepsy among the relatives decreased (6.4% to 1.5%) as the age at onset of seizures in the patient increased (0-1 year to over 30 years).

In 1960, Lennox examined the records of 2,053 patients to determine the relationship of the age of the patient at the onset of seizures to the incidence of epilepsy among the families. As with the influence of age on the number of affected relatives, Lennox demonstrated that the familial incidence of epilepsy decreased as the age of the patient at the time of the first seizure increased. However, the percentual differences for the incidence of epilepsy among families (46.8% at ages 0 to 1 year and 18.1% after 30 years of age) were less marked than the corresponding differences among the relatives (6.4% and 1.5%, respectively). The ratio of the spread for the group of relatives was 4.2 to 1, whereas the spread for the group of families was 2.6 to 1. In the tabulation of familial epilepsy, Lennox reported that the percentage in the organic group (24 per cent) was three-fourths that of the non-organic group (31 per cent).

Lennox investigated 18,837 near relatives to determine which members of the patient's family were affected. Seventy-eight per cent (14,773) of these near relatives were related to patients with metabolic epilepsy. His findings for the total series (metabolic plus symptomatic) are as follows: fathers, 3.4 per cent; mothers, 3.6 per cent; siblings, 3.2 per cent; and children, 3 per cent.

This investigator calculated the incidence of epilepsy among the relatives of his male and female patients and found the incidence to be higher among the relatives of the female patients (4.1%) than among the relatives of the male patients (3.6%). Lennox's findings relative to the distribution of epilepsy in the various members of the family and his findings regarding the incidence of epilepsy among the relatives of the male and female patients are in disagreement with a number of recent, significant studies.

Lennox investigated 225 pairs of twins, 42.2 per cent of which were monozygotic and 57.8 of which were dizygotic, and reported his findings in 1960. This author found that:

(1) the concordance among all monozygotic twins was 62.1 per cent; the concordance among all dizygotic twins was 14.6 per cent. The ratio was 4.2 to 1.

(2) in all monozygotic twins with metabolic (nonorganic) epilepsy concordance was 84.5 per cent; in all dizygotic twins with metabolic epilepsy concordance was 15.9 per cent. The ratio was 5.3 to 1.

(3) the corresponding percentages for twins with organic (symptomatic) epilepsy were 27 per cent and 13.4 per cent. The ratio was 2 to 1. Lennox stated that ". . . (as a cause of epilepsy), in this group of patients, heredity is twice as important as an acquired brain lesion."

Lennox concluded that "the high degree of concordance in one-egg twins without brain injury leaves no doubt that heredity is very important in the etiology of epilepsy."

Lennox studied 121 pairs of twins with nonorganic epilepsy (58 monozygotic pairs and 63 dizygotic pairs) to determine the degree of concordance with respect to the type of seizure. He reported that grand mal seizures appeared concordantly in 82.3 per cent of monozygotic and in 15.4 per cent of dizygotic twins. The corresponding figures for psychomotor seizures were 38.5 per cent and 5.3 per cent. Concordance in petit mal, combined grand mal and petit mal, and combined grand mal and psychomotor was 75 per cent, 76.9 per cent and 27.3 per cent, respectively. Concordance in petit mal, combined grand mal and petit mal, and combined grand mal and psychomotor was not demonstrated among the dizygotic twins.

The first comprehensive investigation of the hereditary aspects of the electroencephalographic pattern in association with epilepsy was carried out by Lennox and the Gibbses. In 1940, these authors reported that electroencephalographically demonstrated abnormalities are more frequent among relatives of epileptics than in the general population. They examined 183 near relatives (parents, siblings and offspring) of ninety-four epileptics who showed pronounced electroencephalographic abnormalities. These workers reported that about 60 per cent of these relatives presented abnormal electroencephalographic recordings as compared with but 10 per cent in a "normal" control series. Lennox and co-workers concluded that the electroencephalographic dysrhythmia of epilepsy is inheritable, and when demonstrable may be considered as an indication of the existence of a latent predisposition to epilepsy.

In those cases where both parents were investigated, the electroencephalograms of both father and mother were found to be abnormal in 35 per cent; only one was abnormal in 60 per cent; and both were normal in 5 per cent.

These investigators determined that dysrhythmia was more frequent among the relatives of female patients (65%) than among those of male patients (56%), and more frequent among the female relatives (65%) than among the male relatives (54%). They also reported that a large proportion of the electroencephalographically dysrhythmic relatives presented various mental anomalies.

Lennox and the Gibbses reported a high incidence of cerebral dysrhythmia among the relatives of patients with symptomatic epilepsy and suggested that the epileptic seizures in such cases also develop on the basis of an existing hereditary predisposition. These workers reported that the incidence of dysrhythmia among the relatives of the patients with symptomatic epilepsy was not significantly different from that of the relatives of patients with cryptogenic epilepsy. On the results of their 1940 investigation, Lennox and the Gibbses proposed that cerebral dysrhythmia discloses the epileptic genotype which is inherited as a monomeric dominant character.

In 1943, Lennox and the Gibbses investigated and evaluated the interseizure electroencephalograms of 1,260 epileptic patients and 1,000 "normal" controls with no form of seizure disorder and no known lesions of the central nervous system. They reported the occurrence of paroxysmal activity in only 0.9 per cent of the control group, in 29.3 per cent of patients over twenty years of age and in 51.3 per cent of patients under twenty years of age.

In 1947, Lennox reported the occurrence of some degree of electroencephalographic abnormality in 50 per cent of his series of 470 near relatives as compared to 16 per cent among his adult control group.

In 1945, Lennox and the Gibbses reported on the influence of hereditary factors on the electroencephalographic pattern as revealed by a series of twins. These authors studied fifty-five pairs of normal monozygous twins and their findings revealed a very pronounced similarity, both with respect to the general character of the electroencephalogram and to the occurrence of abnormalities. In forty-seven of the fifty-five monozygous twin pairs both twins presented practically identical electroencephalograms; in six, the similarity was doubtful; and, in two the records differed considerably. In eighteen of the nineteen pairs of dizygous twins, however, the electroencephalograms were markedly dissimilar.

In 1951, Lennox reported his results of a study of sixty-one pairs of monozygous twins, of whom at least one partner had epilepsy and dysrhythmia. He found almost identical electroencephalographic records for the co-twins in thirty-seven cases (61%). The concordance was dependent upon the nature of the electroencephalographic abnormality. The greatest frequency of concordance was observed at simple changes in the basal rhythm (74%) and at three per second spike and wave forms (37%). Only three of forty dizygous twin pairs showed electroencephalographic concordance.

In his recent book (1960) Lennox stated that he investigated eighty-five of 121 pairs of twins with non-organic epilepsy to determine concordance of electroencephalographic patterns. He concluded that "the seizure discharges vary in their value as genetic indicators. Electroencephalographic evidence of heredity as shown by certain brain wave patterns is handicapped by the tendency of their abnormalities to subside with time."

METRAKOS AND METRAKOS

In 1961, Metrakos and Metrakos presented the results of their second study in a series of investigations concerning the genetics of convulsive disorders. In their search for genetic factors involved in convulsive disorders, these workers studied centrencephalic patients, because "this group can be identified on the single objective criterion of the electroencephalogram. Furthermore, the typical centrencephalic electroencephalogram is so characteristic that there is almost universal agreement among electroencephalographers as to its presence or absence from a particular record." The typical centrencephalic patient, according to these authors, has a "paroxysmal bilaterally synchronous 3-per-second wave-and-spike," and the atypical centrencephalic patient has a "slight variant of this."

These investigators obtained 211 patients with typical or atypical centrencephalic epilepsy from the Convulsive Disorders Clinic of the Neurology Service of The Montreal Children's Hospital. Each of these patients suffered with recurrent petit mal and/or grand mal seizures, had a centrencephalic electroenceph. alogram and presented "no obvious neuropathology to account for their seizures."

Their control series consisted of 112 patients from The Montreal Children's Hospital who had no history of convulsions, whose illness at the time of examination was "not considered to be neuropathologic" and whose electroencephalogram was "within normal or borderline normal limits." The centrencephalic probands were compared with the control group for parental age, ethnic origin, socio-economic status, sibship size and parity, and these investigators could demonstrate no significant differences.

Metrakos and Metrakos obtained information regarding age, medical history, cause of death and convulsive disorders for 7,377 relatives of the centrencephalic probands and for 4,026 relatives of the control probands. These authors found the incidence of individuals with convulsions for the total group of relatives of the centrencephalic probands to be 3.88 per cent; the corresponding incidence for the total group of relatives of the control probands was 1.76 per cent. The incidence of persons with convulsions among the relatives of the centrencephalic group, therefore, was 2.2 times greater and significantly higher than the corresponding figure for the relatives of the control group.

These investigators reported that 13.5 per cent of the parents, 12.7 per cent of the siblings, 4.2 per cent of the aunts and uncles, 2.6 per cent of the grandparents and 1.5 per cent of the cousins of the centrencephalic probands presented a history of convulsions.

The corresponding percentages for the control relatives were 1.3 per cent of the parents, 4.7 per cent of the siblings, 3.1 per cent of the aunts and uncles, 0.7 per cent of the grandparents and 0.7 per cent of the cousins. Metrakos and Metrakos concluded that "the data clearly demonstrate a familial distribution for convulsions, for, as the genetic distance between the relative studied and the proband increases, the prevalence of affected individuals decreases . . . in the case of the centrencephalic group but tends to fluctuate within narrower limits around 2 per cent for each class of relative in the control group."

These investigators also determined that the distribution of near relatives with convulsions was essentially the same for both the typical and atypical centrencephalic probands.

In contrast to the findings of some other investigators, Metrakos and Metrakos did not find a higher prevalence of affected near relatives of female probands (3.84%) than of male probands (3.93%).

Metrakos and Metrakos investigated the prevalence of electroencephalographic abnormalities in 223 siblings of centrencephalic patients and 103 siblings of control probands. In the former group, 53.4 per cent of the siblings presented some form of electroencephalographic abnormality, whereas only 28.2 per cent of the siblings of the control group had an abnormal electroencephalogram. When only epileptiform dysrhythmias were considered, the number of siblings who presented such an abnormality in the centrencephalic group (46.2%) was three times greater than the number of such siblings in the control group (15.5%). The incidence of siblings with centrencephalic electroencephalograms in the centrencephalic group was 36.8 per cent; the corresponding figure for siblings in the control group was 8.7 per cent.

Electroencephalographic investigation of 195 parents of the centrencephalic probands revealed an incidence of 7.7 per cent (15 parents) with a centrencephalic electroencephalogram. However, only 2.4 per cent (2 parents) of eighty-four parents of the control probands revealed such an electroencephalographic abnormality. It is of interest that the incidence of electroencephalographic abnormalities was higher among the parents of the control group (14.3%) than among the parents of the centrencephalic group (13.3%).

Metrakos and Metrakos analyzed the effect of the age of the siblings and parents on their electroencephalographic data and concluded that "if due allowance is given to the variability of age at onset of the centrencephalic type of electroencephalogram and also to its tendency to disappear in later years," their data are compatible with the hypothesis that an autosomal dominant gene, with the unusual characteristic of a very low penetrance at birth which rises rapidly to near complete penetrance for ages 4½ to 16½ years and declines gradually to almost no penetrance after the age of 40½ years, is responsible for the centrencephalic electro-encephalogram.

HARVALD

Harvald's comprehensive electroencephalographic investigation of the hereditary aspects of epilepsy was published in 1954. His study group consisted of 237 epileptic patients (120 males and 117 females) and 901 relatives. His control series was composed of 693 healthy young (the great majority between 18 and 21 years of age) male applicants for aviation training. The epileptic disorder was "probably of a symptomatic nature" in thirty-four patients; in the remaining 203 patients, the epilepsy was "probably cryptogenetic."

Harvald attempted to prove or disprove the electroencephalographic results of Lennox and the Gibbses and to investigate the feasability of guidance with regard to the genetic prognosis on the basis of electroencephalographic examinations of the patient and his relatives.

Harvald calculated the morbid risk for the relatives in the total series as 2.65 per cent; when cases of a doubtful epileptic nature were included, the risk was increased to 3.2 per cent.

The morbid risk for near relatives (parents, siblings and offspring) of the patients with cryptogenetic epilepsy was calculated to be 4.2 per cent; the morbid risk for the near relatives of patients with symptomatic epilepsy was found to be 1.0 per cent.

The risk for relatives of patients with cryptogenetic epilepsy was found by Harvald to be 3.0 per cent; this was significantly higher than the risk found for the relatives of the patients in the symptomatic group, 0.3 per cent.

The morbid risks for near and distant relatives of patients with marked non-focal electroencephalographic abnormalities were calculated to be 4.3 per cent and 2.6 per cent; the morbid risks for near and distant relatives of patients with focal electroencephalographic abnormalities were found to be 3.7 per cent and 1.2 per cent.

The morbid risk in the individual family groups was found to be about twice as high for near relatives (4.2%) as for distant relatives (2.4%). Harvald found no significant difference between the risks for parents and siblings.

Harvald found the incidence of epilepsy among the relatives of male patients to be 3.4 per cent, and among the relatives of the female patients to be 1.9 per cent. This finding is in contrast with that of Lennox who found that the incidence of epilepsy among the relatives of his male patients was lower than that among the relatives of his female patients.

Harvald compared the incidence of electroencephalographic abnormalities in the male relatives of his patients with that of the control group and found a significant difference—23.5 per cent for the former group and 17.3 per cent for the latter group.

Harvald compared the results of his electroencephalographic study with those reported by Lennox and co-workers in 1945 and stated that the "incidence of abnormalities was higher among the relatives in the American series than in the present." Some of the other results of these two studies are shown in Table 17.

TABLE 17

Comparison of the Electroencephalographic Data for Near Relatives in Harvold's Series and in the Series of Lennox, Gibbs and Gibbs (1945) *

| EEG | Harvald | | Lennox, Gibbs and Gibbs | |
	Near Relatives	*Control Group*	*Near Relatives*	*Control Group*
Normal	63.8%	82.7%	49.5%	84.2%
Slightly abnormal	26.7%	13.3%	36.4%	13.8%
Markedly abnormal	9.5%	4.0%	14.1%	2.0%

*Modification of Table 28 shown in, Harvald, B.: *Heredity in Epilepsy.* Copenhagen, Munksgaard, 1954, page 77.

In 1940, Lennox and co-workers reported that dysrhythmia occurs as frequently among relatives of patients with symptomatic epilepsy as among relatives of patients with cryptogenic epilepsy, suggesting that the seizures in the cases in the former group also develop on the basis of an existing hereditary predisposition. Harvald, however, reported that "this view has not been confirmed through the investigation here reported." He compared the electroencephalographic data of the relatives of patients with cryptogenetic epilepsy with those of the relatives of patients with symptomatic epilepsy and found that electroencephalographic abnormalities were significantly more frequent among the relatives in the former group. Harvald also found that the frequency of dysrhythmia among the relatives of patients with focal abnormalities did not exceed that found in the control group.

Harvald stated that he could not statistically confirm or disprove Lennox's theory that electroencephalographic dysrhythmia discloses the epileptic genotype which is inherited as a monomeric dominant character. Harvald demonstrated that epileptic patients show no absolute correlation between the electroencephalographic abnormality and the frequency of seizures and concluded that "the problem of the inheritance of epilepsy is not finally solved with the solution of the question of hereditary dysrhythmia, as first supposed by Lennox." After examining the electroencephalograms of twenty-nine suspected carriers of epilepsy, Harvald concluded that "this procedure is unfit for disclosing carriers, as only eight of these had markedly abnormal electroencephalograms, while sixteen had quite normal tracings."

This investigator stated that "there is much evidence to suggest that epilepsy in most cases is due to additive action of several genes. In a few cases, however, the disease seems to depend on a single dominant or recessive factor." He advanced the hypothesis that "mutually independent hereditary factors may be responsible for a tendency to spontaneous cerebral paroxysms and for a tendency to transition of even inconsiderable paroxysms into generalized epileptic seizures." Harvald found that only carriers with a pronounced tendency to spontaneous paroxysms can be disclosed electroencephalographically.

In 1940, Lennox and the Gibbses suggested the possibility of explaining, on an electroencephalographic basis, a genetic relationship between epilepsy, migraine, psychopathy, etc., as different forms of manifestation of a hereditary cerebral dysrhythmia. Harvald found that psychogenic psychosis, psychopathy, criminality, suicide, oligophrenia, schizophrenia and manic-depressive psychosis did not occur more frequently among the relatives of epileptics than in the general population. Harvald also reported that generalized convulsions in infancy (spontaneous or febrile), syncopes with epileptic stigmata and migraine were not more frequent among the relatives of epileptics than in the general population.

Harvald drew the following conclusions from his exhaustive electroencephalographic investigation:

"(1) Epilepsy seems to depend in part on hereditary factors, the morbid risk for the relatives of the patients being significantly higher than for the general population. The genetic prognosis is generally good. The morbid risk for the nearest relatives of the patients with cryptogenetic epilepsy is on an average only about 4 per cent.

(2) The presence of a hereditary predisposition to epilepsy may in some cases manifest itself solely by an abnormal EEG. The frequency of dysrhythmia is greater among the relatives of epileptics than in the general population, especially among the relatives of patients who themselves present pronounced non-focal abnormalities. Dysrhythmia is twice as frequent among female relatives as among male, possibly owing to sex-limited manifestation.

(3) Electroencephalographic examination is unfit as a general method for disclosing unaffected carriers, as some of these proved to have perfectly normal records.

(4) Epilepsy bears no genetic relation to generalized convulsions in infancy, febrile convulsions, syncopes, migraine, psychogenic psychosis, psychopathy, criminality, suicide, oligophrenia, schizophrenia, or manic-depressive psychosis.

(5) Epilepsy is no genetic entity. The inheritance is probably in most cases polymeric with additive gene action.

The results achieved by Lennox, Gibbs, and Gibbs have in the main been confirmed, except that there has not been found sufficient evidence to support Lennox' theory of dysrhythmia as a monomeric dominant trait. The conditions seem rather complicated and will probably remain so until a more exact knowledge of the mosaic of genes and enzymes enables us to determine the modes of inheritance of the individual monomeric characters."

ALSTRÖM

Alström investigated 897 epileptic patients and 5847 relatives and reported his results relative to the clinical, social and genetic aspects of the epileptic disorder in 1950.

Alström reported that the incidence of epilepsy found in the different groups of relatives of his probands varied somewhat, but that the figures were "remarkably low." The mean incidence of epilepsy in the three groups (parents, siblings and offspring) was 1.5 ± 0.18 per cent. The percentual incidence of epilepsy for parents, siblings and children of the patients in this study were 1.3 per cent, 1.5 per cent and 3.0 per cent, respectively. No difference was found in the incidence of epilepsy among relatives of the mentally affected patients with epilepsy of unknown origin (Group U) compared with the relatives of the other patients. These results are tabulated in Table 18; the figures in parenthesis represent the adjusted percentual frequency when cases of single seizures which did not intrinsically warrant a diagnosis of epilepsy are added.

This investigator calculated the incidence of epilepsy for the proband siblings and proband offspring in the U group (patients with epilepsy of unknown etiology) when they have passed the military call-up age, twenty-one years, as 0.9 per cent and 0.7 per cent for male and female relatives, respectively. These figures seem to be in accord with the reported frequency of epilepsy among conscripts in the United States during World Wars I and II.

Alström investigated the incidence of oligophrenia and mental diseases (schizophrenia, manic-depressive psychosis, senile and presenile psychoses) among the relatives of his patients and found good agreement with the figures reported for the general population in Sweden.

TABLE 18

Percentual Incidence of Epilepsy for Parents, Siblings and Children of Patients with Epilepsy of Unknown (U), Probable (P), and Known (K) Etiology*

The figures in parenthesis are the increased percentages after the addition of cases with single epileptic fits. The standard errors were computed on the basis of weighted numbers.

	U	P	K	All Groups	U Mentally Changed
Parents	1.5 ± 0.36 (1.7)	1.1 ± 0.63 (1.8)	0.8 ± 0.55 (1.2)	1.3 ± 0.27 (1.7)	1.4 ± 0.70
Siblings	1.6 ± 0.32 (1.9)	1.2 ± 0.60 (1.2)	1.3 ± 0.58 (1.5)	1.5 ± 0.25 (1.7)	1.5 ± 0.61
Children	3.1 ± 1.16 (4.0)	3.6 ± 2.51 (5.4)	1.6 ± 1.58 (3.2)	3.0 ± 0.93 (4.1)	2.7 ± 2.60
All Said Relatives	1.7 ± 0.24 (2.0)	1.2 ± 0.43 (2.0)	1.1 ± 0.39 (1.5)	1.5 ± 0.18 (1.9)	1.5 ± 0.46

*Modification of Tables 20 and 21 shown in, Alström, C. H.: *A Study of Epilepsy in its Clinical, Social and Genetic Aspects.* Copenhagen, Munskgsard, 1950, pages 118 and 119.

Alström determined that the incidence of consanguineous marriages among the parents of the probands was 2.7 per cent for the entire series, with small random variations for the different groups. He stated that this finding is in agreement with the corresponding figure for the general rural population in Sweden.

Alström attempted to apply various genetic hypotheses—simple monohybridism (recessive and dominant), inhibition of manifestation, dominant monohybridism and modifying polygenes, polyhybridism, a physiological seizure threshold determined by multiple additive genetic factors, and multiple allelism—to explain the epileptic manifestation as a genetically determined trait. However, he concluded that "none of these hypotheses gives a perfectly satisfactory explanation of the existing facts. And they can scarcely be said to do so even if very far-reaching auxiliary hypotheses are introduced in the equation. The hypothesis of a dominant main gene and modifying polygenes determining the epileptic manifestation in general seems to show the best agreement with the results of this investigation. This hypothesis, however, is at present not susceptible of proof, nor can it be entirely disproved."

Alström's group of patients contained sixteen pairs of twins, of which two pairs were monozygotic. Neither of the twin partners suffered from or had a history of convulsive seizures. This finding is in disagreement with the studies of Conrad and Lennox, who, according to Alström, found epilepsy in about 80 per cent of the monozygotic twin partners in their series. Alström is familiar with an unselected sample of four Scandinavian pairs of monozygotic twins in which the proband, but not the twin partner, suffered from epilepsy. Alström stated that the probability of getting such a sample at random is less than 0.002 if the "degree of manifestation" were to be the same as in Conrad's and Lennox's series. He concluded that "this probability is so small that some other factors than random variation must reasonably be responsible for the difference . . . ."

Alström called attention to the fact that in Lennox's series of sixty-six pairs of twins, 2/3 were monozygotic twins; however, only 1/3 of all twin births in the general population of the United States are monozygotic twins. Also, Lennox reported a preponderance of female twins, which he interpreted to indicate that epilepsy is genetically conditioned to a greater extent among females than among males. Alström analyzed Lennox's data and concluded that these differences "can scarcely be conditioned by chance. The most probable cause is a bias of some kind or other."

Alström reported that the epileptic manifestation appeared to be a symptom in a genetically determined monohybridical disease in only about one per cent of the 897 probands—eleven probands belonging to eight families. He stated that the mode of transmission was probably recessive in four and dominant in seven probands. Alström was unable to elicit support for the assumption of a uniform monohybrid mode of transmission in epilepsy in the remainder of the 897 families. Cases with epilepsy other than in the proband were lacking in 92 per cent of the families of the probands.

Alström took exception to the conclusion of Lennox, Gibbs and Gibbs that "the dysrhythmia of epilepsy is inheritable and when demonstrable, may represent a predisposition to epilepsy or some allied disorder." The Gibbses and Lennox reported that the incidence of electroencephalographic abnormalities in the relatives of their study groups was ten times that of epilepsy in the population. These workers asserted that it is possible by use of the electroencephalograph to definitely find support for the assumption of a monohybrid, dominant mode of transmission in cerebral dysrhythmia. Manifest epilepsy develops in about five per cent of individuals with cerebral dysrhythmia and the remainder are considered to be latent bearers of the trait. In a number of cases some contributory factor is necessary in addition to the presence of this trait; Lennox and co-workers designated such epilepsy as "acquired." In the majority of instances, approximately 75 to 80 per cent, the trait alone appears to be sufficient and epilepsy develops without any contributory factor; Lennox and co-workers designated such epilepsy as "genetic." Alström summarized his objections to Lennox's theory as follows:

"1. The incidence of 'cerebral dysrhythmia' of this kind is estimated to be approximately 10 per cent in the general population. This would explain why epilepsy only develops in a minority of individuals who have sustained head injuries. This does not tally—amongst other things—with the fact that with cerebral tumors the incidence of epilepsy is higher and varies with the localization of the tumor. Nor can it be reconciled with the fact that all individuals can react to electro-shock treatment with epileptic fits.

"2. A theory of multiple allelism can neither be proved nor entirely disproved. If, however, all the known facts are taken into consideration, it is scarcely reasonable.

"3. Further, 'there are still different views about the significance of an abnormal EEG in epilepsy' . . . It is as yet too early, without further investigations, to make this heterogeneous phenomenon the basis of a genetic hypothesis. An extensive genetic analysis is also required.

"4. The risk for confusion when mixing concepts from three different fields of observation—clinical, electroencephalographic and genetic—" is great.

"5. The classification of epilepsy into focal and nonfocal is not satisfactory from a logical point of view. If a focus is found, well and good. But if it is impossible to find any focus by means of EEG, it is not justified on these grounds alone to designate the case as non-focal epilepsy in the true meaning of the term. Epilepsy without known focus is the reasonable term.

"6. The paroxysmal dysrhythmia of the type '3 per second waves' is assumed by Lennox to be proof of a general cerebral dysrhythmia with its origin in all the ganglion cells. He calls this type of epilepsy 'idiopathic.' It is thus assumed to be non-focal in nature and to exist on a genetic basis. No support for the latter statement that is tenable from a genetic viewpoint is forthcoming."

Alström introduced the findings of Penfield, Jasper and co-workers to argue against Lennox's classification of 3 per second spike and wave dysrhythmia as non-focal. He stated that these workers have shown that, with great probability, the characteristic 3 per second spike and wave dysrhythmia may have a definite focal origin and that, therefore, it does not differ essentially in nature from other focal epilepsy.

Alström reported that electroencephalographic data are unable to indisputably support the theory that epilepsy can be interpreted as a uniform genetic phenomenon. He was of the opinion that "from a genetic aspect, 'cerebral dysrhythmia' is, to say the least, somewhat controversial as a manifestation of a simple dominant hereditary trait."

From the results of his very comprehensive study, Alström hypothesized that "epilepsy, even that in a so-called 'nuclear group,' is not a disease *sui generis*, but is to be interpreted as an unspecific neurological clinical symptom of a pathological irritation of the central nervous system, focal in origin. The focus or foci may be regarded as 'pacemakers.' This symptom may occur in a large number of basic cerebral diseases, of known or unknown etiology, as the only symptom or together with several other symptoms. The more serious the basic disease is, the worse its prognosis is, and the easier it is, on an average, to diagnose it with the clinical methods at present available. The basic diseases may be hereditary—i.e., gene determined, rare neuropsychiatric disorders—or, and most commonly, they may be diseases not determined by genes, but by injuries, infections, etc. This would then explain the fact that no uniform mode of hereditary transmission is found for a symptom of so general a nature."

EISNER, PAULI AND LIVINGSTON

(The Johns Hopkins Hospital Epilepsy Clinic)

The hereditary aspects of epilepsy were studied in our clinic and the results were reported in 1959. I believe that this study is particularly significant because the various groups of epileptic patients were compared with a control population which was comparable to the patient group in all significant factors. A total of 669 epileptic patients with 3362 close relatives were included in the test series and 470 patients (from four clinics at The Johns Hopkins Hospital) with 2858 close relatives, were included in the control series.

Our findings in this study do not allow a definite answer to the question of whether or not epilepsy is inherited. Hereditary transmission of epilepsy could not be demonstrated, but it could not be ruled out. We were unable to demonstrate familial aggregation of epilepsy in any type of seizure except idiopathic major motor epilepsy. The types of epilepsy in which we found no evidence of familial aggregation were:

Organic Major Motor Epilepsy—83 probands, 469 close relatives;

Focal Epilepsy—89 probands, 466 close relatives;

Petit Mal Epilepsy—34 probands, 130 close relatives;

Minor Motor Epilepsy—31 probands, 120 close relatives; and,

Psychomotor Epilepsy—11 probands, 61 close relatives.

We were unable to demonstrate familial aggregation in idiopathic major motor epilepsy when seizures started after fifteen and one-half years of age.

In those patients with mixed epilepsy, we were unable to demonstrate familial aggregation of any type of epilepsy other than major motor.

The data relative to focal epilepsy, petit mal epilepsy, minor motor epilepsy, psychomotor epilepsy and mixed epilepsy are presented in Table 19. No significant differences were found in the first three groups upon comparison with the control group either in the number of relatives with seizures of any type or the number of relatives with major motor convulsions; none of the close relatives in the psychomotor epilepsy group had seizures. We found a significantly higher prevalence of major motor seizures among relatives in the mixed epilepsy group than in the control series. The major motor plus psychomotor category apparently accounts for most of the familial aggregation of major motor epilepsy found in the mixed epilepsy group. Although the prevalence of major motor seizures among the close relatives in both the major motor plus petit mal and the major motor plus minor motor categories was higher than in the control group, the differences were not significant.

The idiopathic major motor epilepsy group consisted of 321 probands and 1658 close relatives. We were able to demonstrate a small but significant familial aggregation of idiopathic major motor epilepsy in this group of patients. However, we were unable to demonstrate familial aggregation when the age of onset was over fifteen and one-half years. The familial aggregation in the idiopathic major motor group appeared to vary with the age of onset of the proband's epilepsy (Table 20). This finding is in agreement with that reported by Ounsted in 1955. We found the incidence to be highest when the proband's epileptic disorder

TABLE 19

DIFFERENT TYPES OF EPILEPSY COMPARED WITH CONTROLS FOR INCIDENCE OF CONVULSIONS AMONG CLOSE RELATIVES*

Type of Epilepsy	Test Group		Major Motor Convulsions			Convulsions of Any Type		
	Number of Probands	Number of Close Relatives	Per Cent Affected Relatives		Standard Error of Difference	Per Cent Affected Relatives		Standard Error of Difference
			Test	Control		Test	Control	
Focal	89	466	2.17	1.75	0.75	2.70	2.77	0.85
Petit mal	34	130	0.66	1.93	0.82	1.37	3.07	1.28
Minor motor	31	120	0.42	1.94	0.88	1.22	3.10	1.47
Psychomotor	11	61	0			0		
Major motor + petit mal	30	135	3.95	1.75	1.79	3.95	2.80	1.80
Major motor + minor motor	42	189	4.60	1.95	1.49	6.19	3.13	1.74
Major motor + psychomotor	28	133	6.50	1.81	1.96	6.50	2.85	1.97
All mixed epilepsy	100	457	4.65	1.53	1.01	5.24	2.69	1.05

*Modification of Table 9 shown in, Eisner, V., Pauli, L. L., and Livingston, S.: Hereditary Aspects of Epilepsy. *Bull. Johns Hopkins Hosp.*, *105*:256, 1959.

TABLE 20

Idiopathic Major Motor Epilepsy, by Age of Onset of Epilepsy.
Comparison with Control Series*

Age of Proband at Onset of Epilepsy	Number of Case-	Number of Relatives	Adjusted Per Cent of Relatives with Major Motor Epilepsy, Test Group	Adjusted Per Cent of Relatives with Major Motor Epilepsy, Control Group	Standard Error of Difference
0–3	136	622	8.29	2.17	1.11
4–9	85	390	4.26	1.76	1.06
10–15	66	382	5.75	1.74	1.22
16+	34	264	3.36	1.56	1.10

*Modification of Table 5 shown in, Eisner V., Pauli, L. L. and Livingston, S.: Hereditary Aspects of Epilepsy. *Bull. Johns Hopkins Hosp.*, *105:*252, 1959.

started between the ages of 0 and three and one-half years, and nine and one-half and fifteen and one-half years. The highest incidence of familial aggregation of major motor convulsions was found in the group with onset from 0 to three years. The group with onset from ten to fifteen years revealed a higher prevalence of major motor convulsions than did the group with onset from four to nine years. We could find no evidence for familial aggregation of epilepsy in those instances where the proband's seizures started at sixteen or more years of age; however, because of the small number of patients in this group, it is impossible to state definitely that familial aggregation does not exist.

We further divided the idiopathic major motor epilepsy group by other criteria to determine if these criteria would separate subgroups which differed in the familial incidence of convulsions. Sex, economic level of home address, occupation of head of family, race and income, presence or absence of mental retardation in the proband and the electroencephalographic findings had no demonstrated effect on the prevalence of convulsions among family members. We could find no relationship between electroencephalographic findings and the incidence of convulsions among relatives in this group. In addition to presence or absence of generalized electroencephalographic abnormalities, we examined specific abnormalities and various combinations of them, but were unable to demonstrate significant differences.

We tested our data revealing familial aggregation against some mathematical models of genetic transmission (single dominant gene hypothesis, single recessive gene hypothesis, the binomial hypothesis, the number of consanguineous matings, Haldane's test of recessive inheritance) and were unable to demonstrate that the aggregation followed any theoretical pattern of simple genetic inheritance.

We then attempted to explain the familial aggregation by means of a non-genetic hypothesis. We assumed that if a given event in the perinatal period is the cause of the familial aggregation observed in major motor epilepsy, then if the families of those probands who experienced the event are grouped together, these families will present a higher prevalence of epilepsy than the remaining families. We found no significant differences when the families were divided according to the proband's length of gestation, type of delivery, type of anesthesia used at the delivery, length of labor, cyanosis noted at birth or a history of miscarriage in the proband's mother. In addition, no significant differences could be demonstrated when divisions were made by age of onset of the proband's epilepsy and these criteria.

When other perinatal abnormalities such as signs of fetal distress, signs or a history suggesting mechanical trauma during delivery, and maternal toxemia or hypertension are examined, the situation is different. Families in which the probands revealed one of these abnormalities presented a significantly higher incidence of major motor epilepsy among close relatives than families in which no such abnormalities were recorded. We concluded that familial aggregation of idiopathic major motor epilepsy may be due to familial aggregation of perinatal injury, to inheritance or to a combination of these factors.

Lennox studied a large series of twins and reported a high concordance for epilepsy among monozygotic twins and a much lower concordance among dizygotic twins. We cannot agree that inheritance is the only possible explanation for the combination of familial aggregation and high concordance among monozygotic twins. A familial tendency to an epileptogenic trauma occurring before or during birth might also explain the observations, and it has been demonstrated by Lilienfeld and Pasamanick that there is an association between perinatal injury and epilepsy. In addition, Yerushalmy and Sheerar have shown that like-sexed twins show higher stillbirth, prematurity and perinatal mortality rates than unlike-sexed twins. This may be interpreted to mean that perinatal injury is more common in monozygotic than in dizygotic twins.

TABLE 21

PER CENT RISK OF MAJOR MOTOR EPILEPSY FOR CLOSE RELATIVES OF PROBAND WITH IDIOPATHIC MAJOR MOTOR EPILEPSY*

(This table shows the chance at birth of developing major motor epilepsy if the child survives to the age shown)

		Age of Onset of Proband's Epilepsy			
Age	Control	0–15½	0–3½	3½–9½	9½–15½
4½	0.66	3.22	5.60	0.81	1.92
9½	1.08	4.25	6.57	2.35	2.54
14½	1.22	5.06	7.05	2.68	4.26
19½	1.43	5.50	7.61	3.43	4.26
29½	1.96	6.54	8.66	4.78	5.14
39½	2.27	7.53	9.35	6.02	6.27
49½	2.43	8.21	—	7.10	7.07

*Modification of Table 12 shown in, Eisner, V., Pauli, L. L. and Livingston, S.: Hereditary Aspects of Epilepsy. *Bull. Johns Hopkins Hosp.*, *105:*262, 1959.

We developed risk tables which may be used to estimate the chances of a given person developing epilepsy. The highest risk we found was to close relatives of probands who developed major motor epilepsy before three and one-half years of age (Table 21): 7.6 per cent of these relatives may be expected to develop major motor epileptic seizures by nineteen and one-half years of age and 9.4 per cent by thirty-nine and one-half years of age. Comparable control risks were 1.4 per cent and 2.3 per cent. It is of interest to note that Ounsted found that the risks to siblings of patients whose first seizure occurred during the ages of one to three and one-half years are substantially higher than the risks when the patient's first seizure occurred after three and one-half years of age.

DISCUSSION

I have summarized the findings of the genetic studies conducted by some of the physicians who are considered to be experts in the fields of epilepsy and/or genetics. An analysis of the results of these investigations reveals considerable differences, not only in the statistical data per se, but also in regard to the genetic significance of this data. Because of inherent or resultant biases or prejudices, each of these studies, including the investigation carried out in our clinic by Eisner and co-workers, is subject to criticism. In many instances, specific aspects of the various genetic studies cannot be directly compared because of significant biases present in the respective investigations.

Some of the factors responsible for the conflicting findings of the various genetic investigations are as follows:

(1) Disagreement as to the definition of epilepsy;

(2) Disagreement as to the classification of seizures;

(3) Age of the proband;

(4) Age of the patient at the onset of epilepsy;

(5) Use of a control group not comparable to the patient group in all significant aspects;

(6) Disagreement as to the incidence of epilepsy in the general population;

(7) Disagreement in the interpretation of electroencephalograms;

(8) Non-representative patient groups resulting from biased methods of selection;

(9) Unreliability of results obtained from the questioning of relatives;

(10) Disagreement as to the definition of concordance in twin studies;

(11) Exclusion of the effect of prenatal and perinatal factors in the etiology of epilepsy.

When one considers the many pitfalls besetting a study of the hereditary aspects of the epileptic disorder, it is not difficult to understand the lack of agreement in the findings.

Some of the earlier studies (Conrad, 1935; Lennox—1947, 1951; Lennox, Gibbs and Gibbs—1939, 1940, 1945) revealed findings which were interpreted by the investigators as evidence favoring inheritance as a predominant etiological factor in epilepsy. However, the results of some of the more recent investigations (Alström, 1950; Eisner and co-workers, 1959; Harvald, 1954) are not in complete accord with the findings reported in the earlier studies. For example, the assumption that electroencephalographic abnormalities are genetically the same as epilepsy, while an attractive hypothesis, has not been proved. Many hypotheses regarding a mode of hereditary transmission for epilepsy have been offered, but proof has been generally lacking.

Protagonists of the theory that heredity is a major etiological factor in epilepsy base their opinions primarily on the following findings:

(1) A higher incidence of electroencephalographic abnormalities in the relatives of epileptics than in the relatives of a control group;

(2) A higher incidence of epilepsy in the relatives of epileptics than in a control group (or the general population); and,

(3) The high degree of concordance with regard to epilepsy in monozygotic twins.

The significance of the relationship between electroencephalographic abnormalities and the incidence of epilepsy has not been established. Harvald could not statistically confirm or disprove the theory that electroencephalographic dysrhythmia discloses the epileptic genotype which is inherited as a monomeric dominant character. Harvald was unable to demonstrate a parallelism between the incidence of epilepsy and the incidence of electro-encephalographic abnormalities in his series and concluded that electroencephalographic examination is unfit for disclosing unaffected "carriers" of epilepsy.

It is reasonable to assume the hereditary transmission of a characteristic if it can be demonstrated that it occurs more frequently among the relatives of those with the characteristic than among the relatives of a comparable group of people without the characteristic. However, to validate the conclusion, it must be demonstrated that the difference is greater than would be expected by random distribution, and that any conditions, other than heredity, which might influence the distribution of the characteristic operate equally in the families of those with the condition and in the families of the group with which they are compared. Alström was unable to demonstrate familial aggregation of epilepsy and we were able to demonstrate familial aggregation only in association with idiopathic major motor epilepsy.

It was generally accepted that if a condition is entirely hereditary, it can be demonstrated in: (1) both or neither of a pair of monozygotic twins, and (2) both of a pair of fraternal twins as often as it can be shown in both of two siblings who are not twins. The greater the influence of heredity, the more closely these conditions will be fulfilled.

Significant criticisms regarding the selection of cases in the twin studies of Conrad and Lennox have been presented by various investigators such as Alström, Eisner and co-workers and Harvald. For example, Harvald was of the opinion that since Lennox collected his twin patients through reports of practicing neurologists, the number of concordant cases was too great; he classified Lennox's series of twins as "hardly representative." According to Harvald, Lennox regarded as concordant, twins one of whom had epilepsy and the other perhaps only convulsions in infancy or isolated convulsive fits.

It is also of interest to note that the genetic value of the results obtained from studies of twins has recently been attacked by Morton, who stated that ". . . twin studies have seemed to some students to hold forth the promise of separating the contributions made to family resemblance by heredity and environment. An entire journal is devoted to this so-called 'twin method,' but the assumptions required for estimation of heritability from twin studies are so little subject to proof that they have taken on the character of articles of faith, to which few of the younger geneticists adhere. . . . Not only are twin studies incapable of elucidating complex genetic situations, but they are of limited value in simple cases. . . . In conjunction with other family data, twin concordances are of circumstantial and qualitative value in assessing the role of genetic factors."

CONCLUSIONS

When one studies all of the significant investigations relative to heredity and epilepsy, including the one carried out in our clinic, it becomes obvious that a genetic mode of transmission of epilepsy has not been established. The genetics of epilepsy is a wide open field and much work has yet to be done to solve this problem. I believe it is fair to state that most authorities in the field today are of the opinion that the inheritability of epilepsy has not been proved and that the data compiled to date indicate that the genetic factor in epilepsy is slight.

In view of the data which are available today, what advice should be given to the epileptic patient in answer to the following question: "Should I marry and have children?" Also, the parents of an epileptic child very frequently ask the following questions: "Should we have additional children? What are the chances that we will have another epileptic offspring?"

Throughout the medical literature, the figure most frequently encountered as representing the calculated risk that the offspring of a marriage of an epileptic and a non-epileptic will develop epilepsy is one in forty. Epilepsy is a relatively common disorder; its occurrence in the general population has been estimated to vary from one in fifty to one in 200. In view of this relatively high incidence of epilepsy in the general population, it is obvious that all individuals are subject to a definite risk of having an epileptic offspring. I do not believe that any investigator has significant data which would enable him to specifically calculate the chances of epilepsy developing in the offspring of any marriage, including the commonly quoted figure of one in forty.

I base my decision in regard to marriage and children for epileptics primarily on the frequency of the patient's seizures and his or her physical and mental ability to raise a family. My decision is not influenced to the slightest degree by the possibility that a marriage between an epileptic and a non-epileptic may produce an epileptic offspring.

The following are the attitudes of some other physicians who have had considerable experience with epilepsy.

Lennox (Epilepsy and Related Disorders, 1960, page 574): "Many considerations enter into the question of marriage. We believe that most epileptics who wish to marry and rear children should be encouraged to do so."

Metrakos and Metrakos: In their publication (1961) these investigators did not offer any genetic advice in regard to marriage and children. They stated, "What possible factors may be operating to precipitate clinical seizures in a child with a centrencephalic electroencephalogram and what the significance of this is in genetic counselling will . . . be considered in a subsequent paper."

Ounsted (1955): "The role of the geneticist and the eugenic counsellor is necessarily large in the epilepsies of childhood. This is evident from the fact that genetic ideas enter in any discussion of these diseases. What answers can we give? I think the answers can be generally of a positive and cheerful nature. The general risk that the child of an adult epileptic will himself, when adult, be also an epileptic lies between 2 and 4 per cent: a low risk. To impose a general bar on procreation for epileptics seems, therefore, likely to be dysgenic."

Harvald (1954): "The present as well as previous investigations have consistently shown that the risk of developing epilepsy is comparatively low for the relatives of epileptics, and that the risk of mental disorders of different kinds hardly exceeds that in the general population. In general there is accordingly no reason to advise patients with epilepsy against marrying and having children."

Alström (1950): At the time of this writing the law in Sweden relative to the marriage of epileptics was "The individual who suffers from epilepsy that is due mainly to endogenous causes shall not contract marriage." Alström bitterly attacked this law, stating: "It is not based on scientific facts. It is built on an antiquated conception of the problems of epilepsy. That this conception is directly inaccurate appears to be the most reasonable interpretation of— amongst other matters—the results of the present study of an unselected sample of Swedish epileptics. . . . The most reasonable result should be for this Law to be abolished."

In conclusion, there is little evidence for making eugenic recommendations to the parents of an epileptic child. It is generally considered that estimates of risk to siblings of an epileptic patient are not of sufficient magnitude to warrant advising against future pregnancies.

BIBLIOGRAPHY

Alström, C. H.: *A Study of Epilepsy in Its Clinical, Social and Genetic Aspects*. Copenhagen, Munksgaard, 1950.

Conrad, K.: Erbanlage und Epilepsie: Untersuchungen an einer Serie von 253 Zwillingspaaren. *Ztschr ges Nurol. u. Psychiat.*, *153:*271, 1935.

Eisner, V., Pauli, L. L., and Livingston, S.: Hereditary Aspects of Epilepsy. *Bull. Johns Hopkins Hosp.*, *105:*245, 1959.

Harvald, B.: *Heredity in Epilepsy*. Copenhagen, Munksgaard, 1954.

The Genuine Works of Hippocrates. Translated by Francis Adams. New York, Wood, Vol. II, p. 338, 1929.

Kanner, L : The Folklore and Cultural History of Epilepsy. *Medical Life*, *37:*167, 1930.

Lennox, W. G.: Marriage and Children for Epileptics. *Human Fertil.*, *10:*97, 1945.

...........: Sixty-six Twin Pairs Affected by Seizures. *A. Res. Nerv. & Ment. Dis.*, *Proc.*, *26:*11, 1947.

...........: The Genetics of Epilepsy. *Am. J. Psychiat.*, *103:*457, 1947.

...........: The Heredity of Epilepsy as Told by Relatives and Twins. *J.A.M.A.*, *146:*529, 1951.

...........: Epilepsy and Related Disorders. Boston, Little, Brown & Co., 1960.

Lennox, W. G., Gibbs, E. L., and Gibbs, F. A.: The Inheritance of Epilepsy as Revealed by the Electroencephalograph. *J.A.M.A.*, *113:*1002, 1939.

...........: Inheritance of Cerebral Dysrhythmia and Epilepsy. *Arch. Neurol. & Psychiat.*, *44:*1155, 1940.

...........: The Brain-Wave Pattern, An Hereditary Trait. Evidence from 74 "Normal" Pairs of Twins. *J. Hered.*, *36:*233, 1945.

Lilienfeld, A. M., and Pasamanick, B.: Association of Maternal and Fetal Factors with Development of Epilepsy. *J.A.M.A.*, *155:*719, 1954.

Metrakos, K., and Metrakos, J. D.: Genetics of Convulsive Disorders. *Neurology*, *11:* 474, 1961.

Morton, N. E.: in *Methodology in Human Genetics* (Burdette, W. J., Editor), San Francisco, Holdan-Day, Inc., 1962.

Ounsted, C.: Genetic and Social Aspects of Epilepsies of Childhood. *Eugenics Rev.*, *47:*33, 1955.

Preuss, J : *Biblisch-Talmudische Medizin; Beitrage Zur Geschichte Der Heilkunde und der Kultur Uberhaupt*. Berlin, S. Karger, 1923.

Yerushalmy, J., and Sheerar, S. E.: Studies on Twins; On Early Mortality of Like-Sexed and Unlike-Sexed Twins. *Human Biol.*, *12:*247, 1940.

Ziskind, E., and Sommerfeldt-Ziskind, E.: Inadequacy of Evidence for Hereditary Predisposition. *Am. J. Psychiat*, *95:*1143, 1939.

Chapter 17

PROGNOSIS OF EPILEPSY

CONTROL OF EPILEPTIC SEIZURES

WHEN I first started working with epileptic patients some twenty-six years ago, the number of patients who could be satisfactorily controlled of their seizures was not too great. At that time the only effective antiepileptic drugs which were available were bromides and phenobarbital.

In 1946, Bridge and co-workers reported that 17.4 per cent of a group of epileptic patients who had been followed in our clinic for at least fifteen years had been seizure free for more than five years.

We are currently in the process of determining the outcome of our present group of approximately 15,000 epileptic patients. Although we have not completely finished this study as yet, I can state that complete seizure control was obtained in approximately 60 per cent of the cases; the number of seizures in another 25 per cent were reduced in frequency to the extent that they should not cause the patient a significant handicap; in the remaining 15 per cent of the patients, the seizures were refractory to all forms of antiepileptic therapy.

The improved outlook for the control of epileptic seizures which has occurred during the past several decades is due to many factors. Prior to 1939, the only available antiepileptic drugs of any value were bromides and phenobarbital. However, since 1939, a number of new therapeutic agents have been introduced and successfully employed for the control of epileptic seizures, such as Dilantin (1939), Tridione (1944), Mysoline (1952) and Zarontin (1961).

Improved technique in the administration of the ketogenic diet regimen has also contributed to the better outlook for the epileptic, at least in our clinic. This latter therapeutic regimen is only of value in the control of epileptic seizures in young children.

The introduction of electroencephalography as a diagnostic adjunct in detecting epilepsy has also played a great part, since early diagnosis and early institution of therapy are very important in the obtention of control of seizures. In my experience, the longer the epilepsy exists, the more difficult it is to control the seizures. Certainly, it is much more difficult to satisfactorily control a patient who has had fifteen to twenty seizures than one who has had only two or three seizures. A possible explanation for this finding has been postulated by some physicians in the past: "the brain gets into the habit of having convulsions in those patients who have frequent seizures." There may be some validity to this statement since it is generally known that, by and large, the longer any habit persists, the more difficult it is to control.

When I began to work with epileptic patients it was the general policy of our clinic to continue medication for periods of not much longer than one year after the patient's last seizure. During the subsequent years, the period of duration of therapy was increased to much longer periods of time and at present it is our policy that medication be continued for at least four years after the patient's last seizure, and in many instances, particularly adults, for the rest of their lives. We observed a considerable reduction in the number of patients who have had a recurrence of seizures when the duration of therapy was increased from one to two to three to at least four years of freedom from seizures. I believe it is unquestionable that the longer anticonvulsant therapy is continued in any epileptic patient, the less likely it is that he will experience a recurrence of seizures after the therapy is discontinued.

My earlier observations have taught me the importance of the gradual withdrawal of antiepileptic medication in order to maintain freedom from seizures. This is particularly true in the case of major motor seizures. It has been my experience that it is frequently very difficult to control a recurrence of seizures precipitated by a sudden withdrawal of antiepileptic medication.

Although the surgical treatment of epilepsy, in my experience, has not been of significant value for the overall epileptic population, good results have been obtained in selected cases.

Improvement in the control of epilepsy is related to the general factors heretofore mentioned. However, in predicting the specific outcome of the seizures in any individual patient, the following factors must also be taken into consideration: the type of epileptic seizure, the duration of the epileptic disorder, the presence or absence of well-defined precipitating factors, and the presence or absence of emotional disturbances. This present discussion is confined to the first of these factors, the type of epileptic seizure. The relationship of the duration of the epileptic disorder to the outcome of the seizures has already been briefly mentioned in this section and is also discussed in more detail in the section of this book entitled Medical Treatment of Epilepsy (Chapter 8) under the specific title of General Principles of Drug Therapy. The relationship of the presence or absence of precipitating factors and emotional disturbances is discussed in Chapters 5 and 12.

Many patients have asked me if a family history of epilepsy has any bearing on the control of epileptic seizures. A study reported by Bridge and co-workers from our clinic in 1946 revealed that "it is evident that the intensity of the hereditary . . . factors has no relationship to the outcome of the seizures of the individual patients." My subsequent experiences relative to the importance of a familial history of epilepsy in prognosticating the outcome of the seizures in any given case have been in accord with the findings reported by Bridge and co-workers. In fact, I believe it is reasonable to assume in many instances that if an epileptic patient should have an epileptic offspring, the outcome of this offspring may be more favorable than that of an epileptic patient whose parents are free of epilepsy. I express this opinion because an epileptic parent should be able to cope with the disorder better than a non-epileptic parent. Also, since the epileptic parent generally has a good understanding of the nature of the disorder of epilepsy, the child would be less subject to mismanagement and other environmental factors which adversely affect the emotional and social progress of the epileptic.

Type of Seizure

1. Major Motor (Grand Mal) Seizures

Major motor seizures may make their initial appearance at any period of life, and are encountered much more frequently than any other type of epileptic seizure. Approximately 80 per cent of my patients suffered with this form of epilepsy.

Although a major motor seizure is generally the most disturbing and distressing type of epileptic seizure (both to the patient and the observer) because of its violent clinical manifestations, it is generally the easiest to control. It has been my experience that the seizures can be completely controlled or greatly reduced in frequency in the vast majority of patients who suffer with pure grand mal epilepsy. However, I have observed that, by and large, when these seizures begin during the first few years of life, particularly before the first year, they are sometimes quite resistant to antiepileptic therapy.

The question as to whether or not major motor seizures can cause irreversible brain damage is discussed in another section of this chapter entitled Do Convulsions Cause Permanent Brain Damage?

2. Petit Mal Seizures

Petit mal epilepsy, in my experience, is a disorder limited entirely to children (patients under 21 years of age). This disturbance usually makes its initial appearance between the ages of four and eight years. In fact, I cannot recall an instance of petit mal epilepsy commencing after the onset of adolescence.

A follow-up study which we are currently conducting on a large group of patients with petit mal epilepsy who have been followed in our clinic for many years indicates that this form of epilepsy only rarely continues much after the patient passes through adolescence. Before the introduction of effective anti-petit mal therapeutic agents such as Tridione and Zarontin, it was a well established fact that, in many instances, petit mal epilepsy disappeared spontaneously when the child reached puberty. The details of our current follow-up study have not been tabulated as yet, but the findings which were on hand at the time of this writing indicate that the majority of our patients with pure petit mal epilepsy were relieved of their spells. It seems quite evident that the antiepileptic therapeutic regimens were responsible for the cessation of seizures in most of these patients. However, one cannot be absolutely certain that the antiepileptic drugs were completely responsible for the cessation of spells, since it is well known that in many instances petit mal epilepsy disappears spontaneously when patients reach puberty.

It is important to note, however, that many patients who initially suffer with petit mal epilepsy subsequently develop other types of epileptic seizures, especially grand mal seizures. The most common age at which these other seizures appear is at adolescence. The details of the current follow-up study on our group of patients with petit mal epilepsy will be reported at a later date. However, the figures which we had at the time of this writing indicate that approximately 60 per cent of these patients developed major seizures.

3. Psychomotor Seizures

Psychomotor seizures occur mostly in adults, but this form of epilepsy is also encountered in children.

By and large, psychomotor epileptic seizures are very resistant to antiepileptic therapeutic regimens. We have employed all of the available antiepileptic drugs in the treatment of our patients and have also submitted some of our patients to surgical investigation. Our findings indicate that approximately 25 per cent of our patients, both children and adults, have been benefited by the available antiepileptic therapeutic regimens.

4. Minor Motor Seizures

Minor motor epilepsy is limited entirely to children. These seizures generally make their initial appearance very early in life, most commonly around three or four months of age. In my experience, none of the available antiepileptic drugs are effective in controlling these seizures. We have obtained some favorable results relative to seizure control with the ketogenic diet regimen. By and large, however, it has been my general experience that minor motor seizures continue to recur with some brief remissions during the first four or five years of life. In most instances, minor motor seizures disappear spontaneously after this age. However, many patients subsequently develop other types of epileptic seizures, particularly grand mal seizures.

Minor motor epilepsy is the most serious of all the epilepsies. The most serious hazard of this form of epilepsy is not necessarily the seizures themselves, but the associated mental retardation.

The degree of mental retardation found in patients with minor motor epilepsy varies from mild to severe; in most instances, however, it is severe.

It is important that the parents of children with minor motor epilepsy be informed about the most likely outcome of the condition, so that they can prepare themselves for the future and also make suitable arrangements for the care of the child. In many instances, institutional care is the only logical recourse.

DO CONVULSIONS CAUSE PERMANENT BRAIN DAMAGE?

The question as to whether or not convulsions per se cause irreversible brain damage is a controversial one, especially those which occur in association with epilepsy. My opinions relative to this problem, based on follow-up studies of thousands of patients who suffered with convulsions associated with various disorders, are as follows.

Epileptic Seizures

My observations, based on follow-up studies of hundreds of patients with recurrent epileptic seizures of short duration, indicate that such seizures rarely, if ever, cause demonstrable irreversible brain damage. On the other hand, a few of my epileptic patients who had normal intelligence and who also had revealed negative neurological examinations, manifested evidence of permanent brain damage (mental retardation and/or neurological abnormalities) immediately after they had experienced a prolonged epileptic seizure or status epilepticus. It therefore appears that these seizures may have been responsible for the organic brain damage in these patients. However, it is important to note that I have seen many patients who maintained normal intellectual levels and did not present neurological abnormalities in spite of the fact that they had suffered with frequent episodes of prolonged convulsions.

There are physicians who question whether convulsions of any duration are the sole cause of irreversible brain damage. They argue that it is quite possible that the convulsion and also the subsequent brain damage may be due to the same underlying brain disease. Certainly, I do not believe that this hypothesis has been definitely disproved.

I may add that we have performed postmortem examinations on the brains of some of our epileptic patients who had suffered with frequent seizures of various durations and who also presented marked electroencephalographic abnormalities. The pathologist was unable to demonstrate anatomical cerebral defects in some of these patients. Certainly, this is conclusive evidence that at least all patients who have seizures and electroencephalographic abnormalities do not have macroscopic or microscopic anatomical evidence of brain damage. In those patients in whom the pathologist was able to demonstrate organic brain damage, he could not be sure whether these changes existed before the onset of the epileptic disorder or were a result of the convulsive episodes.

Hypoglycemic Convulsions

It is a well established fact that irreversible brain damage does occur in some individuals, particularly young children, who suffer with hypoglycemic convulsions. I do not believe that it has been definitely proved that the brain damage in these instances is due solely to the convulsions themselves. It is quite likely that the brain damage may be caused by the hypoglycemia or a combination of the convulsion and the hypoglycemia or by unknown factors.

Simple Febrile Convulsions

Simple febrile convulsions rarely, if ever, cause irreversible brain damage. I have followed many patients who suffered with simple febrile convulsions and did not observe that these convulsions caused brain damage in any of these patients. The disorder of simple febrile convulsions is discussed in detail in another section of this book entitled Disorders Simulating Epilepsy (Chapter 6).

Breath-holding Spells

Some young children have frank convulsions in association with breath-holding spells. I have not encountered the slightest indication that convulsions associated with breath-holding spells caused brain damage in any of my patients. In fact, I have always been impressed with the fact that many children with breath-holding spells have exceedingly high intellectual levels. Breath-holding spells are discussed in detail in another section of this book entitled Disorders Simulating Epilepsy (Chapter 6).

Other Convulsions

Brain damage is frequently encountered in patients who have convulsions in association with disorders such as encephalitis, meningitis and degenerative disorders of the brain. However, it is reasonable to assume that the brain damage which occurs in association with these disturbances is due to the underlying brain disorder and not to the convulsive episode.

INJURIES AND LONGEVITY RELATIVE TO EPILEPSY

Many patients live in a constant state of fear that they may injure themselves or even die as a result of a seizure.

As far as injuries are concerned, the patient must realize that there is a calculated risk of injury, particularly if he should be in a precarious position at the time of occurrence of a seizure.

Epileptic seizures, in many instances, are immediately preceded by an aura. Most auras are of very short duration, usually lasting several seconds or so. However, in some instances, auras last for longer periods of time. In such instances, sufficient time may elapse between the onset of the aura and the occurrence of the frank seizure to permit the patient to protect himself from a fall which may result in an injury. A discussion of auras is presented in another section of this book entitled Classification of Epileptic Seizures (Chapter 4).

There is one form of epilepsy, known as minor motor epilepsy, which occurs only in the very young child and is associated with a relatively high incidence of personal injuries. During a minor motor seizure, a standing child will very frequently fall to the ground, striking his forehead or his chin. Some young children with this form of epilepsy will have as many as 50 to 100 such spells daily. I can mention many instances where it was necessary to rush the patient either to a hospital or to a physician in order to suture a laceration of the forehead or chin which resulted from a fall to the ground. These injuries can be prevented by having the patient wear a helmet, such as is shown in Figure 11, when he is in the upright position, that is, when he is walking about or playing. Minor motor epilepsy is discussed in detail in another

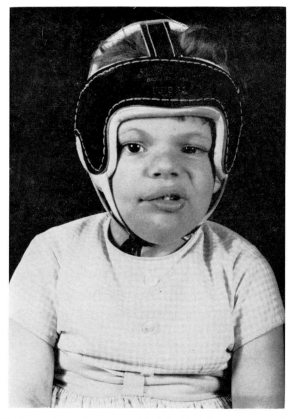

Figure 11. Photograph of a four year old girl with minor motor epilepsy wearing a helmet to protect her against injuries to the head. This particular helmet does not give protection to the chin. In those instances where patients have sustained injuries to their chins in falls associated with seizures, a military chin piece can be attached to the strap so that the helmet is held on the head by the chin piece. (This helmet is manufactured by Stall and Dean Manufacturing Co., 95 Church Street, Brockton, Mass.)

section of this book entitled Classification of Epileptic Seizures (Chapter 4).

I do not believe that one can obtain accurate statistics in regard to the incidence of personal injuries in the epileptic population at large. However, I can definitely state that I have not been impressed with a significantly large number of injuries in my group of patients who suffered with epilepsy other than those who

suffered with minor motor epilepsy. I definitely question whether
the incidence of accidents is greater among epileptics than among
the so-called normal population.

It has been my experience that most epileptics realize the
nature of their disorder and are generally exceedingly cautious
when performing actions such as walking across the street and
other activities which require that they be on the alert. I cite the
following as an example.

This is the case of a forty-two year old male who has been
working for the past seven years in a brick factory. His duties
are essentially those of a laborer and consist primarily of carrying
bricks from one part of the building to another. The path that he
must take in transporting the bricks crosses over an open space in
the floor which measures one foot square by six feet deep. He must
cross over this opening many times a day. "When I come to the
opening in the floor," he told me, "I stop, think and then step
over." I was informed by this patient that one of his fellow-workers,
who performs similar duties, recently stepped into the opening
while carrying bricks and broke his leg. The patient said that
newcomers to the factory frequently ridicule him for his cautious
procedure in negotiating the opening in the floor. However, he
usually replies, "I've been walking over this hole for seven years
and I've never fallen in."

It is also of significance to note that this patient has never been
late for work and has missed only an average of two days per year.
These absences were due to situations totally unrelated to his
epileptic disorder. He has been having on the average of one or
two seizures per year and has never sustained an injury of any
type while at work.

A recent study made by Dr. Harry Sands, Program Director
for the United Epilepsy Association, revealed that sneezing and
coughing on the job cause more than twice as many industrial
accidents as do epileptic seizures. This survey was based on New
York State Workmen's Compensation Board records. An analysis
of closed compensation cases for the thirteen year period, 1945-
1957, showed that compensated industrial accidents resulting from
epileptic seizures averaged out to 8.1 cases per year. In contrast,
the seven year period, 1951-1957 (for which data was available),

showed compensated cases due to sneezing and coughing averaging out at 20.2 cases per year.

Other examples of the low accident rate of epileptics are presented in other sections of this book entitled Employment for the Epileptic (Chapter 15) and Automobile Driving and Epilepsy (Chapter 15).

As far as longevity is concerned, the patient should definitely understand that epilepsy per se rarely causes death and that there is no reason why an epileptic should not live "as long as he would if he did not have epilepsy." The evidence for this statement is based on the observations which I have made in the follow-up of my group of epileptic patients (approximately 15,000), on the reports of the Metropolitan Life Insurance Company and on the findings of Schwade and Otto, Alström and others.

In a bulletin published by the Metropolitan Life Insurance Company in August, 1951, it is stated that "Epilepsy is only a minor cause of death. Just under 2,000 deaths were ascribed to it in the United States in 1948, the death rate being 1.3 per 100,000 population."

Schwade and Otto investigated and evaluated the mortality of epileptics in the State of Wisconsin for the year 1953. The Wisconsin State Board of Health recorded seventy deaths in Wisconsin in 1953 in which the cause of death was coded as "due to epilepsy." The total number of deaths in Wisconsin from all causes was 34,839 in the same year. According to the State Board of Health, deaths attributable to epilepsy were 0.2 per cent of all deaths or 2 per 100,000 in the population. It is of interest to note that deaths due to diabetes in Wisconsin for the same year totaled 682; this figure represents 2 per cent of all deaths or 19.3 per 100,000 in the population. It is readily observed that the number of deaths ascribed to diabetes in Wisconsin in 1953 was ten times that caused by epilepsy.

Schwade and Otto analyzed the data supplied by the Wisconsin State Board of Health and separated the seventy deaths attributed to epilepsy into four categories as follows:

(1) Deaths caused directly by epilepsy (in the course of status epilepticus)—fourteen deaths, or 20 per cent of the total;

(2) Deaths that were the accidental consequence of seizures,

such as drowning, suffocation, asphyxiation and severe brain injuries as a result of trauma—twelve deaths, or 17.2 per cent of the total;

(3) Cases in which it did not appear that death was properly related as a natural or accidental consequence of epilepsy, such as death due to coronary thrombosis, pulmonary edema, cerebral hemorrhage, purulent bronchitis and pneumonia—twenty-two deaths, or 31.4 per cent of the total;

(4) Cases in which the additional data was insufficient to permit a decisive opinion as to the cause of death, such as diagnoses of influenza, rheumatoid arthritis, cerebral arteriosclerosis, cardiac failure, cerebral damage and fetal erythroblastosis—twenty-two deaths, or 31.4 per cent of the total.

These authors recommended that epilepsy should be listed as a cause of death only when the terminal condition is the proximate or accidental consequence of seizures. They concluded that epilepsy was the cause of death in only twenty-six (37.2%) of the seventy cases and that forty-four (62.8%) of the deaths attributed to epilepsy were not, in fact, "due to epilepsy." The twenty-six deaths attributed to epilepsy represented less than 1 per 100,000 in the population.

Alström investigated the mortality of the epileptic in his group of 897 patients and reported his results in 1950. He divided the patients into three groups, the guiding principle of the division being the possibility of establishing the cause of the seizures— unknown (U), probable (P) and known (K) cause. The 897 patients were distributed as follows: Group U—606; Group P— 150; and Group K—141.

The mortality in this series of out-patients was computed with "the method of the calculated numbers" and was calculated for the time during which the patients were under observation. For the purpose of his mortality study, Alström further divided his patients into two groups: mentally healthy and mentally changed.

The mentally healthy patients of Groups U and P presented an insignificant excess mortality; the ratios between the observed and the calculated (on the basis of the general population) number of deceased were 1.0 for Group U and 1.6 for Group P. Alström stated, "It is not possible to demonstrate any significant excess mortality in the case of the numerically largest group, i.e., the mentally unaffected patients in the U group. It seems on the whole in agreement with the mortality in the general population. This also appears to apply to the corresponding patients in the P group."

My general observations are in complete agreement with the findings of the heretofore mentioned studies. I am currently in the process of securing definite statistical data relative to the mortality rate among my overall group of epileptic patients. However, I can state that the figures which I have on hand at the present time indicate that the mortality rate in my group of patients, exclusive of those with minor motor epilepsy, is not significantly higher than that found in the general population. For the purpose of this writing, I can definitely state that I am in complete agreement with the statement by Schwade and Otto that "the epileptic, under adequate medical control with patient and critical guidance and understanding of his problem, is substantially a mortality risk no greater than the average normal person."

However, the information obtained from a follow-up study conducted in our clinic on 622 patients who suffered with definite clinical evidence of brain damage in addition to seizures of the type classified as minor motor epileptic seizures indicates that the incidence of death in this group of patients should be considered as significant. This finding is in accord with that of Alström who also reported an excess mortality rate in his patients who presented clinical evidence of brain damage.

We found that twenty-three of these 622 patients died before the age of six: four deaths were due to an injury associated with seizures, three due to status epilepticus, ten were found dead in bed and six died of acute infections. These findings indicate that premature death is not uncommon in patients who suffer with so-called minor motor epilepsy, although a direct relationship of death to seizures per se in the patients heretofore mentioned could be established in only seven cases. In view of the fact that minor motor epilepsy is relatively rare and constitutes a very small percentage of the overall epileptic population, the apparent relatively high death rate in this form of epilepsy does not materially alter the death rate of epilepsy per se.

There are certain situations which could make an epileptic who is still having seizures more prone to fatal injuries or death, and I would like to emphasize that it is important that the patient be cognizant of these situations. For example, an uncontrolled epileptic should not perform activities such as climbing to high altitudes, driving an automobile or swimming alone.

I also believe that the uncontrolled epileptic should be warned against bathing in a bath tub unless he is observed. In those instances where it is not feasible or practical for the patient to be observed while in the bath tub, he should be instructed that the level of the water in the tub should not exceed a height of several inches or so. Patients should be warned against lying flat in the bath tub. It is probably better for most epileptic patients to resort to a shower instead of a bath for bathing purposes.

There are instances of epileptic patients having been found dead in bed with their heads "buried" in a pillow. It was thought, although one cannot be completely certain, that they suffocated by pressing their heads into the pillow during a spell. It is best for epileptics, particularly those who have nocturnal seizures, to sleep without a pillow or to use a firm pillow.

There is one form of epileptic disorder, so-called status epilepticus, which is sometimes fatal and must be treated as a medical emergency. The entity of status epilepticus is discussed in detail in another section of this book entitled Classification of Epileptic Seizures (Chapter 4). When death does occur in association with status epilepticus, it is usually due to disturbances such as cerebral edema, infection or cardiac or pulmonary arrest.

In conclusion, the epileptic should be made to understand that epilepsy per se should not shorten his life's span. He should realize that there are certain activities which he should not perform. The epileptic who conducts himself in the proper manner can get some encouragement from the realization that sometimes "it is good" for a person to have a "minor handicap." Many such individuals take better care of themselves and do not take unnecessary risks. It is well known that many handicapped people live a healthier, longer, happier and a more productive life than so-called "perfectly normal people."

BIBLIOGRAPHY

Alström, C. H.: Mortality in Mental Hospitals with Especial Regard to Tuberculosis. *Acta Psych. et Neurol.*, Suppl. XXIV., 1942.

Alström, C. H.: *A Study of Epilepsy in its Clinical, Social and Genetic Aspects*. Copenhagen, Munksgaard, 1950.

Bridge, E. M., Kajdi, L., and Livingston, S.: A Fifteen Year Study of Epilepsy in Children. *Proceedings of Association for Research in Nervous and Mental Disease*, Vol. XXVI, 1946.

Livingston, S., Eisner, V., and Pauli, L.: Minor Motor Epilepsy, Diagnosis, Treatment and Prognosis. *Pediatrics*, 21:916, 1958.

Metropolitan Life Insurance Company: Progress in the Control of Epilepsy, *Statistical Bulletin*, 32:8, 1951.

Sands, H.: *Epilepsy News*, Vol. VII, No. 1, 1961.

Schwade, E. D., and Otto, O.: Mortality in Epilepsy. *J.A.M.A.*, 156:1526, 1954.

SPECIAL BIBLIOGRAPHY

This bibliography contains a list of books and some pamphlets and periodical publications dealing with epilepsy. These latter writings marked with asterisk (*) were written primarily for lay reading.

Ajmone-Marsan, C., and Ralston, B. L.: *The Epileptic Seizure—Its Functional Morphology and Diagnostic Significance.* Springfield, Ill., Thomas, 1957.

Alström, C. H.: *A Study of Epilepsy in its Clinical, Social and Genetic Aspects.* Copenhagen, Munksgaard, 1950.

Baldwin, M., and Bailey, P., Editors: *Temporal Lobe Epilepsy.* Springfield, Ill., Thomas, 1958.

Barrow, R. L., and Fabing, H. D.: *Epilepsy and the Law.* New York, Hoeber, 1956.

Bridge, E. M.: *Epilepsy and Convulsive Disorders in Children.* New York, McGraw-Hill, 1949.

*Bryant, J. E.: *Genius and Epilepsy.* Concord, Mass., Old Depot Press, 1953.

Cadhilac, J.: *Hippocampe et Epilepsie.* Montpelier, Imprimerie Paul Dehan, 1955.

Chao, D. H., Druckman, R., and Kellaway, P.: *Convulsive Disorders of Children.* Philadelphia, Saunders, 1958.

Chavany, J. A.: *Epilepsie: Etude Clinique, Diagnostique, Physiopathogenique, et Therapeutique.* Paris, Masson et Cie, 1958.

*Children's Hospital, Los Angeles; Jerry Price Seizure Clinic. *Brochure for Parents.* Los Angeles, The Clinic, n. d. 10 p.

de Haas, L. (Editor): *Lectures on Epilepsy.* Amsterdam, Elsavier Press, 1958.

*Epilepsy and The School Child, Epilepsy Information Center, Inc., Room 204, 73 Tremont Street, Boston 8, Massachusetts.

Fairfield, L.: *Epilepsy—Grand Mal, Petit Mal Convulsions.* London, Gerald Duckworth & Co., 1954.

Gastaut, H.: *The Epilepsies.* Springfield, Ill., Thomas, 1954. Translated by Mary A. B. Brazier.

Gibbs, F. A., and Stamps, F. W.: *Epilepsy Handbook.* Springfield, Ill., Thomas, 1958.

Gowers, Sir Wm. R.: *Epilepsy and the Other Chronic Convulsive Diseases: Their Causes, Symptoms and Treatment.* 2nd edition. London, Churchill, 1901.

Grunspun, H.: *Disturbios Psiquiatricos Da Crianca.* Fundo Editorial Procienx, Sao Paulo, Brasil, 1961.

Harvald, B.: *Heredity in Epilepsy.* Copenhagen, Munksgaard, 1954.

Kanner, L.: Folklore and Cultural History of Epilepsy. *M. Life, 37:*167, 1930.

*Leonard, J. T.: *Diagnosis—Epilepsy—A Guide for Parents.* The Parents Committee on Epilepsy, Family Health Association, Inc., 3300 Chester Ave., Cleveland 14, Ohio, 1962.

*Lennox, W. G.: *Science and Seizures.* 2nd edition. New York, Harper, 1946.

Lennox, W. G.: *Epilepsy and Related Disorders.* 2 vols. Boston, Little, Brown and Co., 1960.

Livingston, S.: *Diagnosis and Treatment of Convulsive Disorders in Children.* Springfield, Ill., Thomas, 1954.

Livingston, S.: Convulsive Disorders in Infants and Children, in *Advances in Pediatrics.* Chicago, The Year Book Publishers, Inc., 1958.

*Miers, E. S.: *Why Did This Have To Happen?* National Society for Crippled Children and Adults, Inc., 2023 West Ogden Avenue, Chicago 12, Illinois.

*National Institute of Neurological Diseases and Blindness: *Epilepsy—Hope Through Research.* Washington, D. C.: Govt. Printing Office, 1962.

Penfield, W., and Erickson, T. C.: *Epilepsy and Cerebral Localization.* Springfield, Ill., Thomas, 1941.

Penfield, W., and Jasper, H.: *Epilepsy and the Functional Anatomy of the Human Brain.* Boston, Little, Brown and Co., 1954.

Penfield, W., and Kristiansen, K.: *Epileptic Seizure Patterns.* Springfield, Ill., Thomas, 1951.

*Putnam, T. J.: *Convulsive Seizures: How to Deal with Them.* Philadelphia: J. B. Lippincott, 1943. 160 p.

*Putnam, T. J.: *Epilepsy: What It Is: What To Do About It.* Philadelphia, J. B. Lippincott, 1958. 190 p.

Roger, A. R.: *Contribution a l'etude experimentale de l'epilepsie partielle.* These p. Doctorat en medecine—Medical Faculty of Marseille, Laval, Impr. Barneoud, 1955.

Sakel, M.: *Epilepsy.* New York, Philosophical Library, 1958.

Sauerbrei, H-U.: *Kinder mit Krampfanfallen.* Dustri-Verlag, Remscheid-Lennep, 1956.

Schwartz, P.: *Cerebral Apoplexy: Types, Causes and Pathogenesis.* Springfield, Ill., Thomas, 1961.

Services for Children with Epilepsy, The American Public Health Association, 1790 Broadway, New York, 19, N. Y., 1958.

Taylor, J., Editor: *Selected Writings of John Hughlings Jackson.* Vol. I. London, Hodder and Stoughton, 1931.

Temkin, O.: *The Falling Sickness.* Baltimore, Johns Hopkins Press, 1945.

Terry, G. C.: *Fever and Psychoses.* A Study of the Literature and Current Opinion on the Effects of Fever on Certain Psychoses and Epilepsy. New York, Hoeber, 1939.

The Child With Epilepsy. Children's Bureau, U. S. Department of Health, Education and Welfare, Order from: U. S. Gov't. Printing Office, Washington 25, D. C.

The Person With Epilepsy At Work. Group for the Advancement of Psychiatry Publications Office, 1790 Broadway, New York 19, New York.

Thomas, J. C., and Davidson, E. McL.: *Social Problems of the Epileptic Patient.* Montreal, Montreal Neurological Institute, 1949.

Torrent, J. G.: *Tratado de Electroencefalografia y estudio fundamental de las Epilepsias.* Madrid, Minerva Medica, 1955.

Total Rehabilitation of Epileptics. U. S. Department of Health, Education and Welfare, Office of Vocational Rehabilitation, Washington, D. C., January, 1962.

Tower, D. B.: *Neurochemistry of Epilepsy.* Springfield, Ill., Thomas, 1960.

Walker, A. E.: *Posttraumatic Epilepsy.* Springfield, Ill., Thomas, 1949.

Wallis, H. R. E.: *Masked Epilepsy.* Edinburgh and London, E. & S. Livingstone Ltd., 1956. 51 p.

Wright, G. N.: *Epilepsy Bibliography—Jan. 1956-Jan. 1960.* Chicago, National Epilepsy League. 1960. 24 p.

*U. S. Children's Bureau: *The Child with Epilepsy.* (Children's Bur. folder no. 35.) Washington, D. C., Govt. Print. Off., 1952. 15 p.

*Yahraes, H.: *Now—A Brighter Future For The Epileptic.* Public Affairs Pamphlets, 22 East 38th Street, New York 16, New York.

APPENDIX 1

FILMS ON EPILEPSY

WITH the exception of the last film, the following data was taken from the book entitled *Total Rehabilitation of Epileptics*, U. S. Department of Health, Education, and Welfare, Office of Vocational Rehabilitation, Washington, D. C., January, 1962. (Permission granted by Maurice A. Melford, National Director of the National Epilepsy League, Inc., 203 N. Wabash Avenue, Chicago 1, Illinois.)

Films listed below are currently available for loan. Significant information about each is given to assist in making appropriate selections. No rental charge is made by the loaning agencies. These agencies are coded as follows:

N.E.L. — National Epilepsy League, 203 North Wabash Ave., Chicago 1, Illinois.

U.E.A. — United Epilepsy Association, 111 West 57th Street, New York 9, N.Y.

E.I.C. — Epilepsy Information Center, 73 Tremont Street, Boston 8, Mass.

A.E.F. — American Epilepsy Federation, ℅ Kansas City Epilepsy League, 1601 East 57th Street, Kansas City, Mo.

C.E.S. — California Epilepsy Society, 1904 West 48th Street, Los Angeles 62, Calif. (Loan in California only.)

FILMS

Blueprint for Epilepsy
Shows Epi-Hab (epilepsy workshop) in Los Angeles, discussion on the disorder, vocational case histories. Made for Ciba Laboratories. For all adult audiences; 16 mm. black and white, sound; 30 minutes. Available from N.E.L., E.I.C., A.E.F., C.E.S.

Boy in a Storm

Shows an unhappy, deserted high-school boy, his examination in a hospital, his adoption, simulated convulsions. Made for TV. For all adult audiences; 16 mm. black and white; sound; 25 minutes. Available from N.E.L., C.E.S.

Modern Concepts of Epilepsy

Shows various types of seizures, causes, diagnoses, treatment by drugs and by surgery, effect of drugs, patient interviews, simulated convulsions. Made for Ayerst Laboratories. For professional audiences only; 16 mm. color; sound; 24 minutes. Available from N.E.L., E.I.C., C.E.S., and from Ayerst Laboratories, 22 East 40th Street, New York 16, N.Y.

People Apart

Shows interviews with epileptic adults and their feelings about employment and other difficulties, simulated convulsions. Made for British Epilepsy Association. For professional and lay audiences; 16 mm. black and white; sound; 30 minutes. Available from E.I.C., A.E.F., C.E.S.

Second Class Citizen

Shows job problems of a young woman with epilepsy who is married and works, and her courageous struggle to find acceptance by society. Made for TV program "Mr. Citizen." For all adult audiences; 16 mm. black and white; sound; 30 minutes. Available from N.E.L., A.E.F., C.E.S.

Seizure

Shows a veteran and his difficulties following onset of seizures, his diagnosis, treatment, brain surgery, job-finding problems and despair. Made by Veterans' Administration. For all adult audiences; 16 mm. black and white; sound; 45 minutes or 21 minutes (short version). Available (short version) from E.I.C., A.E.F., C.E.S.; (long version) local VA.

The Dark Wave

Shows a 12-year-old girl having simulated petit mal seizures, threat of exclusion from school, parents' shock, misunderstanding by playmates—with happy ending through improved attitudes.

Made by 20th Century Fox. Suitable for all audiences. Cinema-Scope (for flat screen required adapter lens available from local camera supply store), 16 mm. color; sound; 26 minutes. Available from E.I.C., U.E.A., A.E.F., C.E.S.

The Exceptional Child—Program Eleven

Shows epileptic teenagers in group discussion about their feelings toward marriage, driving, employment, and general life goals. Made for educational television for lay audiences; 16 mm. black and white; sound; 29 minutes. Available from E.I.C.

A Case of Reflex (Sonogenic) Epilepsy

Shows a 4-year-old boy with reflex epilepsy. Prepared by R. C. MacKeith M.D., London. For professional audiences; black and white; silent; 2 minutes. Available from Association of American Medical Colleges, 2530 Ridge Ave., Evanston, Ill.

A Certain Time—A Certain Darkness

This Ben Casey TV drama shows the disaster of parental over-protection and secrecy in the life of a young married woman, and how she overcomes the shroud of fear. 16 mm. black and white; sound; 50 minutes. Available from N.E.L.

APPENDIX 2

FOURTEEN AND SIX PER SECOND POSITIVE SPIKE ELECTROENCEPHALOGRAPHIC PATTERN

IN 1951, Gibbs and Gibbs reported the occurrence of a cerebral electrical discharge which they designated as 14 and 6 per second positive spikes in 6 per cent of a group of 5,000 patients who suffered with epilepsy or who were suspected of having epilepsy. Many of these 5,000 patients presented symptoms referrable to the autonomic nervous system, such as dizzy spells, syncopal attacks, attacks of nausea and vomiting and abdominal pain. They also reported that this 14 and 6 per second discharge occurred in the electroencephalograms of approximately 2 per cent of 300 control subjects.

Since that time numerous reports have appeared in the literature relative to this cerebral electrical pattern. It has been reported in patients who presented a wide variety of disturbances and abnormal performances, among which may be mentioned abdominal pain, fainting spells, syncopal attacks, headaches, hyperkinesis, larceny, bad check writing, juvenile delinquency, defective hearing, enuresis, loss of interest in school, behavior disorders of various types and criminal tendencies. In fact, it has been reported in patients who have presented many of the symptoms of thalamic or hypothalamic dysfunction.

Some investigators carried out controlled studies and in each instance the incidence of 14 and 6 per second positive spike pattern was found to be higher in patients with symptoms of the type heretofore mentioned than in the so-called normal controls.

In 1961, Dr. Woods presented a paper in the medical literature relative to the "6 and 14 dysrhythmia" and murder. This article was subsequently publicized in newspapers throughout the country and also in *Time Magazine* (Vol. LXXIX, No. 1, Jan. 5, 1962, page 48). In the *Baltimore Sun*, December 22, 1961, this article was summarized with the title headlined "Brain Wave Pattern Seen Crime Cause, Abnormality Found in Some Teen-Agers Who Commit Murder." The parents of several of my patients, in whom electroencephalographic studies revealed 14 and 6 per second positive spikes, became quite disturbed upon reading these newspaper and magazine reports. I reassured them that this electroencephalographic finding has in no way been proved to be diagnostic of criminal tendencies. I told them that I was in complete agreement with Dr. Frederic A. Gibbs, who took exception to some of Dr. Wood's comments and stated in a subsequent issue of *Time Magazine* (Vol. LXXIX, No. 3, Jan. 19, 1962, page 7), "My wife and I are the discoverers of what has been referred to as '6 and 14 dysrhythmia,' and we have been recording for many years electroencephalograms on normal children, epileptics, and children with behavior disorders, including all the famous child murderers in northern Illinois. We can assure you that there is not a significant correlation between murder and 14 and 6 per second positive spikes."

It is true that the 14 and 6 per second positive spike electroencephalographic discharge has been found in many patients who presented symptoms which are of the type associated with thalamic and hypothalamic dysfunction. However, after reviewing the medical literature, it is my definite impression that much more extensive work, including studies with adequate controls, has to be carried out before the clinical significance of this electrical aberration can definitely be established.

BIBLIOGRAPHY

Cutts, K. K., and Jasper, H. H.: Effect of benzedrine sulfate and phenobarbital on behavior problem children with abnormal electroencephalograms. *Arch. Neurol. & Psychiat., 41*:1138, 1939.

Garneski, T. M.: Six and fourteen per second spikes in juvenile behavior disorders. *E.E.G. and Clin. Neurophysiol., 12*:505, 1960.

Garneski, T. M., and Green, J. R.: Recording the fourteen and six per second spike phenomenon, *E.E.G. and Clin. Neurophysiol., 8*:501, 1956.

Gibbs, F. A.: Subjective complaints and behavior disturbances associated with fourteen and six per second positive spikes. *E.E.G. and Clin. Neurophysiol., 7*:315, 1955.

..............: Clinical correlates of 14 and 6 per second positive spikes (1865 cases). *E.E.G. and Clin. Neurophysiol., 8*:149, 1956.

Gibbs, E. L., and Gibbs, F. A.: Electroencephalographic evidence of thalamic and hypothalamic epilepsy. *Neurology, 1*:136, 1951.

Gibbs, F. A., and Low, N. L.: Symposium on laboratory tests and special procedures: electroencephalography in children. *Pediat. Clin. North America, 2*:291, 1955.

Hughes, J. R.: The 14 and 7 per second positive spikes—a reappraisal following a frequency count. *E.E.G. and Clin. Neurophysiol., 12*:495, 1960.

Jasper, H. H., Solomon, P., and Bradley, C.: Electroencephalographic analysis of behavior problem children. *Am. J. Psychiat., 95*:641, 1938.

Kellaway, P., Moore, F. J., and Kagawa, N.: The "14 and 6 per second positive spike" pattern of Gibbs and Gibbs. *E.E.G. and Clin. Neurophysiol., 9*:165, 1957.

Kellaway, P., Crawley, J. W., and Kagawa, N.: A specific electroencephalographic correlate of convulsive equivalent disorders in children. *J. Pediat., 55*:582, 1959.

Low, N. L., and Dawson, S. P.: Electroencephalographic findings in juvenile delinquency, *Pediatrics, 28*:452, 1961.

Millen, F. J., and White, B.: Fourteen and six per second positive spike activity in children, *Neurology, 4*:541, 1954.

Mills, W. B.: Paroxysmal 14 and 6/sec. spike discharges and clinical cases, including a teenage murder. *E.E.G. and Clin. Neurophysiol., 8*:344, 1956.

Niedermeyer, E., and Knott, J. R.: On the significance of 14 and 6 per second positive spikes in the E.E.G. *Arch. Psychiat. Nervenkr., 202*:266, 1961 (Ger.).

Poser, C. M., and Ziegler, D. K.: Clinical significance of 14 and 6 per second positive spike complexes. *Neurology, 8*:903, 1958.

Presthus, J., Refsun, S., Skulstad, A., and Ostensjo, S.: Fourteen and six per second positive spikes; an electroencephalographic and clinical study; preliminary report. *Acta. Psychiat. et Neurol. Scandinav., 31*:166, 1956.

Schwade, E. D., and Geiger, S. G.: Matricide with electroencephalographic evidence of thalamic or hypothalamic disorder. *Dis. Nerv. System, 14*:18, 1953.

Schwade, E. D., and Geiger, S.: Behavior disorders of the impulsive-compulsive type with consistent abnormal EEG findings. *E.E.G. and Clin. Neurophysiol., 7*:473, 1955.

Schwade, E. D., and Geiger, S.: Abnormal electroencephalographic findings in severe behavior disorders. *Dis. Nerv. System, 17*:307, 1956.

Schwade, E. D., and Otto, O.: Homicide as manifestation of thalamic or hypothalamic disorder with abnormal electroencephalographic findings, *Wisconsin M. J., 52*:171, 1953.

Stephenson, W. A.: Intracranial neoplasm associated with fourteen and six per second positive spikes. *Neurology, 1*:372, 1951.

Taterka, J. H., and Katz, J.: Study of correlations between electroencephalographic and psychological patterns in emotionally disturbed children. *Psychosom. Med., 17*: 62, 1955.

Walter, R. D.: Some clinical correlation of 14 and 6 per sec. spiking activity, *E.E.G. and Clin. Neurophysiol., 9*:377, 1957.

Winfield, D. L., and Ozturk, O.: Electroencephalographic findings in matricide: A case report. *E.E.G. and Clin. Neurophysiol., 9*:570, 1957.

Woods, S. M.: Adolescent violence and homicide. *Arch. Gen. Psychiat., 5*:38, 1961.

APPENDIX 3

GLOSSARY

This glossary was prepared for the convenience of the non-medical reader.

Ablate—To remove, especially by cutting.

Acidosis—Acid intoxication of the body.

Afebrile—Without symptoms of fever.

Agranulocytosis—An acute disease characterized by marked leukopenia and neutropenia and which is frequently associated with ulcerative lesions of the throat and other mucous membranes, the gastrointestinal tract and the skin.

Albuminuria—The presence of albumin in the urine.

Alkalosis—A clinical term commonly used to indicate an increased alkalinity of the blood.

Allele—One of two or more contrasting genes situated at the same locus in homologous chromosomes, which determine alternative characters in inheritance.

Alopecia—Baldness; deficiency of hair, natural or abnormal.

Amblyopia (toxic)—Dimness of vision, without detectable organic lesion of the eye due to poisoning as from tobacco or alcohol.

Amyotrophic Lateral Sclerosis—A serious disease marked by a hardening of the lateral columns of the spinal cord with muscular atrophy.

Aneurysm—A sac formed by the dilatation of the walls of an artery or of a vein and filled with blood.

Anomaly—Marked deviation from the normal standard.

Anorexia—Loss of appetite for food.

Anoxia—reduction of oxygen in body tissues below physiologic levels.

Aphasia—Any partial or total loss of the power of articulate speech which is not due to defects in the peripheral organs but to disorder in some of the cerebral centers connected with this function.

Aplasia—incomplete or defective development of tissue.

Aplastic Anemia—Deficiency of blood cell formation associated with aplasia of the bone marrow, deficiency of hemoglobin in red cells, deficiency of leukocytes, and predominance of lymphocytes.

317

Arteriosclerosis—The thickening and hardening of the walls of an artery.

Aspiration—The act of breathing or drawing in some foreign substance or object into the lungs.

Ataxia—irregularity in muscular action through failure of muscular coordination.

Atrophy—to cause to waste away or wither.

Automatism—The performance of non-reflex acts without conscious volition.

Autosomal—Pertaining to an ordinary paired chromosome as distinguished from a sex chromosome.

Bronchiectasis—A chronic dilatation of the bronchi or bronchioles marked by fetid breath and paroxysmal expectoration of matter containing mucus and pus.

Calcification—The process by which organic tissue becomes hardened by a deposit of calcium salts within its substance.

Carious—Affected with ulceration and decay.

Cataract—An opacity of the crystalline eye lens or of its capsule.

Cerebral—Pertaining to the main portion of the brain.

Cerebral Hemisphere—Either lateral half of the brain.

Cerebral Lesion—Any pathological or traumatic discontinuity of the brain tissue.

Cerebrospinal Fluid—The fluid contained within the brain cavities, subarachnoid sinus and the central canal of the spinal cord.

Consanguineous Marriage—Marriage between blood relatives.

Chromosomes—Characteristic, deeply staining bodies found in the nucleus of a cell during cell division that contain the genes or determiners of heredity.

Clinical—Pertaining to or founded on actual observation and treatment of patients, as distinguished from theoretical or experimental.

Clonic—Characterized by spasms in which rigidity and relaxation alternate in rapid succession.

Congenital—Born with; existing from birth; existing at, and usually before birth.

Convulsive Threshold—The level above which convulsions occur; the resistance to convulsions.

Cortex (of the brain)—The outer layer of the brain as distinguished from its inner substance.

Cortical—Pertaining to or of the nature of a cortex.

Craniotomy—Any operation on the cranium.

Cutaneous—Pertaining to the skin.

Cyanosis—Any bluish discoloration of the skin; a disordered condition of the circulation causing a livid bluish color in the skin.

Cysticercosis—The condition of being infested with a form of larval tapeworm.

Defervescence—The period of disappearance of fever.

Dermatological—Pertaining to the skin and its diseases.

Diplopia—The seeing of single objects as double or two.

Diuretic—A drug which stimulates the secretion of urine.

Diurnal—Done in or pertaining to the daytime.

Dizygotic—Pertaining to or derived from two separate eggs.

Dominant Character—A character from one parent that manifests itself in offspring to the exclusion of a contrasted (recessive) character from the other parent.

Dominant Gene—One which produces an effect in the organism, regardless of the state of the corresponding allele.

Drug Intoxication—Drug poisoning; the state of being poisoned by a drug.

Dysarthria—Imperfect articulation in speech.

Dysgenic—Detrimental to the race or tending to counteract race improvement.

Dysrhythmia—Disturbance or irregularity in rhythm.

Ecchymosis—A discoloration, as a black and blue spot, resulting from the rupture of small blood vessels by a blow or contusion.

Eclampsia—Convulsions and coma occurring in a pregnant or puerperal woman, associated with hypertension, edema and proteinuria.

Edema—The presence of abnormally large amounts of fluid in the intercellular tissue spaces of the body.

Encephalitis—Inflammation of the brain.

Encephalopathy—Any disease of the brain.

Enuresis—Incontinence of urine; involuntary discharge of urine.

Enzyme—An organic compound, frequently a protein, capable of accelerating or producing by catalytic action some change in its substrate for which it is often specific.

Epileptiform—Resembling epilepsy or its manifestations.

Epileptogenic Focus—The area of the cortex responsible for causing epileptic seizures, as revealed in the electroencephalogram.

Epistaxis—nosebleed.

Erythema Bullosum Malignans—A severe disease, one of the manifestations of which is the occurrence of many blister-like lesions scattered over the greater part of the body.

Etiology—The study or theory of the causation of any disease.

Eunichism—The condition of a castrated male.

Euphoric—Characterized by an abnormal or exaggerated sense of well-being.

Exfoliative Dermatitis—A serious disease characterized by very extensive falling cff of the skin in scales.

Extracranial—Outside of the skull.

Fetal—Pertaining to the developing young in the human uterus after the end of the second month.

Flexion—The act of bending.

Focal Seizures—Seizures that are predominantly one-sided or local or present localized features.

Focus—The chief center of a morbid process.

Functional—Of, or pertaining to a function; affecting the functions, but not the structure.

Gamete—A mature reproductive or germ cell, either male (sperm) or female (ovum).

Ganglion—Any collection or mass of nerve cells that serves as a center of nervous influence.

Gene—The unit of inheritance which is transmitted from one generation to another in the gametes and controls the development of characters in the new individual.

General Anesthetic—A drug for producing general loss of feeling and sensation, such as ether and nitrous oxide, as compared to a local anesthetic, whose action is limited to an area of the body around the site of application.

Generalized—Not local; affecting many parts or all parts of the organism.

Genetics—The study of heredity.

Genitourinary—Pertaining to the genital and urinary organs.

Genotype—The internal genetic or hereditary constitution of an organism without regard to its external appearance.

Gestation—Pregnancy.

Gingival Hyperplasia—The abnormal increase in the number of normal cells in the gum tissue; enlargement of the gums from quantitative increase produced by cell division.

Hemapoietic—Pertaining to or affecting the formation of blood cells.

Hematologic—Pertaining to the blood and blood-forming tissues.

Hematoma—A tumor containing effused blood.

Hematuria—The discharge of blood in the urine.

Hemiplegia—Paralysis of one side of the body.

Hemispherectomy—The operation of resecting a cerebral hemisphere.

Hemorrhagic Erythema Multiforme—A disturbance of the skin consisting of hemorrhagic lesions of various sizes and shapes and usually caused by blood disorders.

Hepatic—Pertaining to the liver.

Hepatitis—Inflammation of the liver.

Homologous Chromosomes—A pair of chromosomes having relatively similar structure and value, one from each parent.

Hormonal—Pertaining to or of the nature of hormones.

Hormone—A chemical substance secreted into the body fluids by an endocrine gland, which has a specific effect on the activities of other organs.

Hydatid Cyst—The cyst stage of an embryonic tapeworm, in which the cyst contains daughter cysts.

Hydrocephalus—A condition characterized by abnormal accumulation of fluid in the cranial vault, accompanied by enlargement of the head and prominence of the forehead.

Hyperkinetic—Pertaining to or characterized by abnormally increased motor function or activity.

Hypernatremia—Excessive amount of sodium in the blood.

Hyperplastic—Pertaining to or characterized by an abnormal increase in the number of normal cells in a tissue.

Hypersensitivity—A state of altered reactivity in which the body reacts to a foreign agent more strongly than normal; abnormally sensitive.

Hypertension—Abnormally high blood pressure.

Hypertrichosis—An abnormally excessive growth of hair.

Hyperventilation—Prolonged, rapid and deep breathing, frequently used as a test procedure in epilepsy.

Hypocalcemia—Reduction of blood calcium below normal.

Hypoglycemia—Reduction of concentration of glucose in the blood below normal.

Idiopathic—Of unknown causation.

Insulin Reaction—Insulin shock: A condition of circulatory insufficiency resulting from overdosage with insulin which causes too sudden reduction of blood sugar.

Intracranial—Within the skull.

Irreversible—Incapable of being reversed.

Jaundice—A disorder characterized by excess red bile pigment in the blood and deposition of bile pigment in the skin and mucous membranes with resulting yellow appearance of the patient.

Kernicterus—A severe cerebral form of jaundice associated with erythroblastosis fetalis in which there are degenerating changes and pigmentation of the brain and spinal cord with bile pigments.

Ketone Bodies—Intermediates in fat metabolism: acetone, acetoacetic acid and beta-oxybutyric acid.

Ketonuria—The presence of ketones (ketone bodies) in the urine.

Ketosis—A condition characterized by excessive formation of ketones in the body.

Kilogram—One thousand grams or approximately 2.2 avoirdupois pounds.

Leukopenia—Reduction in the number of leukocytes in the blood, the count being 5,000 or less.

Localized—Not general; restricted to a limited area of the body.

Lumbar—Pertaining to or situated near the loins.

Lumbar Puncture—The tapping of the subarachnoid space in the lumbar region.

Lymphadenopathy—Disease of the lymph glands.

Lymphoma—Any tumor composed of lymphoid tissue.

Maculopapular—Consisting of both discolored spots on the skin not elevated above the surface and small circumscribed, solid elevations of the skin.

Malaise—A vague feeling of body discomfort.

Manic-Depressive Psychosis—An affective-psychosis, chiefly marked by emotional instability, striking mood swings, and a tendency to recurrence.

Megaloblastic Anemia—Anemia marked by the presence in the blood of primitive red blood corpuscles of large size.

Meningeal—Of, pertaining to, or situated near the membranes enveloping the brain and spinal cord.

Meninges—The membranes (dura mater, pia mater and arachnoid) enveloping the brain and spinal cord.

Meningitis—Inflammation of the enveloping membranes of the brain.

Menopause—Change of life; final cessation of the menses.

Metabolic—Relating to the chemical and physical processes by which living organized substance is produced and maintained.

Monohybrid—The offspring of parents differing in one character.

Monoplegia—Paralysis of one part of the body.

Monozygotic—Pertaining to or derived from one egg.

Morbilliform—resembling measles.

Myasthenia Gravis—A syndrome of fatigue and exhaustion of the muscular system marked by progressive paralysis of muscles with sensory disturbance or atrophy.

Myocardial—Pertaining to the muscular tissue of the heart.

Neoplasm—Any new and abnormal growth, such as a tumor.

Neurological—Pertaining to the nervous system.

Neurosis—A disorder of the psychic or mental constitution.

Neutropenia—Deficiency of neutrophil leukocytes in the blood.

Neutrophil—A cell or structural element, particularly a leukocyte, stainable by neutral dyes.

Nystagmus—An involuntary rapid movement of the eyeball which may be horizontal, vertical, rotary or mixed (of two varieities).

Occipital—Pertaining to the back part of the head; pertaining to the lower back part of the head or to the occipital bone.

Ophthalmologist—A specialist in diseases of the eye.

Opisthotonus—A form of tetanic spasm in which the head and heels are bent backward and the body bowed forward.

Orchidectomy—excision of one or both testicles.

Organic—Of, pertaining to, or affecting an organ or organs.

Otitis Media—Inflammation of the middle ear.

Pancytopenia—Deficiency of all the cell elements of the blood.

Paranoia—Chronic mental (personality) unsoundness; dementia with delusions.

Paraplegia—Paralysis of the lower half of the body.

Parenteral—Pertaining to administration other than intestinal, as intravenous, intramuscular or subcutaneous.

Paresthesias—Morbid or perverted sensations; abnormal sensations, as burning.

Paroxysmal—Pertaining to a periodic attack of disease, or to sudden and violent excitement or emotion; pertaining to a sudden recurrence or intensification of symptoms.

Pathogenesis—The development of morbid conditions or of a disease.

Periarteritis Nodosa—An inflammatory disease of the coats of the small and medium sized arteries of the body with inflammatory changes around the vessels and marked by symptoms of systemic infection.

Perinatal—Pertaining to, or occurring at, the time of birth.

Periorbital Edema—Swelling of the tissues immediately surrounding the eye; edema of the eye socket.

Peripheral—Of, or pertaining to, the outer surface of a body or organ.

Perseveration—Continuance of any activity after cessation of the causative stimulus.

Pertussis—Whooping cough.

Petechiae—Small, pinpoint, non-raised, round, purplish red spots caused by intradermal or submucous hemorrhage, which later turn blue or yellow.

Phenylketonuria—A congenital faulty metabolism of the amino acid, phenylalanine, because of which phenylpyruvic acid appears in the urine. It is often associated with mental defects.

Phenylpyruvic Oligophrenia—A hereditary mental deficiency characterized by the excretion of phenylpyruvic acid in the urine.

Photic Stimulation—Stimulation with light.

Photophobia—Abnormal intolerance of light; aversion to or intolerance to light.

Platelet—A circular or oval disc found in the blood of all mammals, which is concerned in coagulation of the blood and in contraction of the clot.

Polyarthropathy—A disturbance of more than one joint.

Polydipsia—Excessive thirst.

Polyhybrid—An offspring whose parents differ from each other in more than three characters.

Polyuria—The secretion and discharge of an excessive quantity of urine.

Precipitant of Epileptic Seizures—A substance or situation which "triggers off" an epileptic seizure.

Premonitory—An actual warning of something yet to occur.

Prenatal—Before birth; existing or occurring before birth.

Proband—The original person presenting a mental or physical disorder who serves as the basis for a genetic or hereditary study.

Prognosis—A prediction or conclusion in regard to the course and termination of a disease.

Prosthesis—An artificial part; the replacement of an absent part by an artificial one.

Pruritic—Itching.

Psychogenic Psychosis—Psychosis having an emotional or psychological origin.

Psychopathy—Any disease of the mind.

Psychoses—The deeper, more far-reaching and prolonged behavior disorders, such as dementia precox.

Psychotic—Pertaining to, characterized by, or caused by psychosis.

Psychotherapy—Treatment aimed at removing or ameliorating abnormal constituents of the mind or abnormal mental or emotional processes.

Puberty—That period in life at which a person of either sex becomes functionally capable of generation, generally considered to be about 14 years in males and 12 years in females.

Puerperium—Pertaining to, resulting from, or following childbirth; the period or state of confinement after labor.

Pulmonary—Pertaining to the lungs.

Purpuric—related to or resembling livid spots on the skin.

Renal—Pertaining to, of, affecting, or situated near the kidneys.

Retina—The inner coat of the eye, which receives the optical image.

Roentgenographic—Photography by means of x-rays.

Roentgenological—Pertaining to x-rays.

Scarlatiniform—A scarlet eruption or rash resembling that of scarlet fever.

Sibling—Another offspring of the same parents as the person of reference.

Sibship—Relationship by blood.

Spasmodic—Of the nature of an involuntary sudden, violent contraction of a muscle or group of muscles.

Spike Focus—A localized cerebral electrical discharge which takes the form of a spike on the electroencephalogram.

Subdural Hematoma—A blood tumor situated beneath the dura.

Subdural Puncture—The introduction of a needle into the subdural space.

Symptomatic—Pertaining to, of the nature of, a symptom.

Syncopal—Pertaining to a sudden faintness or swooning with loss of sensation, motion, and consciousness.

Temporal Lobe—The most inferior of the lobes of the brain, lying below the parietal and in front of the occipital lobe.

Temporal Lobectomy—Excision of the temporal lobe of the brain.

Thrombocytopenia—Decrease in the number of blood platelets.

Tics—Neurotic spasms or twitchings of muscles.

Tonic—Rigid; unrelaxing.

Toxemia of Pregnancy—A series of pathologic conditions, essentially metabolic disturbances, occurring in pregnant women.

Toxoplasmosis—Infection with, or a condition produced by the presence of, parasites of the genus Toxoplasma.

Trachea—The windpipe; the duct composed of membrane and cartilage, by which air passes from the larynx to the bronchi and the lungs.

Trauma—A wound or injury; an injury caused to the body by violence.

Tuberous Sclerosis—A familial disease characterized by acne-like lesions predominantly on the cheeks, nose and chin, convulsions and roentgenological evidence of areas of calcification in the brain.

Unilateral—Relating to or affecting one side only.

Untoward—Causing annoyance or hindrance.

Urticarial—Pertaining to or resembling a disease of the skin characterized by evanescent rounded elevations attended by intense itching.

Vascular—Of, pertaining to, consisting of, or containing vessels or ducts, as blood vessels.

Vascular Accident—A rupture of a blood vessel.

Vascular Anomalies—Abnormalities of the system of blood vessels of the body.

Vascular System—The system of blood vessels of the body.

Vertigo—A sensation as if the external world were revolving around the patient, or as if the patient himself were revolving in space.

INDEX

327

educational training for, 234-236

emotional difficulties and, 191, 214

Epi-Hab, Inc., 220-222

industrial injuries, 216-217, 220-221, 300-301

in Maryland, 219

misconceptions regarding characteristics of epileptics, 216-217

objections of major industries to, 214, 216-217

occupations suitable for patients with infrequent seizures, 215

occupations unsuitable for patients with infrequent seizures, 215

patients and their problems regarding, 213

preparation for of controlled epileptic, 213-214, 234-236

preparation for of patient with seizures, 213

rehabilitation of patient who must change jobs, 214

Roman Catholic priesthood, 215, 235-236

school teacher

  as profession for epileptic, 215, 235

  as vocational counselor, 213-214, 234-236

statement regarding in *J.A.M.A.*, 211

study of employability by Hibbard, 211-212

study of job injuries, 217

study of sickness and accident rate, 217

unacceptability due to misconceptions of disorder, 211

vocational rehabilitation, *See* Vocational Rehabilitation Centers

vocational counseling of students, 213-214, 234-236

Environment

as precipitating factor, 49-52

case histories, 49-51, 51-52

indications for change of, 52

Epamin, *See* Dilantin sodium

Epanutin, *See* Dilantin sodium

Epelin, *See* Dilantin sodium

Epi-Hab, Inc., 220-222

awards received, 221-222

defined, 220

description of program, 221

locations of, 220

objectives of program, 221

origin of, 220

safety performance of employees, 221

services performed, 221

Epilepsy, *See also* Seizures

age of onset, 9-10

attempts to conceal, 11-12, 190-191

case histories, 11-12

causes of, hypotheses, 8-9, 42

classification of, 6

current use of term, 5

decrease in stigma attached to, 12

definition, 5-6

derivation of term, 5, 202

disorders simulating, 61-76

  brain tumors, *See* Brain tumors

  breath-holding spells, *See* Breath-holding spells

  cataplexy, 73

  congenital and degenerative diseases of the brain, 75

  emotional (functional) disturbances, *See* Emotional disturbances

  hypoglycemic convulsions, *See* Hypoglycemic convulsions

  narcolepsy, 72-73

  simple febrile convulsions, *See* Simple febrile convulsions

  tetany, 72

explanation of by parent to child, 204-205

explanation of by teacher to students, 208-210

explanation of to child, 202-203

explanation of to teen-agers, 203

explanation of to parents by physician, 201-203, 204

  of emotional difficulties, 202

  of meaning of word epilepsy, 202

  of stigmas attached to disease, 202

  to avoid feelings of guilt, 204

explanation to relatives and friends, 206-207

explanation to teacher and school authorities, 207-208

F